good health guide

A handy, quick reference guide, written in plain English, to the multitude of services and help available to anyone in Hastings & Rother with a mental health problem.

Important Note

It must be stressed that Hastings Mind, which publishes this *Guide,* cannot be assumed to endorse any of the organisations or individuals listed. Readers may be guided by the professional bodies to which various practitioners belong.

This *Guide* is dedicated to the people of Hastings & Rother.

Mind
The Mental Health Charity

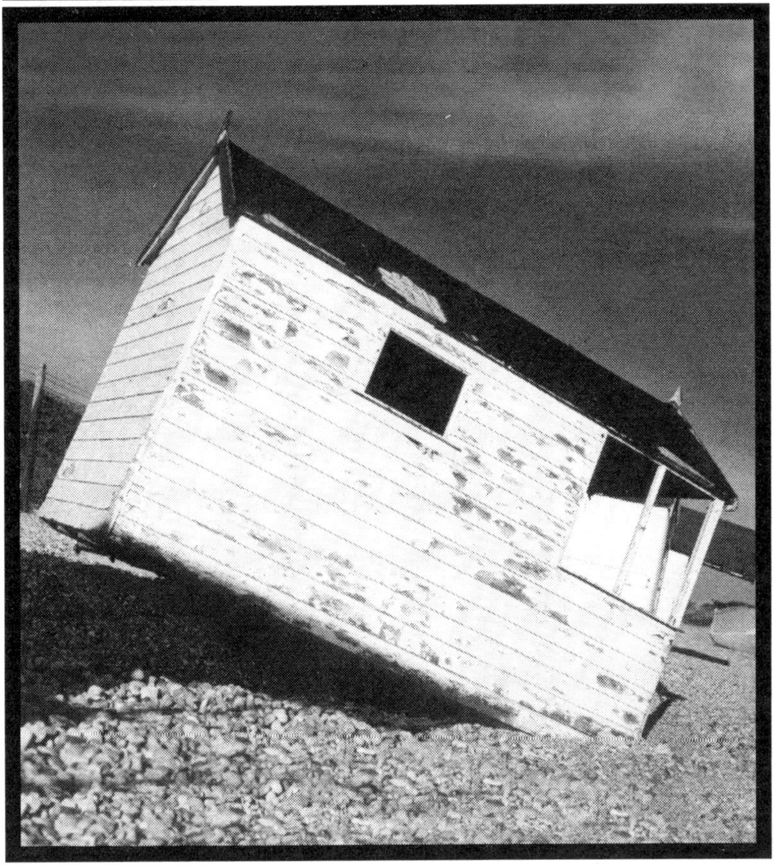

good health guide

Hastings Mind, 2000

Hastings Mind

good health guide

First published 2000 by Hastings Mind.

ISBN 0-9538761-0-1

Printed and bound in Great Britain by Cox & Wyman Ltd, Reading, Berkshire.
Impression number 10 9 8 7 6 5 4 3 2 1

For further copies of the good health guide, please contact the publishers at the following address: Hastings Mind, St Peter's Place, 32/33, St Peter's Road, St Leonards, Sussex, TN37 6JQ.

Cover photograph by Richard Matthews.

HASTINGS MIND

good health guide

Contents

problems

help

alternative help

nhs & social services

references & index

Introduction

Mental health problems

Mental health problems of one sort or another probably affect most households. Where do people turn when they have a problem? Usually to their GP or to friends or even yellow pages.

We understand how difficult it is to know what to do, and where to go for help and information, if you are suffering from mental distress. This guide aims to help people to pinpoint the services which can best help them, make clear their rights and support them through the matrix of mental health service provision.

There are literally hundreds of different organisations, centres, clinics, individual practitioners, self-help groups, and other organisations in the voluntary, public and private sectors involved with mental health.

For someone confronting this task for the first time it can be a very disheartening and daunting task just trying to find out basic information. We have tried to include and present this information in an easy to find, and easy to understand format. We have tried to use only plain English, and where technical words are used they are explained in the text where they first occur.

How to use the *Guide*

There are three main routes into this guide. The easiest way is to look up the subject matter in the Index. We have tried to make the index as thorough as possible: all subjects are included as are all the various people mentioned in the main text. The other methods are to use the 'Contents' list at the beginning or simply browse through the chapters - arranged in alphabetical order by subject.

What is included?

A brief glance at the 'Contents' page will show how wide the area of 'mental health' is. If you had a mental health problem, what would you want to know? Presumably, you would want to know more about the illness you thought you had, where you could get help, what you would do in an emergency, what specialist organisations there were that could help you, what support groups there were, what your rights were, and a thousand other things. We have tried to include all of this here in this guide.

Who the Guide was written for

It is hoped that GPs, mental health professionals, and others working in the mental health field will use this guide. But above all it is for people who actually have a mental health problem, i.e. anyone who is suffering from any kind of mental distress, and of course their carers, friends and families who often become as intimately involved as the person with the actual problem.

Areas covered

Battle, Bexhill, Brede, Broad Oak, Burwash, Cooden, Crowborough, Etchingham, Fairlight, Guestling, Hastings, Hawkhurst, Little Common, Ninfield, Northiam, Ore, Pett, Robertsbridge, Rotherfield, Rye, Sedlescombe, St Leonards, Three Oaks, Ticehurst, Wadhurst, Westfield, Winchelsea.

Acknowledgements

A great many people and organisations have contributed to the material in this guide. Much appreciation too, to all the people who took the time and trouble to answer our endless queries by post, phone and e-mail.

Funding

Funding for the editorial research, typesetting, printing and distribution of the *Guide* was generously provided by East Sussex County Council, Social Services; Bexhill & Rother Primary Care Group; and Hastings & St Leonards Primary Care Group.

Editorial assistance

We would like to express our sincere thanks for the generous help received from the following people and organisations who provided invaluable and expert editorial assistance and other help with various chapters:

Alan Mooncie, Hastings & Rother Manic Depression Fellowship Self-Help Group, *(Manic Depression).*

Andrew Partington, East Sussex Brighton & Hove Health Authority *(Health Authorities & NHS).*

Ann Cox, author, broadcaster and founder of EDRS *(Eating Disorders).*

Anna Barnes, Mental Health Project Worker, Hastings & Rother NHS Trust, *(for invaluable general editorial help).*

Anna Parikh, National Society for Epilepsy *(Epilepsy).*

Anne Dawson, The Advocacy Centre, *(Advocacy).*

Anne Guildford, Threshold Women's Mental Health Initiative, Brighton, *(Women).*

Barbara Hardcastle, ESBHHA Health Promotion, *(Information; NHS).*

Ben Edwards, autogenic therapist and medical herbalist, *(Autogenic Therapy; Herbalism).*

Bobette Newell & Scope *(Cerebral Palsy)*

Candice Miller, Information Officer, ESCC. *(Social Services).*

Chris Chinery, Roebuck Surgery, *(Doctors).*

Christine Lockwood, Community Link Nurses, Woodlands, *(Care Programme Approach, Rehabilitation).*

Claire Power, HCDUFA, *(Children & Young People).*

Clive Looker, Cavendish Clinic *(Smoking).*

Colin Barton, ME Association, *(Chronic Fatigue Syndrome).*

David Harding, solicitor, *(Legal Matters).*

Debbie Rimmer, occupational therapist, Westwood House, *(Occupational Therapy).*

Dee Heyfron, *(Epilepsy).*

Elizabeth Downs, Aromatherapist, *(Aromatherapy).*

Ellen Harley, Senior Community Mental Health Nurse, Westwood House, *(Racial Issues).*

Focus on Mental Health, *(User Groups).*

Francesca Inskipp, counsellor, *(Counselling & Therapy).*

Franco Di Francesco, Manager, Hastings Day Centre, *(Day Centres).*

Frank Clark, Trinity Project, *(Substance Misuse).*

Gladys Stewart, Hastings & District MS Society, *(Multiple Sclerosis).*

Jacqui Wilson, Senior Clinical Nurse & colleagues at Woodlands, *(Hospitals: Woodlands)*

Jan Cackett, Crossroads Care Attendant Scheme, *(Carers).*

Jenny Hart, *(special thanks for careful proof-reading of all chapters).*

Jill Miles, Xpress *(Advocacy).*

John Evans, Seaview Projects, *(Drop-in & Day Centres).*

John Milsom, Brighton Community Support Services, *(Hearing Voices).*

John Reading, Community Alcohol Team, *(Alcohol).*

Judith Guest, AD/HD Support Network, *(Attention Deficit / Hyperactivity).*

Karen Sedgewick, Housing Policy & Resources, Hastings Borough Council, *(Housing).*

Kate Griffiths, Publications Officer, Social Services, *(Social Services).*

Katy Burbridge, Hastings & Rother Federation of Information Providers, *(for general help)*

Linda Mooncie, Cruse bereavement counsellor, *(Bereavement).*

Lynne Jenkins, of Hastings APCMI, *(Befriending).*

Madeleine Iddison, Service Manager, Social Services, *(Community Mental Health Teams).*

Madeleine Mayhew, Communications Department, ESBHHA, *(Media Issues; Health Authorities).*

Margaret Moss, Focus on Mental Health, *(User Groups).*

Margaret Taylor, art therapist, *(Art Therapy).*

Mary Cairns, psychotherapist, *(Counselling & Therapy).*

Mary Dawson, Family Support Practitioner, Hastings & Rother NHS Trust, *(Alternative therapies; Children & Young People; Family Problems).*

Mary Locke, Department of Clinical Psychology, *(Psychology).*

Matt Fribbens, Crisis Response Service, *(Crises).*

Michael Birkett, Consultant Psychiatrist, Rural Rother, Hastings & Rother NHS Trust, *(Psychiatry).*

Mike Cornish, Service Manager, Social Services, *(Social Services)*

Mirna Honeyman, Obsessive Action, *(Obsessions).*

Nick Casey, ESBHHA Health Promotion, *(Substance Misuse).*

Pam Thompson, National Society for Epilepsy, *(Epilepsy).*

Pauline Tensythoff, The Migraine Trust, *(Migraine).*

Peter Baker, Head Psychologist, Community & Learning Disability Service, *(Learning Disabilities).*

Peter Howard, Hastings Sheltered Workshop, *(Employment & Training).*

Phil Gander, East Sussex Social Services, *(Social Services).*

Phillippa Erasmus, Sussex Autistic Society, *(Autism).*

Rose Austen, Volunteer Bureau, *(Voluntary Work).*

Roy Holland, Survivor's Poetry, *(Alternative Therapies: Poetry & Writing).*

Sandra Garner, Citizens' Advice Bureau, Hastings, *(Advice).*

Sandy Lazarus, Care for the Carers, *(Carers).*

Sarah Holmes-Smith, Hastings & Rother NHS Trust, *(for general help).*

Shakil Malik, consultant psychiatrist, Hastings, *(Psychiatry).*

Steve Loynes *(Care Programme Approach).*

Steve Metcalf, East Sussex Social Services, *(Social Services).*

Su Barnicoat, *(Rural Rother).*

Sue Ryan, PD Network, Henderson Hospital, *(Personality Disorder).*

Susie Lyle, Holistic Health Centre, *(Alternative Therapies).*

Toni Wilkinson, Chief Executive, Hastings & St Leonards Primary Care Group, *(Primary Care Groups).*

Trudy Allen, *(Learning Difficulties & Disabilities).*

Additional thanks

Additional thanks to Chris Monk of Yellowduck Design; Mary Shoesmith; Mike Hayles; Mike O'Sullivan of Mind In Barnet; Paul Elmes; Richard Matthews, (for cover photograph); Richard Neale of *Hastings & St Leonards Observer,* and Val Greenwood.

Errors

We have done our best to ensure that the information contained in this guide is correct as at the time of going to press. It is inevitable however that there will be irritating mistakes which have escaped detection.

For these we apologise and would ask that any errors and suggestions for improvement be reported to the Editor in order that the next edition, due to be published in the summer of 2001 may be corrected.

Please send any amendments, updates, corrections or comments to: The Editor, Good Health Guide, Hastings Mind, St Peter's Place, 32/33, St Peter's Road, St Leonards-on-Sea, Sussex, TN37 6JQ. Your help is greatly appreciated, thank you.

HASTINGS MIND

good health guide

problems

This first part of the Guide gives descriptions of many mental health and other problems, together with appropriate information about local and national organisations which can provide help. For a quick overview of this section, please see the Contents on page 6

Alcohol

It is estimated that in the UK, 1 in 20 people aged 16 to 64 are dependent on alcohol to function. Many more regularly abuse alcohol by exceeding accepted safety limits. Have *you* got an alcohol problem? [5202]

Alcohol is probably the oldest drug known to man - our ancestors discovered that fruit left in the corner of a cave underwent a process of change, which in turn led to a change in the effect of the fruit on human beings! We have since learned the effects of yeast on sugars through a process of fermentation that produces alcohol. [5202]

Effects of alcohol

Alcohol problems vary in intensity. They are often referred to by other descriptions, e.g. alcohol dependence, alcoholism and alcohol abuse. The simple fact is that heavy drinking has many effects on the human body.

Liver disease

Heavy alcohol intake is the most common cause of liver damage in the United Kingdom. Approximately 90% of heavy drinkers have a fatty liver, 40% develop alcoholic hepatitis (inflammation of the liver) and many of these will develop alcoholic cirrhosis of the liver after many years of drinking, usually a fatal condition.

Digestive problems

Peptic ulceration, gastritis (inflammation of the stomach) and pancreatitis (inflammation of the pancreas) are all associated with heavy drinking. In fact, 42% of deaths from acute pancreatitis are associated with alcohol.

Heart disease

Drinking above the recommended safe limits is a common cause of high blood pressure, which in turn increases the risk of heart disease and strokes. A condition known as cardiomyopathy, where heart muscle is damaged, can be caused by alcohol and may be fatal.

Sexual issues

Men who are heavy drinkers complain of more impotence problems, whilst heavy drinking in women may be a factor in unwanted pregnancies.

Cancer

Certain cancers are more evident in heavy drinkers, e.g. mouth and throat cancers.

Brain damage

Severe damage can occur in the brain during the process of alcohol withdrawal. This can be acute and may cause permanent damage or even death. Over long periods of time alcohol contributes to brain cell death, which in turn contributes to loss of memory and related illnesses. [5202]

Help

It is recommended for those experiencing problems with excessive alcohol consumption to first make an appointment to see a general practitioner (GP).

Addiction to alcohol is becoming much more common in the UK and a GP can help in various ways. Initially he or she may talk about alcohol consumption and indicate some of the damage that it may be causing. Depending upon local facilities, the GP may then decide to offer treatment directly, perhaps with the help of the Community Alcohol Team (CAT) or other local facilities.

Occasionally a GP may decide to refer a patient to a psychiatrist, who is more experienced in treating people with alcohol problems.

Whatever decision the GP makes, that first visit to a GP is the biggest step that someone can take in recognising a problem and starting on the road to making a full recovery. *Alcoholism is an illness* and can be treated with specific methods tailored to individuals' needs. [5202]

Mental health
Alcohol plays havoc with emotions. In those who are already anxious, alcohol can contribute in the long term to increased levels of anxiety. In those who are unhappy or sad, depression may plunge to new depths. The rate of suicide has long been acknowledged to be extremely high in alcohol abusers and alcohol dependent individuals. [5202]

How many people drink?
It is estimated that in the UK 1 in 20 people (aged 16-64) are dependent on alcohol to function. Many more regularly abuse alcohol by exceeding the accepted safety limits of 14 units per week for women and 21 units for men.

Contrary to popular belief, whilst the older population is at risk, it is the young, particularly men, between the ages of 16 to 24 years of age who are most at risk. [5202]

Medication

Medication such as chlordiazepoxide *(Librium)* may be prescribed to help prevent withdrawal effects caused during adaptation to an alcohol free situation. This period, often referred to as detoxification or medically assisted withdrawal, will take around a week and might be conducted at home if circumstances are suitable, or in hospital.

Do you have a problem?

If there is need for concern about your own levels of consumption or that of a friend or a family member, there are some frequent symptoms that might suggest that the alcohol intake is excessive. These may include:

Sleep problems - difficulty in getting off to sleep if insufficient alcohol has been consumed at night.

Gastritis - nausea, vomiting, stomach pain or just plain 'indigestion'.

High blood pressure - possibly giving rise to headaches or nose bleeds.

Trauma - ranging from an increasing number of bruises from domestic incidents to serious injuries in a road traffic accident.

Emotions - increased fear, anxiety, sadness, depression - as outlined above.

Questions to ask yourself:

1. Have you ever felt you should cut down on your drinking?
2. Have people annoyed you by criticising your drinking?
3. Have you ever felt bad or guilty about your drinking?
4. Have you ever had a drink first thing in the morning to steady your nerves or to get rid of a hangover? [5202]

It is important to have psychological support during this time and afterwards. At this point, a patient may experience the urge or desire to drink, often referred to as craving.

During the last three years a new medication has been developed to help reduce these cravings, which is called acamprosate *(Campral)*. In clinical trials it has been shown to double patients' abstinence rates compared to counselling alone. It is taken as a tablet and is now prescribed by many doctors to help people overcome the cravings they experience.

Other medicines may be used to assist in recovery such as disulfiram *(Antabuse)*, which has been used by some doctors for many years, or naltrexone, which is not licensed in the UK for use in alcohol related problems, but may be prescribed under certain circumstances for heavy drinkers. [5202]

Treatment

Alcohol dependence is 'a state of suffering which can very usefully be described and treated as an illness.' (So states the opening sentence in Clouds' description of its treatment model and philosophy). It continues 'To do so does not in any way exclude proper consideration of social or personal factors which may have a bearing on a person's present health.'

How much should you drink?

Sensible drinking guidlines are:

Men: If you drink between 3 and 4 units a day or less - there are no significant risks to health.

Women: If you drink between 2 and 3 units a day or less - there are no significant risks to health.

It is important to note that these guidlines are per day, and should not be 'saved up' for say, a binge at the weekend. [5202]

Individuals bear some responsibility for doing what they can to improve their health. They can best do so if given appropriate help. Abstinence, while essential for severely dependent people, is not an end in itself but a necessary step on the way to improving overall health and well-being.

People with alcohol and drug dependency tend to invite others to treat them badly. We resist this invitation as essential to breaking a vicious circle. People can change and become healthier if given the right conditions in which to realise their desire to do so. These conditions include: care trust, respect, understanding, empathy, support, warmth. Information and skilled help must be provided.

While focusing primarily on the dependence, we look at a variety of other issues which may individually or in combination threaten recovery. [5072]

Paying for treatment

The method of getting access to the substance misuse services (for alcohol or drugs) depends on whether you are paying for yourself or not.

If you are able to fund yourself, access is relatively simple. You ring up the relevant unit and staff will arrange to see you to undertake an assessment to see if they can help you. However, if you need financial assistance, you will require a Community Care Act Assessment to determine whether you are eligible for the assistance. This means a social worker has to assess whether you are in the top priority for assistance, and whether the budget is sufficient to pay for your care.

The Community Alcohol Team, the DDU and the Trinity Project can arrange for a social worker to do this assessment. Even if you are funding yourself, it is still useful to contact these services for their help because their attached social worker can help you plan your rehabilitation programme once you are detoxed.

In the future it is proposed to link these substance misuse services to the CMHTs so that access is simplified. [5344]

Independent clinics

There are a number of independent healthcare providers in the UK, such as Clouds and Priory Healthcare, which run intensive, structured rehabilitation programmes within residential units, and these have very good success rates in returning individuals to alcohol free lives.

Whatever the chosen treatment it will be confidential, and will be handled with respect by trained and experienced staff who simply want to help you get better. Please see 'Clouds' and 'Priory Healthcare' pages 17 and 18. [5202]

Training courses

Please see under 'ADCESBH' below.

Local Organisations

ADCESBH

The Alcohol & Drugs Council for East Sussex and Brighton and Hove runs training courses. They are intensive non-residential introductions to substance misuse and interventions. The courses cover alcohol, volatile substances, prescribed and over-the-counter medicines as well as illegal drugs. *Address:* ADCESBH, Centenary House, The Avenue, Eastbourne, East Sussex, BN21 3XT. [5019]

Alcoholics Anonymous

Please see under 'National Organisations'

Al-Anon Family Groups

Please see under 'National Organisations'

Community Alcohol Team

The Community Alcohol Team (CAT) is an independent non-profit making organisation that exists to help those who are experiencing problems with alcohol. A free and confidential service is offered to anyone who is concerned with their own or someone else's drinking. [5400]

CAT Counselling Service: What is counselling? Counselling is a joint activity, and on the first session you and your counsellor will concentrate on your drinking and other areas of your life you may want to change.

Talking things through and knowing you will be listened to in a safe setting will help. It is up to you how much you want to share with your counsellor, and you will make a plan together to carry out the changes you decide upon.

We appreciate that sometimes we need to change other areas of our life to bring about changes in our drinking. You will be able to discuss options and the possible solutions with your counsellor.

Your first session will last about an hour. It is possible that you may want someone else who is important to you to come with you. They are welcome to do so. Counsellors are not experts or advisors. They won't tell you what to do or what not to do. Their skills are based around helping you to help yourself. Monday to Friday, 9.00am to 5.00pm. 5401

CAT Eastbourne: Address: Community Alcohol Team Projects, 41a, Susans Road, Eastbourne, East Sussex, BN21 3TJ. Tel: 01323 419696. Fax: 01323 419610. May 2000

CAT Hastings: Address: Community Alcohol Team, 46, Cambridge Road, Hastings, Sussex, TN34 1DT. *Tel:* 01424 460066. *Fax:* 01424 430874. Jun 2000

DAIS

Drug and Alcohol Information Service Helpline: 01424 220788. Please see main entry in 'Substance Misuse' chapter, p 131.

Phoenix House

A national charity with a base in Bexhill, whose main work involves drug rehabilitation. Please see main entry under 'Substance Misuse', page 136. Jun 2000

Sussex Alcohol Advice Centre

A confidential one-to-one counselling service for anyone concerned about their own drinking, or someone else's. A wide range of information is available about alcohol services in the Sussex area and nationally.

The service also runs short courses and training sessions for the statutory and voluntary sectors. Self referral or professional referral can be made. The Counselling Service is available daytime and some evenings. *Contact:* Mal Thompson. *Hours:* Office: Monday to Friday 9.00am to 5.00pm.

Address: Sussex Alcohol Advice Centre, 60 West Street, Brighton, BN1 2RB. *Tel:* 01273 739147. *Fax:* 01273 773846. Jun 2000

Units of alcohol.

A unit of alcohol is 10ml. of alcohol. To calculate the number of units in a drink, work out the actual amount of pure alcohol in your drink and divide by 10.

Example: a 750ml. bottle of wine of say 12% strength contains 750 x 12% = 90ml. of alcohol. At 10ml. per unit, that is 9 units.

Another example: a 440ml. can of 5% lager contains 440 x 5% = 22ml. of alcohol, which is 2.2 units.

One more example: a 700ml. bottle of Scotch whisky at 40% contains 700 x 40% = 280ml. of alcohol, or 28 units.

Other measures are:

Double whisky, (50ml.): 2.0 units
Single whisky, (25ml.): 1.0 unit
Pint of 4% beer, (568ml.): 2.7 units
Half pint 5% lager, (284ml.): 1.4 units
Bottle of 12% wine, (750ml.): 9 units
Glass of wine, 12% (125ml.): 1.0 unit

National Organisations

Alcoholics Anonymous

Group meetings for clients and anyone who has a desire to stop drinking. Meetings throughout the area provide support and advice from other recovering alcoholics, based on their own experience. Meetings held 7 days a week, in various locations in the Hastings & Rother area. For further information please ring one of the following telephone numbers:

Helpline *tel:* 0345 697555; Help & information *tel:* 01622 751842 (8.30am to 10.30pm & answerphone from 10.30pm to 8.30am local call rate). 5867 Jun 2000

Al-Anon Family Groups

Al-Anon is a worldwide network of self-help groups offering understanding and support for families and friends of problem drinkers, whether the alcoholic is still drinking or not. Alateen, a part of Al-Anon, is for young people aged 12 to 20 who have been affected by someone else's drinking, usually that of a parent.

There are over 900 Al-Anon and Alateen groups throughout the UK and Eire. Meetings last about one and a half hours and there is no charge although, as we are a self-supporting organisation, groups do hold a voluntary collection.

Only first names are used at meetings and everything which is said is held in confidence. In order to protect the anonymity of members, groups are not normally open to people with a professional interest although special arrangements can be made. 5000; 5001; 5002.

Address: Al-Anon Family Groups UK & Eire, 61, Great Dover Street, London, SE1 4YF. *Tel:* 020 7403 0888. *Fax:* 020 7378 9910. *E-mail:* alanonuk@aol.com *Website:* www.hexnet.co.uk/alanon/ Jun 2000

Alcohol Counselling Service

Address: Alcohol Counselling Service, 34, Electric Lane, London, SW9 8JT. *Tel:* 020 7737 3579. Jun 2000

Chemical Dependency Centre

This London centre offers a 48-day out-patient programme which costs £55 per day. It is called the 'Sharp' programme (Self-help addiction recovery programme).

Address: Chemical Dependency Centre, 11, Redcliffe Gardens, London, SW10 9BG. *Tel:* 020 7351 7785 & 020 7352 2552. *Fax:* 020 7351 4498 & 020 7351 4498. 5418 Jun 2000

Clouds

Clouds is a charitable alcohol and drug dependency service offering various services (listed below). Clouds' aim is to offer help, hope and freedom from alcohol and drug dependency by providing interrelated services of the highest quality and effectiveness which have a clear and ethical basis and which meet the real needs of clients.

Clouds House: Clouds House is a residential alcohol and drug treatment centre in Wiltshire, offering first-stage intensive abstinence-based integrated treatment for alcohol and/or drug dependency. Treatment aims to improve overall lifestyle and relationships and change self-destructive patterns in a safe, respectful environment, under the care of a multi-disciplinary team. Chief executive: Nick Barton.

Fees: Six weeks' treatment at Clouds House costs just over £1,000 per week, but about two-thirds of those attending receive statutory funding.

Clouds' services: For full details of the services offered by Clouds, please telephone.

Address: Clouds House, East Knoyle, Salisbury, Wiltshire, SP3 6BE. *Tel:* 01747 830733. *Fax:* 01747 830783.
E-mail: admin@clouds.org.uk
Website: www.clouds.org.uk 5072 & 5823; 6090

Drinkline

Offers advice, information and support to anyone concerned about their own or someone else's drinking. *Hours:* Mondays to Fridays 9am to 11pm; Saturdays & sundays 6pm to 11pm. Outside these hours there is a voicemail system in operation.

Address: Healthwise Helpline, The Drinkline for England & Wales, Cavern Court, 8, Mathew Street, Liverpool, L2 6RE. *Call free on:* 0800 917 8282. Jun 2000

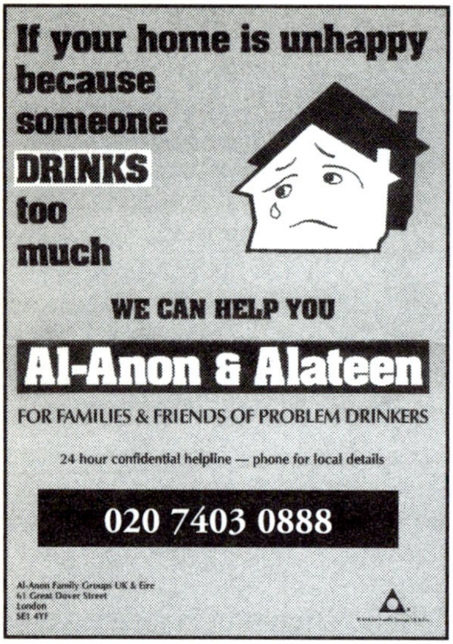

Priory Healthcare

Priory Healthcare operates 14 centres across the country treating alcohol related problems. For further information, or to find the location of your nearest Priory Hospital please telephone 0845 60 50 121; you can e-mail at: prioryhealthcare.co.uk\nottingham or visit the website at: www.prioryhealthcare.co.uk 5202 Jun 2000

Further Information

Health Information Service

The HIS is a free and confidential 24-hour service. You can speak to staff during office hours, and you can listen to any of hundreds of tapes at any time, e.g: *Alcohol: help for families of problem drinkers* (Tape 001); *Alcohol: sensible drinking* (Tape 003); *Alcohol: the facts* (Tape 002); *Cirrhosis of the liver* (Tape 280); *Hangover* (Tape 478).
Address: The College of Health, St Margaret's House, 21, Old Ford Road, London, E2 9PL. *Freephone:* 0800 66 55 44. 5367

See also these chapters ...

Community Mental Health Teams, page 305.
Substance Misuse, page 131.

Anxiety

We all feel anxious at certain times in our lives, perhaps before an important event such as a job interview or exam, or when we're in a difficult or dangerous situation. Although this anxiety can be unpleasant, it rarely lasts long and we usually manage to cope with it. But for some people anxiety is a much more frightening experience which becomes a real problem in their lives.

How it feels

Anxiety of this severe kind can mean feeling overcome with panic, experiencing restlessness, breathlessness, or sweating. It can involve excessive worrying or feeling unable to control disturbing or upsetting thoughts. It can even mean being unable to leave your home because of overwhelming fears, or being unable to keep a job because the anxiety interferes with your concentration.

Everyday life

Anxiety can be described as a feeling of discomfort or unease. Anxiety which continues for a long time can have a serious effect upon your ability to cope with everyday life. You may not be able to identify a specific cause of your anxiety, although feelings of anxiety are often associated with particular places or events.

Adrenaline

The easiest signs of anxiety to recognise are physical changes, such as sweating, a racing heart, palpitations, or rapid breathing. These changes are caused by an increase in adrenaline, the substance which is released by your body to help you get ready to deal with danger. It is quite normal to feel anxious when you are facing something dangerous or difficult, but it is not usual to feel anxious all the time or to feel that anxiety is ruling your life. [5181]

Illness

'Anxiety is a state of fear or worry where your mind is over-active and your body is tense. Most people feel anxious from time to time, but anxiety becomes an illness when it feeds on itself and dominates your life.

Panic attacks

Sometimes people have panic attacks - a rapid build-up of anxiety where your heart pounds, your body sweats and either you start breathing quickly or you find it difficult to breathe.' [0534]

Facts about anxiety

The following information is taken from The Fundamental Facts, published 1999 by the Mental Health Foundation: 'More than one in ten people are likely to have a 'disabling anxiety disorder' at some stage in their life'.

Phobia.

'An estimated 13% of the adult population will develop a specific form of anxiety known as a phobia at some point in their life'. [1571]

Organisations

First Steps to Freedom

Registered charity which aims to help, in a practical way, people who suffer from phobias, obsessional compulsive disorder, anxiety, panic attacks, anorexia and bulimia, and those who wish to come off tranquilisers, and their carers. For more details, please see main entry in 'Phobias' chapter, page 103.

No Panic

A voluntary charity which helps people who suffer from panic attacks, phobias, obsessive compulsive disorders and other anxiety disorders, including those people who are trying to give up tranquilisers. Please see main entry in 'Panic' chapter, page 98.

Further Information

Essential Help for Your Nerves

By Dr Claire Weekes. Many people have suffered from nerves all of their lives and have never attempted to deal with their anxiety. In this new book which combines her previous books *Peace from Nervous Suffering* and *More Help for Your Nerves,* Dr Claire Weekes helps forge an understanding of nervous illness, and creates a recovery programme to instil confidence and happiness. Published by Thorsons, 2000. ISBN: 0-7225-4013-2. 412 pages. Price £8.99. Available from Mind. *Tel:* 020 8221 9666.

5024

Overcoming Anxiety

Written by Helen Kennerley. "Based on clinically proven techniques of cognitive therapy, this book helps you to overcome a whole range of anxieties and fears." Published by Robinson, 1997, 181 pages. ISBN: 1-85487-422-5. Price: £7.99. Available from Mind. *Tel:* 020 8221 9666.

Jan 2000

See also these chapters ...

Phobias, page 103.

Asthma

Local Organisations

Eastbourne Support Group

Contact: Mrs Josie Buxton. *Tel:* 01323 739674. Jun 2000

Brighton Support Group

Contact: Mrs Elaine Lansley. *Tel:* 01273 596103. Jun 2000

National Organisations

Asthma Helpline

The helpline is staffed by asthma nurse specialists who have received further training in listening and counselling skills. They deal with over 18,000 calls per year about asthma and related conditions. The helpline is open from 9am to 7pm from Monday to Friday and calls are charged at local rate. *Tel:* 08457 01 02 03. Jun 2000

Asthma Information Centre

Address: Asthma Information Centre, 14, South Street, St Austell, Cornwall, PL25 4BH. *Tel/Fax:* 01726 616666. 5850

National Asthma Campaign

The National Asthma Campaign is the leading UK charity for people with asthma, with offices in London and Edinburgh, an information centre in St Austell and more than 80 branches throughout the UK. Registered Charity No. 802364.

Aims of the NAC

- to fund research into asthma and related allergy, and to disseminate the results;
- to raise awareness of asthma and related allergy through media work, campaigning, working with MPs and the Government and through public education initiatives;
- to provide information and support to people with asthma, their families and friends, health professionals and the public.

Information and resources

Staff and volunteers at National Asthma Campaign headquarters answer around 40,000 written and telephone enquiries a year. A comprehensive range of literature and resources is available for use both by people with asthma and by health professionals. This includes over 30 factsheets giving detailed advice on specific issues such as housing and dust control products; and 10 different information booklets.

Membership

Over 20,000 people are members of the National Asthma Campaign. Four times per year members receive a copy of *Asthma News* - the magazine for people with asthma and their families and friends. It gives independent advice on how to manage asthma and news about the latest advances in asthma care and research.

Address: National Asthma Campaign, Providence House, Providence Place, London, N1 0NT. *Tel:* 020 7226 2260. *Fax:* 020 7704 0740. *Asthma helpline:* 0845 701 02 03. *Website:* www.asthma.org.uk Jun 2000

Attention Deficit

The full name for this disorder is Attention Deficit/Hyperactivity Disorder, or AD/HD for short.

AD/HD in children

Estimates vary according to the diagnostic measure used. For example, in a UK study, 2% of 7 year old boys had AD/HD; using another definition, 5% of boys between the ages of 6-8 had hyperactivity; and finally, using a third definition, 17% of boys between the ages of 5-11 years had AD/HD. This disorder is a biologically based brain disorder. [1571]

To contact the

HASTINGS & ROTHER ADHD
CHILDREN'S SUPPORT GROUP

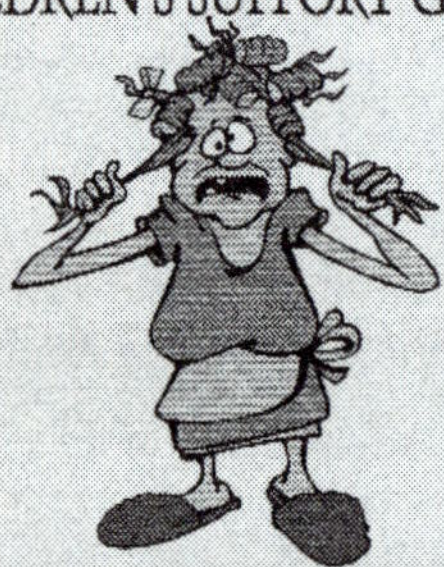

Attention Deficit & Hyperactivity Disorder

TELEPHONE: CARE FOR CARERS

01424 717931

Tell them you need to be put in touch with the Support Group and someone will be in touch with you. Please DO contact and join a Support Group. It is a step in the right direction. Successfully raising a child with ADHD requires lots of support, information and STRONG Mothers!

For Adult Support call: 01424 420767 and speak to Judith.

Local Organisations

Adult Support Network

Adult support network, affiliated to AD/HD Support Group - Sussex, run by Judith Guest and covering all areas of the UK.

The aims of the service are: to disseminate information as widely as possible; educate people from every walk of life about the effects of AD/HD on adult life; ensure that the genetic links of AD/HD are identified so that children of AD/HD adults receive early interventions; listen and understand; offer advice and comfort, especially to mothers. *Address*: Judith Guest, AD/HD Adult Support Network, 75a, Middle Road, Hastings, TN35 5DL. *Tel*: 01424 420767. *Fax:* 01424 202933. *E-Mail:* jguest@200m.co.uk [5445]

Children's Support

Please see panel, this page.

Sussex Support Group

Address: AD/HD Support Group, Sussex, PO Box 50, East Grinstead, RH19 2YE. *Tel*: 01293 428025. *Contact:* Kaz. *Tel*: 01323 642093. [Feb 2000]

Acknowledgements
Our grateful thanks to Judith Guest of AD/HD Adult Support Network, Hastings, for her editorial assistance with this chapter.

Autism

Autism is a complex disorder affecting over 2,800 children in Sussex. It is more common in boys and affects social and communication skills and imaginative activities throughout a person's life.

Some children do not develop speech and those who do often use it in a meaningless and repetitive way. They have difficulty expressing thoughts and desires and cannot understand those of other people.

Chaotic

To children with autism, everything appears chaotic. They behave in unpredictable ways, making normal family life very difficult. Autism varies immensely from child to child, but there are several common signs.

These include displaying indifference, anti-social behaviour, lack of creativity, talking incessantly about one topic and inappropriate laughing or giggling. [From article by Lanie Whiting, May 19 1999]

What is autism?

Autism, which includes Asperger's syndrome, is a developmental disorder affecting especially social and communication skills and imaginative activities. It affects four times as many boys as girls and has no class, creed or racial barriers.

Autism can be found in people of widely differing degrees of mental ability from the severely handicapped to those of above average intelligence. A few show surprising skills in certain areas such as music, drawing or mental arithmetic. No single cause has yet been found for this devastating handicap.[5182]

Speech

Some children with autism do not develop speech and those who do, often use it in a meaningless, repetitive way. They have difficulty in expressing their thoughts, desires, and feelings, and they cannot easily understand those of other people. Everything around them appears chaotic and, consequently, they can behave in bizarre and unpredictable ways. They find comfort in repetitive activities and dislike changes in familiar routines.[5182]

Asperger Syndrome

Asperger syndrome is a form of autism, a disability that affects the way people communicate and relate to others. A number of traits of autism are common to Asperger syndrome including difficulty in communicating, difficulty in social relationships, lack of understanding of the thought processes of others (empathy). Most do not have the accompanying learning disability often associated with autism.

Most people with Asperger syndrome (AS) have a good vocabulary and often speak fluently though their words may sound over-formal and stilted. Whilst often excelling at facts and figures, people with AS find it hard to think in abstract ways. They often develop an all-consuming interest in a hobby or collection.

People with Asperger syndrome realise that they are different to other people and can feel isolated and become depressed. Sadly they can make an easy target for bullying at school or in the workplace. Their social naivety makes them vulnerable to exploitation.

Most people with Asperger syndrome are intelligent, very honest and conscientious. They need help so that they can make relationships and use their skills for the benefit of themselves and society. For help and advice contact the Sussex Autistic Society.

Local Organisations

Sussex Autistic Society

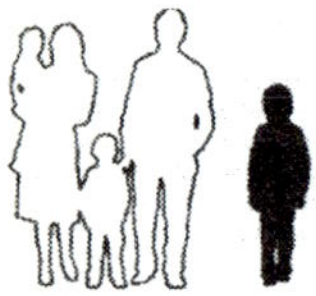

The Sussex Autistic Society was formed in 1980 and is a local self-help group for families of children with autism living in Sussex. The Society and its support groups welcome all parents of children with autism.

The Society's aims & objectives are:

- to provide opportunities for parents to meet, when ideas can be exchanged and problems dicussed;
- to encourage awareness of autism and the special problems that exist for people with autism;
- to encourage professionals in education, health and social services to be more aware of the special needs of people with autism;
- to press local authorities to provide better services for children and adults with autism;
- to provide a range of support services for families and their children with autism.

Contacts: Philippa Erasmus, Administrator, and Amanda Brewis, Family Support Service Co-ordinator. Vi Menzies, Asperger support worker. Mike Stone, Outreach manager.

Address: Sussex Autistic Society, Bridge House, 40, Keymer Road, Hassocks, West Sussex, BN6 8AP. *General enquiries tel/fax:* 01273 846846. *Family support service helpline tel:* 01273 841254 (available Mondays to Thursdays 10am to 12.30pm). *Asperger helpline: tel.* 01273 841408; *fax:* 01273 846846. *E-mail:* admin.sas@virgin.net 5183 May 2000

Sussex Autistic Community Trust

The Sussex Autistic Community Trust runs support groups for adults with Asperger syndrome in East and West Sussex. The groups have weekly meetings in Brighton, Crawley, Hastings and Worthing.

The aims of the groups are:

- to provide mutual support through discussion and conversation;
- to provide opportunities to expand social contact;
- to plan outings to practice skills in social situations;
- to practice skills in meeting people and building friendships.

The groups in each of the different areas are developing differently in response to the wishes of the different members. People are encouraged to express wishes and opinions in a safe and supportive environment.

These social groups offer individuals the opportunity to develop and practice conversation, listening and interaction in this safe environment and to use real life situations to develop skills further.

Activities include social skills games, board games, discussion and debate, planning group outings in social settings.

Being given a diagnosis of Asperger Syndrome can bring a feeling of relief following years of uncertainty. It can also bring feelings of anger, emotional pain and confusion.

Joining a group of people with similar concerns could help you to deal with these feelings in a positive way and to develop ways of coping. *Contact*: Vi Menzies, Asperger Support Worker.

Address: Bridge House, 40, Keymer Road, Hassocks, West Sussex, BN6 8AP. *Tel:* 01273 841408. May 2000

National Organisations

Autism Information Centre

Information Centre for interested professionals, students, general public (tel: 020 7903 3599 Mondays to Fridays 10am to 4pm) drawing on a research database covering all aspects of autism.

National Helpline

National Autism Helpline for parents, carers, families and people with autism (tel: 0870 600 8585, Mondays, Tuesdays, Wednesdays and Fridays 10am to 4pm; Thursdays 10am to 8pm). *E-mail:* autismhelpline@nas.org.uk Jun 2000

National Autistic Society

The National Autistic Society exists to champion the rights and interests of all people throughout the UK with autism and to ensure that they and their families receive quality services appropriate to their needs. It runs schools and adult centres; offers families and carers information, advice and support; works to improve awareness of autism; offers a diagnostic and assessment service; and provides training and promotes research.

Patron: HRH The Princess Royal. President: Jane Asher, the actress. Chief Executive: Paul Cann. Acting Chief Executive: Tony Kay.

Address: National Autistic Society, 393, City Road, London EC1V 1NG. *Tel:* 020 7833 2299. *Fax:* 020 7833 9666. *E-mail:* nas@nas.org.uk *Website:* www.oneworld.org/autism_uk/ May 2000

Peach

PEACH (Parents for the Early Intervention of Autism in Children).

PEACH is a charity advocating and supporting parents who are conducting a home-based behavioural intervention programme as pioneered by Dr Ivar Lovaas for children with autism and related disorders. The pack includes an interview with Dr Lovaas about the inception of Applied Behavioural Analysis.

Peach was started in 1996 by a group of parents who were using home-based behavioural intervention to help their learning-disabled children. What began as a committed few has grown to some 900 members still focused on that original purpose. *Contact:* Carrie Haslett, PEACH President.

Address: PEACH, Behavioural Intervention Programme, School of Education, Brunel University, St Margaret's Road, Twickenham, Middlesex, TW1 1PT. *Tel:* 020 8891 0121. *Fax:* 020 8891 8209. *E-mail:* peachatbrunel.ac.uk *Website:* www.peach.uk.com 5888

Further Information

Health Information Service

The HIS is a free and confidential 24-hour service. You can speak to staff during office hours, and you can listen to any of hundreds of tapes at any time, e.g: *Autism: children* (Tape 267). *Address:* The College of Health, St Margaret's House, 21, Old Ford Road, London, E2 9PL. *Freephone:* 0800 66 55 44. 5367

Back Pain

Organisations

BackCare

Covering all areas of the UK, BackCare helps people manage and prevent back pain by providing advice, promoting self-help, encouraging debate and funding scientific research into better back care. For an information pack (price £3), membership or general enquiries, please contact via the address below or on their website.
Executive director: Emma Tait.

Address: BackCare, 16, Elmtree Road, Teddington, TW11 8ST. *Tel:* 020 8977 5474. *Fax:* 020 8943 5318. *E-mail:* backpain@compuserve.com *Website:* www.backpain.org [5451]

Further information

Audio cassettes

Coping with back pain.
Successful techniques for the relief of all types of back pain; what you can do to cope on a daily basis and how to improve your quality of life. Contains relaxation exercise. Published by Talking Life, tel: 0151 632 0662,

Bereavement

Bereavement refers to the emotional state of being 'bereft', a word which originally meant 'to be torn open'. At no time do we feel more torn open than when we experience what is known as a 'high grief' - a sudden or violent death, a suicide or the loss of a child. [5265]

Bereavement refers to the emotional state of being 'bereft', a word which originally meant 'to be torn open'. At no time do we feel more torn open than when we experience what is known as a 'high grief' - a sudden or violent death, a suicide or the loss of a child.

A 'low grief' death is one which has been expected for a long time, such as that of an extremely elderly person, or a loss for which we have already grieved, such as someone with a terminal illness; or the death of someone to whom we are not particularly attached.

The depth of pain we experience in high or low grief is connected to our degree of attachment to the person and how much he or she was integral to our sense of well-being.

Bereavement is a lengthy process. When the grieving is especially protracted, it might be appropriate to seek bereavement counselling, a specialised type of counselling focussing on a return to a way of life which takes account of the loss experienced.[5265]

Counsellors

The following people offer bereavement counselling. For full details of each person please see 'Counselling & Therapy' chapter.

Julie Askew (Brighton & Hove); Susan Chiswell Jones (Brighton); Lorna Couldrick (Bexhill); Joy Cobban (Eastbourne); Sue Cottrell (Hove); Val Cunningham (KCPU Tunbridge Wells);Jane Dale (Brighton/Hove); Rosemary Dixon-Nuttall (Crowborough); Prue Doherty (Bexhill); Lynn Jackson (Brighton); Graham Molyneux (Brighton); Edna Murdoch (Hove); Genievieve Picquart (Hove); Roger Powe (Brighton); Gillian Rock (Brighton); Janet Seller (Forest Row); Frankie Sidhu (Brighton); John Stedman (Hove); Christine Terris (Ticehurst); Melanie Withers (Brighton).

Local Organisations

Cruse Bereavement Care

The local Cruse office covers Bexhill, Hastings, St Leonards & Rural Rother. Cruse Bereavement Care offers counselling and help to any bereaved person. Counselling is carried out by counsellors specifically trained in the area of bereavement. Anyone may apply to Cruse. Counselling sessions usually take place in the client's own home, although neutral venues can be arranged. All services are free of charge.

Address: Cruse Bereavement Care, 6, Wartling Drive, Bexhill, Sussex, TN39 4QN. *Tel:* 01424 845006 (Charles Croft, for admin and referrals); 01424 732093 (Halina, for referrals). [5629]

St Michael's Bereavement Service

The aim of the Service is to offer individual counselling support. It is intended to be a temporary support during the most difficult period of grief. The counsellors are carefully selected. They have attended a bereavement counselling course and are given further in-service training and on-going supervision. Individual counselling sessions last up to 1 hour, generally once a week or fortnight, over a period of weeks or months.

Office hours are Mondays to Fridays, 8.30am to 5.00pm. *Contact*: Keith Brunger.

Chairman: Mrs Veronica Bishop, Director of Clinical Support Services, St Michael's Hospice 25, Upper Maze Hill, St Leonards, Sussex, TN39 0LB.

Service Co-ordinator: Keith Brunger. *Address:* St Michael's Bereavement Service, Bexhill Hospital, Holliers Hill, Bexhill, Sussex, TN40 2DZ. *Tel:* 01424 755255, ext. 5314. *Fax:* 01424 213250. May 2000

Bexhill

Address: Bereavement Co-ordinator, St Michael's Bereavement Service, Bexhill Hospital, Holliers Hill, Bexhill-on-Sea, East Sussex, TN40 2DZ. *Tel*: 01424 730077. Jun 2000

St Leonards

Address: Bereavement Co-ordinator, St Michael's Bereavement Service, 25, Upper Maze Hill, St Leonards-on-Sea, East Sussex. *Tel*: 01424 445177. Jun 2000

National Organisations

Bereavement Register

If you wish to stop unwanted letters being sent to deceased relatives, contact the Bereavement Register, which specialises in clearing mailshot databases. This is a free service. Helpline: 0870 600 7222 (charged at local rate). *Website*: www.thebereavement-register.org.uk Jun 2000

Child death helpline

Telephone helpline for anyone affected by the death of a child. Call free on 0800 282986. *Hours:* Monday, Wednesday and Friday 10am to 1pm; every evening from 7 to 10pm. Jun 2000

Compassionate Friends

Covering all the UK, an organisation offering support and friendship for bereaved parents and their families by those similarly bereaved. Registered Charity No. 263463. *Contacts:* Mr Jon Gilbody, office administrator; Mrs Pearl Hunt and Mrs Maggie Indelicato, Pastoral assistants.

Address: Compassionate Friends, 53, North Street, Bristol, BS8 1EN. *National helpline*: 0117 953 9639. *Admin. tel:* 0117 966 5202. *Fax:* 0117 914 4368. *E-mail:* info@tcf.org.uk *Website:* www.tcf.org.uk May 2000

Cruse Bereavement Care

Cruse Bereavement Care is the largest bereavement charity in the UK, with 180 local branches. It offers help to people bereaved by death, in any way, whatever their age, nationality or belief. Cruse's help includes a free counselling service for bereaved people, opportunities for contact with others through bereavement support groups and advice or information on practical matters. It is personal and confidential help, backed by a wide range of publications.

For bereaved people who would like to speak to a counsellor on the telephone, a service is available seven days a week during afternoons and evenings; please call 08457 585 565. Or, alternatively, for details of your local branch of Cruse call (020) 8940

4818.

Self-referral is the usual way most people contact Cruse. However, where the bereaved person has given their consent, we may accept referrals from the family, or the various caring professions. Registered Charity No. 208078. [5187]

National office: Address: Cruse Bereavement Care, Cruse House, 126, Sheen Road, Richmond, Surrey, TW9 1UR. *Tel*: (020) 8940 4818. Also: (020) 8332 7227. 24-hour telephone message. *Fax:* (020) 8940 7638. *E-mail:* info@crusebereavementcare.org.uk [Jun 2000]

National Association

The National Association of Bereavement Services (NABS) is a nationwide network of organisations and individuals offering services to bereaved people. Set up in 1988 as a co-ordinating and support organisation, NABS offers its members a wide range of opportunities to gain and share expertise, and to meet with others involved in similar work.

Aims and Objectives

To provide a forum for members of the Association; to initiate and encourage regional support groups for those involved in bereavement services; to arrange training activities for volunteers, counsellors, co-ordinators and other professionals; to undertake and facilitate debate and research on matters related to terminal illness, loss and bereavement, and to disseminate the results; to highlight gaps in provision and press for new services to be established; to offer advice and information, and to promote awareness of matters relating to the terminally ill and their families, and to bereavement; to compile a national database of bereavement services.

NABS members

NABS members offer a range of bereavement support services to people who have experienced the death of someone close; some provide support to those caring for a relative or friend with a life-threatening illness. Other NABS members offer opportunities for social contact to people whose lives have been shattered by bereavement and loneliness. *Hours*: 10am to 4pm Monday to Friday.

Address: National Association of Bereavement Services, 2nd Floor, 4, Pinchin Street, London, E1 1SA. *Helpline/Advice*: 020 7709 9090. *General Enquiries*: 020 7709 0505 *Fax*: 020 7709 0505. [Jun 2000]

Pet Bereavement

This a special service offering support to those who have lost a pet dog or cat or any other companion animal and who are finding it a difficult experience to cope with.

The first call to the helpline by a bereaved animal lover is free, but subsequent calls are charged at the local call rate. The helpline is run jointly by The Blue Cross and the Society for Companion Animal Studies, and is funded by a Lottery grant. The telephone befrienders are trained for up to six months to learn how to offer pet bereavement support.

Address: Jo-Ann Dono, Head of Pet Bereavement Support Services, The Blue Cross, Shilton Road, Burford, Oxfordshire, OX18 4PF. *Tel*: 01993 825539. *Helpline*: 0800 0966606. [6036 Aug 2000]

Further Information

After the Death of Someone very close

"Available only from Cruse Bereavement Care, this is Cruse's best-selling booklet in which a counsellor guides the reader through some of the feelings commonly experienced during the grief of a bereavement. A basic, helpful introduction to bereavement, whatever the circumstances."

Available from Cruse Bereavement Care, 126 Sheen Road, Richmond, Surrey, TW9 1UR. Price: £1.50 including p&p. Or for a free mail order catalogue please send a stamped, self-addressed envelope. [5187]

Companion to Grief

Written by Patricia Kelly. "Grieving is often a solitary process, but with this book you need not feel you are alone." Published by Piatkus, 1997. ISBN 0-7499-1734-2. 176 pages, £5.50. Available from Mind Mail Order Service. *Tel*: 020 8221 9666. [5106]

Health Information Service

The HIS is a free and confidential 24-hour service. You can speak to staff during office hours, and you can listen to any of hundreds of tapes at any time, e.g: *Bereavement* (Tape 088); *Bereavement after suicide* (Tape 243).

Address: The College of Health, St Margaret's House, 21, Old Ford Road, London, E2 9PL. *Freephone*: 0800 66 55 44. [May 2000]

Acknowledgements
Our grateful thanks to Linda Mooncie, bereavement counsellor, for her editorial assistance with this chapter. March 2000

Brain Injury

Local Organisations

Headway Hurstwood Park

Headway Hurstwood Park is a charity dedicated to providing care, advice, information, support and outreach services for people throughout Sussex affected by acquired brain injury. Headway aims to promote understanding of the consequences of acquired brain injury and to campaign for the provision of services.

Based in Newick, Headway Hurstwood Park offers a day centre providing specialist day care and secondary rehabilitation for adults with acquired brain injuries. The emphasis is on helping clients to realise their potential and to nurture self-esteem and confidence.

Headway Hurstwood Park also provides specialised outreach services in certain areas. The emphasis for this service is the development of planned programmes with goals and targets promoting independence through sustainable activities.

An acquired brain injury co-ordinator works throughout East Sussex, ensuring that relevant information and advice is available at every stage of recovery.

Support groups

There are help groups throughout East Sussex. All groups meet from 7.30 to 9.30pm.

Newick - last Wednesday each month at Headway House.

Brighton and Hove - third Thursday each month at Montague House, Montague Place, Brighton.

Hastings, Bexhill and St Leonards - first Tuesday each month at the Moreton Centre, St Leonards.

An Eastbourne group is planned for later this year.

Contacts: Dr Ella Squires, centre manager; Tony Woods, fundraising resources & development manager; Mark Holloway, acquired brain injury co-ordinator; Ann Cummings, chairman & 24 hour support person.

Address: Headway Hurstwood Park, Headway House, Jackies Lane, Newick, East Sussex, BN8 4QX. *Tel:* 01825 724323. *Fax:* 01825 724363. *E-mail:* info@headway-hp.org.uk *Website:* www.headway-hp.org.uk 5867 Jul 2000; 6003 Jun 2000

Ticehurst House Hospital

Private hospital established 1792, specialising in brain injury, behaviour problems, self-harm, etc. For further details, please see main entry in 'Hospitals & Clinics' chapter, page 323.

National Organisations

British Institute

The British Institute of Brain Injured Children (BIBIC) offers a fighting alternative to accepting brain injury as untreatable. Funds from this campaign will help brain injured children nationwide - providing equipment, therapy and awareness of the problems of brain injury in young people. Registered charity 1057635.

Address: BIBIC, Knowle Hall, Bridgwater, Somerset, TA7 8PJ. *Tel*: 01278 684060. *Website:* www.bibic.org.uk May 2000

British Brain & Spine Foundation

The British Brain & Spine Foundation aims to improve the quality of life for people with neurological disorders and to reduce neurological disability by providing national programmes for research, education and information.

The Brain & Spine Helpline is staffed by neurological nurses and is open Mondays to Fridays 9am to 1pm; Wednesdays 10am to

6 pm. Tel: freephone 0808 808 1000.

Chief Executive: John McDonald, Research & Education Manager, Maggie Alexander. Helpline co-ordinator: Angela Collett. Fundraising manager: Leigh Slocombe. Fundraising officer, Claire Petrie. *Contact:* Victoria Murray, Research & Education Officer.

Address: British Brain & Spine Foundation, 7, Winchester House, Kennington Park, Cranmer Road, London, SW9 6EJ. *Tel:* 0207 793 5900. *Fax:* 0207 793 5939. *E-mail:* info@bbsf.org.uk *Website:* www.bbsf.org.uk [5519]

Headway

Brain Injury Association. *Address*: Headway, 4, King Edward Court, King Edward Street, Nottingham, NG1 1EW. *Tel*: 0115 924 0800. *Fax*: 0115 9584446. *E-mail*: enquiries@headway.org.uk *Website:* www.headway.org.uk [Jun 2000]

PAL

This is a division of the British Institute of Brain Injured Children, which helps children suffering from specific learning difficulties. Registered Charity No. 1057635. Marketing & Communications Manager: Pam Brooks.

Address: Parent Assisted Learning Centre, BIBIC, Knowle Hall, Bridgewater, Somerset, TA7 8PJ. *Tel*: 01278 684060. *Fax:* 01278 685573. *E-mail:* info@bibic.org.uk [May 2000]

National Hospital

The National Hospital for Neurology & Neurosurgery. Two million people in the UK suffer from a neurological disorder. The National Hospital for Neurology and Neurosurgery leads the world in research and development and in teaching.

Address: The National Hospital for Neurology & Neurosurgery Development Foundation, Queen Square, London, WC1N 3BG. *Tel*: 020 7829 8724. *Fax*: 020 7278 2252. *E-mail:* paul.meyer@uclh.org [Jun 2000]

Further Information

Information booklets

The British Brain & Spine Foundation publishes a number of free information booklets. Subjects covered include AIDS and the brain; angiogram; back and neck pain; brain tumours; CT scans; dizziness and balance problems; epilepsy; face pain; headache; head injury and concussion; meningitis and encephalitis; MRI scans; multiple sclerosis; neurophysiology; paralysis; Parkinson's disease; speech, language and communication difficulties; stroke; sub-arachnoid haemorrhage; transient ischaemic attacks. See above for address.

Neurophysiology

A guide to brain and nerve electrical function tests. "Being admitted to hospital for tests for a suspected brain, nerve or spine disorder can be a terrifying experience for patients and their loved ones. The implications are so enormous that it is not surprising that many people find themselves with questions left unanswered. The complexity of the tests can provoke even more anxiety. This publication, written by an expert, seeks to make sense of the procedures and their consequences". Booklet published by the British Brain & Spine Foundation, 1999, £4.00, post free from BBSF, Freepost, London, SW9 6BR. [5185]

Bullying

Question: what do Phil Collins, Harrison Ford, Mel Gibson, Tom Cruise, Michelle Pfeiffer and Frank Bruno have in common? Answer: they were all bullied when young. The Anit-Bullying Campaign receives 20,000 calls a year ... [5242, 5244]

If you want to talk to someone, call the *Anti-Bullying Campaign*. You can also e-mail *Bullying Online*, and on the internet there's *Pupiline* and *Kidscape*.

Bullies and victims

The Anti-Bullying Campaign defines a *bully* as someone who is insecure, has low self-esteem, is bullied at home, likes to be in control, thrives on the feeling of power and status, may have learning difficulties, seeks attention, lacks respect towards peers and their teacher, is materialistically minded and is jealous.

A *victim* is defined as someone who lacks power, has low self-esteem, is not so strong, is perceived as different, is a swot, is vulnerable and isolated, is disabled, is perceived as different socially or racially, is kind and considerate to peers, is gentle and loving, puts others' feelings before their own. [5242]

Facts about bullying

Children who have been bullied are at a greater risk of experiencing periods of anxiety, sleep problems, depression and thoughts of suicide. An estimated 25% of junior and middle school pupils are being bullied. [1571]

If you get bullied

What to do ...

Advice given on pupiline.net: *Remember you don't deserve to be bullied, it's the bully's problem!* Talk about it to someone who will listen. Tell a teacher you trust. Stick to facts and bring a witness. Defend yourself if necessary. Stay in a group. Be firm, if they pressure you, shout 'NO!' - it'll get attention.

What not to do ...

Do not ignore the bullying - make a noise about it! Don't confront the bully. Don't fight back, except to defend yourself. Don't get in a slanging match. If you are scared or intimidated get away and get help. Don't fight to keep your stuff - *you* are more important! [5243]

National Organisations

Anti-Bullying Campaign

The Anti-Bullying Campaign was set up in 1985 by Janet Perry after the tragic death of her son Mark who had been a bullying victim. The group received 20,000 calls in 1999. If you want to speak to someone in person, please ring the helpline number below. On offer, throughout the UK, is constructive advice and support to the child victims of school bullying, and their parents, by means of a 'Samaritan' style helpline. Because they do get so many calls, please be patient if you find it hard to get through. Training is given to schools as well as resource material for teachers to use in class.

Address: Anti-Bullying Campaign 185, 185, Tower Bridge Road, London, SE1 2UF. *Tel*: 020 7378 1446. *Fax*: 020 7378 8374. *E-Mail:* anti-bullying@compuserve.com
Website: ourworld.compuserve.com/homepages/ [5242]
May 2000

Bullying Online

Internet help. They try to reply within 24 hours but at busy times priority is given to children in distress.
E-mail: help@bullying.co.uk [5242]

Kidscape

A useful internet site for information, books, posters, leaflets and videos. *Address*: Kidscape, 2, Grosvenor Gardens, London, SW1W 0DH. *Tel*: 020 7730 3300. *Fax*: 020 7730 7081.
Website:www.kidscape.org.uk [5244]

Pupiline

This website to help victims of school bullying was set up by Colchester teenagers Oli Watts and Kate Riddle in February 2000, who suffered at the hands of playground louts. After being featured on tv's *Kilroy* programme, their site has received thousands of visits, over 23,000 on the first day!
Website:www.pupiline.net [5243]

Further Information

Health Information Service

The HIS is a free and confidential 24-hour service. You can speak to staff during office hours, and you can listen to any of hundreds of tapes at any time, e.g. *Bullying* (Tape 377); *Bullying: in the workplace* (Tape 469)

Address: The College of Health, St Margaret's House, 21, Old Ford Road, London, E2 9PL. *Freephone*: 0800 66 5544.
5367

Cerebral Palsy

In recent years there has been a slight increase in the proportion of children who have cerebral palsy. Currently about one in every 400 is affected. [5285]

Cerebral palsy (CP) is not a disease or an illness. It is the description of a physical impairment that affects movement. The movement problems vary from barely noticeable to extremely severe. No two people with CP are the same - it is as individual as people themselves.

Types of cerebral palsy

'Cerebral palsy' includes a variety of conditions. The three main types correspond to injuries to different parts of the brain:

People with *spastic* CP find that some muscles become very stiff and weak, especially under effort. This can affect their control of movement.

People with *athetoid* CP have some loss of control of their posture and tend to make unwanted movements.

People with *ataxic* CP usually have problems with balance. They may also have shaky hand movements and irregular speech. [5285]

What are the effects?

The main effect of CP is difficulty in movement. Many people with CP are hardly affected, others have problems walking, feeding, talking or using their hands. Some people are unable to sit up without support and need constant enabling.

People with CP often have difficulty controlling their movement and facial expressions. This does not necessarily mean that their mental abilities are in any way impaired. Some are of higher than average intelligence, other people with CP have moderate or severe learning difficulties. Most, like most people without CP are of average intelligence. [5285]

How does it happen?

Cerebral palsy is most commonly the result of failure of a part of the brain to develop, either before birth or in early childhood. This is sometimes because of bleeding or blocked blood vessels, complications in labour or extreme prematurity. Infections during pregnancy, e.g. *rubella*, or infancy and early childhood, e.g. *meningitis* or *encephalitis*, can lead to CP. [5285]

Prevalence of cerebral palsy

Improvements in maternity services and neonatal care have meant that fewer babies develop cp as a result of lack of oxygen (from difficulties at birth) or jaundice, but they have also meant that more babies with very low birth weights survive. These babies are more likely to have CP

Currently about one in every 400 is affected. Among these, the percentage of severely and multiply disabled people needing Scope's support is growing. That need will continue throughout their lives. [5285]

Is there a cure?

No, but we do know that correct treatment from an early age can ease the effects of cp. Occasionally children who appear to have cp lose the signs as they get older. Most importantly, having a disability does not mean that someone cannot lead a full and independent life. [5285]

Local Organisations

Buddy Scheme

If you are over 18 and would like to get out more or have company to access community facilities, you could try the 'Buddy Scheme', a partnership project between Scope and SASBAH. Contact: Amber. *Tel:* 01424 200581. 5833 May 2000

Scope East Sussex

The objects of the charity are the care, welfare, interest and advancement of persons with cerebral palsy. The charity employs a welfare officer to visit members regularly and advise the management committee of their needs and requirements. The charity's main source of income is from sale of goods donated to their shop at 5, George Street, Hastings, East Sussex. Shop staff are all volunteers. *Contact:* Mrs Clare Brazier, welfare officer.

Address: Scope, 5, George Street, Old Town, Hastings, East sussex. *Tel:* 01424 428301. 5867 Jun 2000

Scope South East

Scope South East Area Partnership Team. Working together with disabled children & adults, families & carers. Information, advice and support is offered and the organisation has a particular expertise in the field of cerebral palsy. Applications for financial assistance from individuals and groups are considered. *Contact:* Ms Beryl Cross, Community fieldworker - East Sussex, Brighton & Hove.

Address: Scope, SE Area Partnership Team, 22, High Street, Westerham, Kent, TN16 1RG. *Tel:* 01959 564686. *Fax:* 01959 562021.
E-mail:
southeast.scope@ukonline.co.uk Website: www.scope.org.uk Jun 2000

National Organisations

Scope

Formerly the Spastics Society, Scope is a national organisation working for people with cerebral palsy. *Tel:* 020 7619 7100.
Jun 2000

Helpline

Scope's Cerebral Palsy Helpline provides free and confidential information and support seven days a week. The line is open 9am to 9pm weekdays and 2pm to 6pm weekends. CPH Administrator: Jaime Burbridge.

Address: Scope, PO Box 833, Milton Keynes, MK12 5NY. *Helpline:* 0808 800 3333. *Admin:* 01908 321047. *E-mail:* cphelpline@scope.org.uk
Website: www.scope.org.uk May 2000

Further Information

Health Information Service

The HIS is a free and confidential 24-hour service. You can speak to staff during office hours, and you can listen to any of hundreds of tapes at any time, e.g: *Cerebral palsy* (Tape 417). *Address:* The College of Health, St Margaret's House, 21, Old Ford Road, London, E2 9PL. *Freephone:* 0800 66 5544.
5367

Acknowledgments
Our grateful thanks to Scope for permission to use material from their published information sheets.

Children & Young People

Local Organisations

Blagh

Bisexual, Lesbian & Gay Hastings (Blagh) offers support for under 25s who identify as being bisexual, lesbian or gay, or who are questioning their sexuality or have issues around it. Young people can access support via the helpline, one-to-one support and a safe social meeting place.

Address: BLAGH, c/o 31, Cambridge Road, Hastings, East Sussex, TN34 1DJ. *Tel:* 01424 729292. *Fax:* 01424 430485. *E-mail:* hastingssexualhealth@aol.com

See also the 'Sex' chapter, page 119. 5711

Brief Family Therapy Team

This is a special service provided by NSPCC and NCH Action for Children. It offers 'Brief therapy for a wide range of individual, relationship and family problems'. Independent assessment and therapeutic service where there are concerns regarding risks to, or the welfare of, children. *Hours:* Mondays to Fridays 9.00am to 5.00pm. Appointments required for Thursdays.

Address: Brief Family Therapy Team, 2, Sedlescombe Road South, St. Leonards, Sussex, TN38 0TA. *Tel:* 01424 722117. May 2000

Child & Adult MHS

Child & Adult Mental Health Service. *Address:* CAMHS, Hastings & Rother NHS, Eversfield Hospital, West Hill Road, St Leonards, Sussex, TN38 0NG. *Tel:* 01424 710101 and 710110. May 2000

Child Care Advice

A countywide facility (Sussex) offering free, independent advice on child care has been launched by the County Council in November 1999. It aims to make information about child care more easily available.

For information on all child care issues in the form of brochures and data on child minders, nurseries and playgroups call the telephone number below. *Tel:* 0845 6010 777. All calls at local rate. Jun 2000

Childcare Information Service

A free service to enable people to be better informed about childcare options. *Contact:* Helen Standen, manager.

Address: Kites Childcare Information, Eastbourne Central Library, Grove Road, Eastbourne, East Sussex, BN21 4TL. *Tel:* 01323 737294; *local call rate:* 0845 60 10 777. *Fax:* 01323 737411. *E-mail:* cis.eastbourne@easynet.co.uk *Website:* www.childcarelink.gov.uk May 2000

Child & Adolescent Service

A service provided by Hastings & Rother NHS Trust for children, young people and their families, headed by Dr Jon Doe, consultant child and adolescent pyschiatrist.

Other staff include Dr Patricia Rashbrook, consultant child and adolescent psychiatrist; Mrs Maggie de Vos, consultant psychologist; Dr Hugh Milburn, chartered clinical psychologist; Mrs Janis Newcomen, chartered psychologist.

The team is well trained to help adults, children and young people with a wide range of problems that they may face in everyday life. These could be to do with emotions, behaviour, intellectual development or relationships.

Treatment approaches vary fromcase to case and which member of the team you come to see. All the clinical team have experience of a wide range of treatments, from simple explanation and advice, to more intensive individual or joint psychotherapeutic owerk with family members. Medication, and behaviour modification techniquesmay be used or you may be referred to other services.

Address: The Child & Adolescent Mental Health Service, Hastings & Rother NHS Trust, Eversfield Hospital, West Hill Road, St Leonards, Sussex, TN38 0NG. *Tel:* 01424 710101, 710110. *Fax:* 01424 433870. [5427]

Children's Occupational Therapy

Address: Eversfield Hospital, West Hill Road, St Leonards, Sussex, TN38 0NG. *Tel:* 01424 710103 and 710104. [May 2000]

East Sussex Dyslexia Association

Offering support and advice to dyslexics and their families. Support group meetings are held every two months in different areas of the county.The service arranges conferences twice a year, promoting the positive aspects of dyslexia and giving details of help available. Information packs are available at low cost.

Contacts: Mrs Nicky Woodward, Adult & computer co-ordinator & helpliner; Mrs Diane Pearson, Committee member & helpliner.

Address: East Sussex Dyslexia Association, c/o 74, Upper Belgrave Road, Seaford, East Sussex, BN25 3AY. *Tel:* 01323 896542. *E-mail:* nicky@woodward3040.freeserve.co.uk [5867]

Face to Face

Face to Face offers free and confidential counselling to young people aged 16-25. The service provides the opportunity for young people to explore issues that concern them, by talking through their thoughts and feelings.

Through counselling you can discover new strengths and feelings that will help you recover from difficult experiences and become more confident in the future. Young people can apply directly to Face to Face without having to be referred through a doctor or other professional.

They have an assessment interview with the co-ordinator and if both they and the co-ordinator agree a counsellor is appointed. *Hours*: Mondays to Fridays 9.30am to 12.30pm. Initial interviews are held on Wednesdays between 1.30 and 3.30pm and on Thursdays between 3.30 and 5.30pm & 6.00 and 8.00pm. The service is free. *Contact:* Clare Eason, Administrator.

Address: Face to Face, 5, Queens Road, Hastings, Sussex, TN34 1QP. *Tel*: 01424 466366. [May 2000]

Fellowship of St. Nicholas

Please see under 'St Nicholas Centre', page 40.

Helplines

Social Services Information helpline. *Tel:* 01424 434048. [May 2000]

Information Shop

The Hastings Information Shop for Young People provides advice, support and information for young people aged between 11 and 25 years of age, who are experiencing difficulties in housing, education, employment, health, benefits. The project also provides an excellent cross referral system to additional agencies and organisations in Hastings and Bexhill. *Contact:* Nicola Rebokaz.

Address: Hastings Information Shop for Young People, 31, Cambridge Road, Hastings, Sussex, TN34 1DJ. *Tel:* 01424 447033. *Fax:* 01424 430485.
E-mail: hastingsyouth@aol.com [May 2000]

NCH Action for Children

NCH Action for Children is a team of youth support workers working with young people, 16-21 years of age, who are either leaving care or are facing homelessness. Young people may apply through Social Services.

Contact: Mark Richardson, Project Manager. *Hours:* Mondays to Fridays 9.00am to 5.00pm.

Bexhill
Contact: Tim Hemmings. *Address:* Tall Trees Family Centre, 53, Turkey Road, Sidley, Bexhill, Sussex. *Tel:* 01424 730022. *Fax:* 01424 734402. May 2000

Elphinstone Family Centre
Contact: Leslie Hellier. Full details in 'Family Problems' chapter.

St Leonards
Address: NCH Action for Children, Eastbourne & Hastings Youth Support Team, 5, Brittany Road, St. Leonards-on-Sea, East Sussex, TN38 0RA. *Tel:* 01424 446244. *Fax:* 01424 200700. May 2000

NSPCC

National Society for the Prevention of Cruelty to Children. Patron: HM The Queen, HRH The Queen Mother. Counselling services for abused children and their carers.

Counselling services for adults abused as children; and brief family therapy team - *Tel:* 01424 728500. *Hours:* Mondays to Fridays 9.00am to 5.00pm. *Contact:* Ron Fellows, Local Children's Services Manager.

Address: NSPCC, 2, Sedlescombe Road South, St. Leonards-on-Sea, East Sussex. *Tel:* 01424 428833. *Fax:* 01424 718959. *E-mail:* rfellows@nspcc.org.uk Jun 2000

Parent Link

Gives information, advice and support for parents of children with special educational needs.

Parent Link can arrange for a local volunteer to contact parents who can offer support. Age range of children is 0 to 19. Parent Link also supports the Special Educational Needs Parents' Forum which is a group that meets regularly and where parent representatives aim to influence the education authorities on special educational needs. *Contacts:* Mrs Helen Frederick, Parent Link manager; Mike Robinson, admin.assistant.

Contact information: Helpline number *tel.* 01273 481172 and is open Tuesdays, Wednesdays and Thursdays. Messages can be left at other times on answerphone and Parent Link will ring back.

Address: Parent Link, 47, St Annes Crescent, Lewes, East Sussex, BN7 1SG. *Tel/Fax:* 01273 481172. *E-mail:* parentlink@eastsussexcc.gov.uk
Website: eastsussexcc.gov.uk 5867Jun 2000

Sexual Health Project

Set up to provide a sexual health project for young people aged 11 to 25 via drop-in sessions, outreach programmes and structured group sessions. Opportunities will be provided for young people to be able to explore and feel positive about their own sexuality and receive information to enable them to feel in control of their decision making processes.

Provision will be made for personal and social skills workshops as need identifies. Young people can access one-to-one support and counselling, free condoms and pregnancy tests and advocacy support in accessing services. Project manager: Kerry Smith; Sexual health workers: Steve Noakes & Annette Hardy.

Address: Hastings & Bexhill Youth Service, 31, Cambridge Road, Hastings, East Sussex, TN34 1DJ. *Tel:* 01424 447033. *Fax:* 01424 430485. *E-mail:* hastingssexualhealth@aol.com 5711

See also 'Blagh' in this chapter, page 37..

Social Services

Hastings & St Leonards
Address: Ocean House, London Road, St Leonards-on Sea, East Sussex, TN37 6LW. *Tel:* 01424 723000. Jun 2000

Bexhill
Address: 12-14, Buckhurst Road, Bexhill, East Sussex, TN40 1QF. *Tel:* 01424 212666. Jun 2000

Rural Rother

Address: Saxonwood, Market Square, Battle, East Sussex, TN33 0BX. *Tel*: 01424 774355. Jun 2000

Psychiatry Services

Dr Jon Doe and Dr Patti Rashbrook run the adolescent psychiatry service from Eversfield Hospital, see Child & Adolescent Service, page 37. 5668

St Nicholas Centre

Provides various services for children. These include four 'School's Out' clubs across the town; 'Holiday Play Schemes' for school holidays; 'Family Fun Bus' for outreach work in the community.

Personal development

The St Nicholas Centre runs free personal development courses for parents wanting to go back into employment. Free creche facilities are provided.

Children's workshops

The Centre also runs workshops for 10-14 year old children: art and photography are the subjects currently offered. August 2000

Patron: Baroness Foulkes. Contact: Stephanie Edmonds. *Address*: St Nicholas Centre, London Road, St Leonards-on-Sea, Sussex. *Tel*: 01424 423683. August 2000 *E-mail:* fsn@stleonards3.fsnet.co.uk May 2000

XTRAX

Xtrax is a young people's centre offering information, advice and support to young people aged 16-25, and also recreational facilities, entertainment, cheap food, laundry facilities and shower facilities. *Contact name*: Terry Drinkwater. *Hours:*

Monday 2.00pm-10.00pm
Wednesday & Friday . . . . 2.00pm -10.00pm
Sunday 2.00pm-10.00pm

Address: Provincial House, Provincial Yard, Havelock Road, Hast-ings, East Sussex, TN34 1BP. *Tel*: 01424 722524. *Fax:* 01424 204316. *E-mail:* xtrax@tesco.net Jun 2000

Xpress Advocacy Service

Advocacy, advice and information service for children and young people living in East Sussex up to the age of 21 years. For full details of this service please see 'Advocacy' chapter, page 155.

Under 5s Association

For details of playgroups in your area. Special arrangements are made for children with mental health problems. *Contact:* Clair Power.

Address: Hastings County District Under Fives Association, 418, Harold Road, Hastings, Sussex, TN35 5HG. *Tel/Fax:* 01424 431970. *E-mail:* power@hicc.demon.co.uk Jun 2000

YMCA

Youth, community and welfare organisation providing sporting, educational, social and spiritual programmes, mainly for young people, although all ages are welcome. They also offer a full day nursery. Open to all regardless of age, gender, religion or disability.

Currently there is a membership of about 1000 with many more casual users coming on a regular basis. *Contact name*: Richard Britton. The YMCA also runs a charity shop in Queens Road.

Address: YMCA, St. Paul's Road, St Leonards-on-Sea, East Sussex, TN37 6RS. *Tel*: 01424 429677. *Fax:* 01424 722241. Jun 2000

Youth Service

Address: Hastings & Bexhill Youth Service, 31, Cambridge Road, Hastings, East Sussex, TN34 1DJ. *Tel:* 01424 447033. *Fax:* 01424 430485.
E-mail: hastingsyouth@aol.com

See also entries under 'Sexual Health' and 'BLAGH' in this chapter. [5711]

National Organisations

Barnardo's

Address: Barnardo's, Tanners Lane, Barkingside, Ilford, Essex, IG6 1QG. *Tel:* 020 8550 8822. *Fax:* 0208 551 6870. *E-mail:* postmaster@barnardos.org.uk Website: www.barnardos.org.uk [Jun 2000]

Children's Legal Centre

The Children's Legal Centre provides a free legal advice service by letter and telephone and produces a range of publications including Childright, a monthly multi-disciplinary journal. *Contact:* Jane Paxton. Office hours are 10am to 12.30pm and 2 to 4.30pm, Mondays to Fridays, with a 24-hour answerphone at other times.

Address: Children's Legal Centre, The University of Essex, Wivenhoe Park, Colchester, Essex, CO4 3SQ. *Tel*: 01206 872466. *Fax*: 01206 874026. *Advice line*: 01206 873820. [May 2000]

Childline

Helpline for children and young people in danger, distress or with any problem.

Address: Childline, Studd Street, London, N1 0QW. *Tel:* (020) 7239 1000. *Helpline:* 0800 1111. *Minicom*: 0800 400222. *Fax:* 020 7239 100.

E-mail: reception@childline.org.uk *Website:* childline.org.uk [Jun 2000]

National Union of Students

Address: NUS, 461, Holloway Road, London, N7 6LJ. *Tel*: 020 7272 8900. *Fax:* 020 7263 5713.

E-Mail: nusuk@nus.org.uk

Website: www.nus.org.uk [Jun 2000]

NCH Action for Children

Address: NCH Action for Children, 85, Highbury Park, London, N5 1UD. *Tel:* 020 7704 7000. *Fax:* 020 7226 2537.

Website: nchasc.org.uk [Jun 2000]

NSPCC

The National Society for the Prevention of Cruelty to Children is the UK's leading charity specialising in child protection and the prevention of cruelty to children.

The NSPCC exists to prevent children from suffering abuse and is working for a future for children free from cruelty.

To prevent children from suffering significant harm as a result of ill treatment.

To help protect children who are at risk from such harm.

To help children who have suffered abuse overcome the effects of such harm.

To work to protect children from further harm.

Address: 42, Curtain Road, London, EC2A 3NH. *Tel*: 020 7825 2500. *Fax*: 020 7825 2525. *Helpline*: 0808 800 5000. [5017 Aug 2000]

NSPCC Helpline

For anyone concerned about a child at risk of abuse. The helpline is staffed by social work counsellors. Calls are free. *Helpline:* 0800 800 500. [Jun 2000]

PAL

This is a division of the British Institute of Brain Injured Children, which helps children suffering from dyspraxia and dyslexia. *Contacts*: Jane Stewart-Forshaw or Sue Bond.

Address: PAL, Knowle Hall, Bridgwater, Somerset, TA7 8PJ. *Tel*: 01278 684060. *Fax:* 01278 685573. *E-mail:* info@bibic.org.uk

Website: www.info@bibic.org.uk [Jun 2000]

Parenting Forum

The Parenting Forum brings together those concerned with or working in the field of preparation, education and support for parents. It promotes and maintains a high profile for parenting education and support, where education means learning in the fullest sense: of growing in knowledge, skills, understanding and personal development.

The Forum presses for effective policies and practice at local and national level with the aim of serving the best interests of all children and their families.

Address: The Parenting Education & Support Forum, Unit 431, Highgate Studios, 53-79, Highgate Road, London, NW5 1TL. *Tel:* 020 7284 8370. *Fax:* 020 7485 3587. *E-mail:* pesf@dial.pipex.com
5037

Young Minds

YoungMinds is the national charity committed to improving the mental health of all children and young people. Registered Charity No. 1016968.

Children's mental health matters
When they have it they feel good about themselves, enjoy relationships, learn confidently and overcome their difficulties. When they don't - when they are overwhelmed by misery, anger or fear - all kinds of problems can arise.

YoungMinds Parents' Information Service
Provides information and advice for anyone with concerns about the mental health of a child or young person.
Tel: 0800 018 2138. Jun 2000

Leaflets & Booklets
YoungMinds literature is provided to help young people, parents and professionals to understand when a young person feels troubled and where to find help. YoungMinds Magazine is a leading source of up-to-date news and features on a wide range of issues affecting children's lives.

Seminars & Training
YoungMinds seminars and training increase professional understanding of children's mental health and improve joint working based on good practice and research.

Consultancy
Young Minds Consultancy Services works with health, education, social services and the voluntary sector to develop services for children with mental health problems.

Address: Young Minds, 102, Clerkenwell Road, London, EC1M 5SA. *Tel:* 020 7336 8445 (Admin.). *Fax:* 020 7336 8446. *Parents' information service:* 0800 018 2138. *E-mail:*enquiries@youngminds.org.uk *Website:* www.youngminds.org.uk

Director: Peter Wilson; acting chair: Dr Roger Booker; patrons: Dr Anthony Clare, Nick Hornby; president: Prof Fred Stone.
5345 May 2000

Youth Access

Youth Access is a national membership organisation for youth information, advice and counselling (YIAC) agencies. They provide information on and referrals to youth agencies, but do not provide any direct help, advice or counselling. They also offer consultancy, training, publications and support to organisations who are members.

Hours: Monday to Friday 9.30 am to 4.30 pm.

Address: Youth Access, 1-2, Taylors Yard, 67, Alderbrook Road, London, SW12 8AD. *Tel*: 020 8772 9900. *Fax:* 020 8772 9746. *E-mail:* yaccess@dircon.co.uk May 2000

Director: Barbara Rayment; Central services manager: Dianne Jones; Administrator: Amber Collingwood; Quality manager: Carolyn Mumby; Training co-ordinators: Sue Lee, Robert Downes, Foluke Taylor Mohammed; Development Manager - mental health: Catherine Wilson.

Further Information

Factsheet

'Children & Young People and Mental Distress'. Mind Factsheet by Katherine Darton. Available from Mind, price £1.38. *Tel*: 020 8221 9666.

So Young, So Sad, So Listen

By Philip Graham and Carol Hughes. A book on childhood depression mainly for parents, teachers and health professionals but some teenagers might find it useful. Published by the Royal College of Psychiatrists, price £5.00.

Mental Health

Young person's introduction to mental health by Kaaren Cruse. Mind Information Unit, £1.38. Available from Mind Mail Order Service. *Tel*: 020 8221 9666.

Stress

The 'Young Person's Guide to Stress is published by the Depression Alliance. Parents, teachers, lecturers and friends, as well as young people who feel depressed, would find the guide, which is free of charge, useful. To order, telephone the Depression Alliance.

Tel: 020 7633 0557. *E-mail:* information@depressionalliance.org 5350

Website

www.teenagehealthfreak.org

See also these chapters ...

Attention Deficit / Hyperactivity, page 22.
Family Problems, page 67.

Acknowledgements
Our grateful thanks to Mary Dawson, family support practitioners, for editorial assistance with this chapter. May 2000

Chronic Fatigue Syndrome

Chronic Fatigue Syndrome used to be called 'yuppie flu' as it became known by its effect on young active people. Now it is known as Chronic Fatigue Syndrome or simply ME. It affects the brain and central nervous system. [5284]

Recent research, commissioned by ME Association (Sussex), estimates that in Sussex there are over 4,500 adults and children who are affected by the Chronic Fatigue Syndrome known as ME and that 900 of these are housebound. CFS/ME type illnesses, which can follow a viral infection and/or trauma, have appeared in the medical literature since 1750. Indeed, Charles Darwin and Florence Nightingale are thought to have had the illness.

Names

The disease has been known by many names over the decades including Icelandic Disease, Tapunui flu (New Zealand), and Royal Free Disease when ME was reported in *The Lancet* after people were admitted to London's Royal Free Hospital in 1955; the hospital had to be closed as 292 of the medical and nursing staff were disabled by the syndrome.

Neurological disorder

In recent times ME has been classified by the World Health Organisation as a neurological disorder and the Government's Chief Medical Officer has set up a working group of experts to carry out a review and provide best practice guidelines. This work should be completed during 2001.

Local Organisations

Hastings & Rother ME Group

Offering support for sufferers, their families and carers as well as providing support and information to a wider group via a newsletter and connections with other similar groups outside of the area.

The Group is currently creating a helpful directory of information, tips and hints on how to survive this debilitating disease. They meet on the first Friday of each month at the Pinehurst Centre from 2 to 3pm. *Contacts:* Mrs Susie Lyle, co-ordinator; Mrs Ann Brooker, treasurer.

Address: Hastings & Rother ME Support Group, c/o Pinehurst Centre, 3, Avondale Road, St Leonards-on-Sea, East Sussex, TN38 0SA. *Tel:* 01424 423687. [5867]

ME Association Sussex.

Representatives of ME Association (Sussex) are working with the health authorities who are looking at ways to improve provision for CFS/ME patients. In the meantime the role of the ME Association remains profoundly important, informing, supporting and representing patients.

Services

Services include telephone helplines, quarterly newsletters, meetings, library and special interest groups such as Young ME, Yoga, Christian and Social. The organisation keeps in regular contact with support agencies and medical professionals and has eminent doctors as advisors.

Parliamentary group

The group enjoys the support of five patrons including the two Brighton MPs who are members of an All Party Parliamentary Group which works in the interests of CFS/ME patients. Up to 40% of CFS/ME patients may have mental health problems as part of their illness or as a reaction to it.

For information about CFS/ME and the Association please contact Colin Barton of the ME Association, see below.

Address: ME Association (Sussex), 28, Kemp Court, Church Place, Brighton, Sussex, BN2 5JU. *Tel/Fax:* 01273 682345.

May 2000

Further Information

CFS - a doctors' guide

14-page, post free to doctors and professionals. Copies will be sent to others on receipt of four second class postage stamps. Please contact the ME Association; address above. 5283

Acknowledgements

Our grateful thanks to Colin Barton of the ME Association for editorial assistance with this chapter.

Abbreviations

ME Myalgic Encephalomyelitis.
CFS Chronic Fatigue Syndrome.

Compulsions

Compulsive disorders
A form of anxiety known as obsessive compulsive disorder is where the person experiences obsessive thoughts associated with some form of compulsive behaviour. Studies have suggested that around 2.5% of people are likely to experience obsessive compulsive disorder at some point in their life. [1571]

Compulsions
Examples of compulsions are cleaning, washing, checking, counting, measuring, repeating actions or tasks and confessing imaginary sins. [5013]

Shopping Compulsion
Compulsive shopping disorder is becoming recognised as a specific disorder where the person concerned feels compelled to shop, putting the family's budget under severe strain.

Organisations

No Panic
A voluntary charity which helps people who suffer from panic attacks, phobias, obsessive compulsive disorders and other anxiety disorders, including those people who are trying to give up tranquilisers. Please see main entry in 'Panic' chapter, page 98.

Depression

An estimated one in twenty people will have serious or clinical depression at at any one time' [1571]

Most of us get depressed at some time or other and it can be part of a natural grieving process, for example at the end of a relationship. A 'depressive disorder' or 'clinical depression' is when depressive symptoms like apathy, loss of energy, suicidal thougths, sleep and appetite changes persist, or go beyond normal mood changes. [0534]

Signs of depression

People with depression usually have a number of symptoms. Commonly, these include low mood, loss of interest and pleasure, feelings of worthlessness and guilt, tearfulness, poor concentration, reduced energy, reduced or increased appetite and weight, sleep problems and anxiety.

They may look to others as if they are being lazy or difficult, not doing their best to be happy and occupied or to get over a sad life-event. This is not the case. Carers and friends need to be very patient - attempts to make people 'snap out of' depression will fail. They need help and support to overcome a problem that often responds well to treatment.

Recognising and treating depression as an illness can shorten its duration, as well as reduce the risk of relationship breakdown, sickness, accidents, alcohol and drug misuse, job-loss and suicide. [5179]

What is depression?

'Depression' is used to describe a range of moods, from the low spirits that we all experience occasionally, to a severe problem that interferes with everyday life. It is the latter, defined as a "persistent exaggeration of the everyday feelings that accompany sadness", that is explained here. [5179]

Who gets depression?

Any of us can get depression. At any one time, about one in 20 people will have a serious depression, another one in 20 are more mildly affected and one in 10 have some of the symptoms. Men and women of all cultures and ages can get depression, although their ways of expressing it vary.

One thing that can make it hard for doctors to recognise depression is that people may complain of physical problems (commonly headaches, stomach problems or general pain) either because they really are the significant symptom, or because they find it hard to admit to feeling emotionally bad for reasons even they sometimes cannot identify. [5179]

Are you depressed?

Nothing feels good anymore; sleeping too much or too little; lack of interest in food or overeating; feeling down; lack of self-confidence; agitation; great anxiety; difficulty concentrating; feeling guilty about things; feeling tired all the time; feeling life is pointless; lack of sex drive; tearfulness.

If you have experienced three or more of these symptoms, and have felt like this for more than two weeks, go and see your doctor.

People who suffer from depression usually experience persistent sadness with feelings of helplessness and hopelessness. These feelings may make it difficult to carry out normal daily activities.

Depression is an illness with a wide range of physical and psychological symptoms, which sometimes make it hard to recognise and understand. Depression can affect anyone and does not reduce your value as a human being.[5350]

It is important to remember that:

Depression is an illness that can affect anyone at any age. It is not connected with and does not develop into insanity. Depression can be treated. There is no need to cope alone. [5350]

Facts about depression

The following information is taken from The Fundamental Facts, published 1999 by the Mental Health Foundation. Number of people experiencing depression: 'An estimated one in ten people will have some form of depression at any one time'.

Also, 'Estimates for the lifetime prevalence of depression vary, ranging from one in six to one in four. It can occur at any age, but is most common in people aged 25-44 years'. Clinical depression: 'An estimated one in twenty people will have serious or clinical depression at at any one time'. [1571]

Local organisations

Trinity Project

Trained counsellors who can help with depression if it is associated with drug abuse. Please see main entry in 'Substance Misuse' chapter under 'Local Organisations', page 131.

National organisations

Depression Alliance

'Depression can be overcome. Our experience is that you need not fear it. We too have experienced the misery that depression can bring. We are an alliance of people who have suffered from depression, people who have recovered from depression, carers, families and friends.' [5351]

Contact: Anthony Tiernan, campaign manager. *Address*: Depression Alliance, 35, Westminster Bridge Road, London, SE1 7JB. *Tel*: 020 7633 0557. *E-mail:* information@depressionalliance.org. *Website:* www.depressionalliance.org [Jun 2000]

Depressives Anonymous

Support and encouragement to those suffering depression and to those concerned for them. Advice and support for those wishing to form local depression self-help groups. A newsletter is available, plus leaflets, and a pen friend scheme is provided. National meetings are held to give depressives a chance to meet together for mutual support.

A publication list is available upon request, the main pulication being the FDA Newsletter [(Ref. 5999)] which comes out six times a year and includes letters, news items and helpful ideas, as well as news about depression; all information is supplied by members.

Address: Fellowship of Depressives Anonymous, Box FDAI, c/o Self Help Nottingham, Ormiston House, 32-36 Pelham Street, Nottingham, NG1 2EG. *Tel:* 01702 433838. *Fax:* 01702 433843. [May 2000]

Further Information

Coping with depression.

Audio Cassette. 'Simple, effective strategies for coping with all types of depression. Learn how to fight depression using cognitive techniques; how to turn negative thoughts into positive ones; set targets and goals. Recommended by the Depression Alliance.' 'The tape has lots to offer and takes one gently through the minefield of clinical depression, explaining what it is and what you can do about it. Produced by Wendy Lloyd Audio Productions. Price £8.50 (single cassette); £13.99 (two cassette version), incl. p&p. 40 minutes' playing time. Available from Audio Productions Ltd. *Address*: PO Box 1, Wirral, CH47 7DD. *Tel*: 0151 632 0662. [5298]

Anatomy of Depression
By Lewis Wolpert.

Climbing Out Of Depression.
A practical guide for sufferers. Written by Sue Atkinson. Being depressed often leaves you feeling paralyzed and recovery can sometimes seem almost impossible. You need help and that is what this book offers - practical, humane and spiritual help. Lion Publishing, 1993. ISBN: 0-7549-2248-1. 176 pages. Price £7.99. Available from Mind Mail Order Service. *Tel*: 020 8221 9666. [5251]

A Single Step
'Excellent A5 publication full of tips, stories, letters, reviews, diagnostic explanations etc.' A magazine for those who suffer from depression and those who care for them. £2.00 to non-members from Depression Alliance. *Address*: 35, Westminster Bridge Road, London SE1 3JB. [5298]

Cognitive Therapy Of Depression
By Aaron T. Beck, John Rush, Brian F. Shaw and Gary Emergy. Following the 'cognitive revolution', which one of the authors was instrumental in creating, this landmark book, first published in 1979, presents the synthesis of theory, experimental research and clinical experience upon which modern cognitive therapy is founded. Published by Guilford Press, 1985. ISBN: 0-89862-919-5. 434 pages. Price £15.95. Available from Mind Mail Order Service. *Tel*: 020 8221 9666. [5088]

Dealing With Depression
By Trevor Barnes with the Samaritans. Published by Vermillion, an imprint of Ebury Press, £8.99.

Depression & How To Survive It
By Spike Milligan & Anthony Clare. Published by Ebury Press, 1993.

Depression & Manic Depression
Booklet published by Sane, 1993.

Depression, the Way Out
'Depression, The Way Out Of Your 'rison' By Dorothy Rowe. Published by Routledge. 'Price £6.99.

Depression Workbook
A guide for living with depression and manic depression. By Mary Ellen Copeland. Mary Ellen Copeland is a distinguished teacher and lecturer from Vermont and is herself a manic depressive. In moving language and startling honesty she tells her story here. Published by New Harbinger Publications, 1992.

Depression Alliance

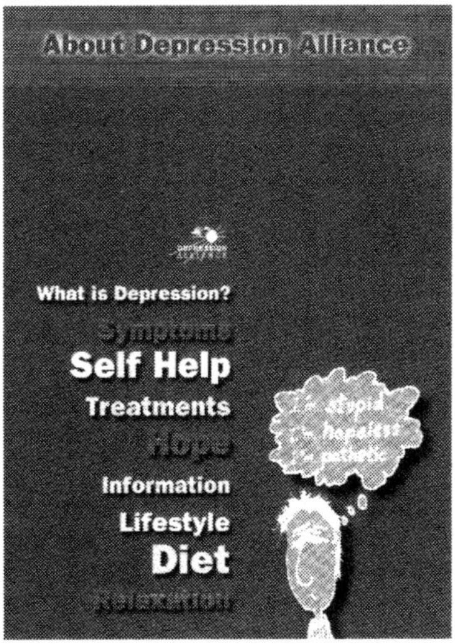

Free, 24 page booklet published by The Depression Alliance - a guide to help you through the misery of depression. Available from Depression Alliance, 35, Westminster Bridge Road, London, SE1 7JB. Tel: 020 7633 9929. [5351]

Feeling Good
Feeling Good, the new mood therapy. By David D Burns. Published by Signet Books, 1980.

Health Information Service
The HIS is a free and confidential 24-hour service. You can speak to staff during office hours, and you can listen to any of hundreds of tapes at any time, e.g: *Depression* (Tape 089 in English; Tape 802 in Bengali-Sylheti dialect; & Tape 902 in Urdu).

Address: The College of Health, St Margaret's House, 21, Old Ford Road, London, E2 9PL. *Freephone:* 0800 66 55 44. 5367

Out Of The Blue
Another Depression Alliance magazine guest-edited by Raj Persaud with contributions by Clare Rayner, Lewis Wolpert and others. Available from Depression Alliance. Price £2.50. *Tel:* 020 7633 0557.

Overcoming Depression
Written by Richard Gillet. "Constructive guide to all different levels of depression and ways of overcoming it." Published by Dorling Kindersley. Price £9.99. 5069

Understanding Depression
Published by 1997 Mental Health Foundation, 20 Cornwall Terrace, London NW1 4QL.

See also these chapters ...
Counselling & Therapy, page 173.
Manic Depression, page 81.

Websites

Mindspring
For a full range of information and specific articles on depression:
www.mindspring.com/~hugman/pendulum

Psycom
www.psycom.net/depression.centra lhtml

Depression Alliance
information@depressionalliance.org

Fightdepression
Fightdepression is an Internet Information Service on depression, which went live Summer 2000. It is a site dedicated to bringing the latest treatment and therapy options available in the UK.

This site aims to cater for those suffering with depression as well as family and others. It is also a service for health professionals, with information on current research, developments and news.

Address: Stephen Clifford, TLC Primary Healthcare, Summer House, 56A, Cranston Ave, Bexhill-on-Sea, East Sussex, TN39 3NN. *Tel:* 01424 220189.
Website: www.fightdepression.co.uk 5157 May 2000

Eating Disorders

Quote: "It's not about food, it's about me." Eating Disorders are not primarily about food, but about underlying emotional turmoil. 5333

There are at least four recognised categories of eating disorder; anorexia nervosa, bulimia nervosa, binge-eating and compulsive overeating. (*Statistics courtesy of the London Centre for Statistical Requirements*).

Anorexia Nervosa

Characterised by the relentless pursuit of thinness through self-starvation and maybe excessive exercise. Each year over 4,500 new cases are diagnosed. Whilst 1% of those ill are women between the ages of 15-30 years, anorexia nervosa manifests itself in all age groups from 8-80 years, and it is estimated that 5 -10% of anorexics are male.

Bulimia Nervosa

Characterised by intermittent binge-eating of large amounts of food, followed by self-induced vomiting and/or purging. Diuretics, excessive exercise, tasting and spitting food out and periods of fasting may also control weight.

Each year over 6,500 new cases are diagnosed. Contrary to media perception, the figures are far higher than for anorexia nervosa; 3% of the general population are considered to be bulimic and 5 -10% of these are males.

Binge-eating

Characterised by intermittent binge- eating of large amounts of food (usually less frequently than in bulimia nervosa) without trying to compensate. An estimated 2% of adult women and 0.2% of adult males are thought to be binge-eaters.

Compulsive overeating

Characterised by high weight and a need to constantly pick at food. Those suffering feel unable to stop eating most of the time and will frequently describe themselves as having no control. Compulsive overeating has often been considered a case of greed in the past, but it is now recognised as having the potential to be a serious eating disorder.

Cases of obesity in the UK are on the increase and are currently at their highest level. Recent statistics suggest 17% of the population are obese, 10% of whom are compulsive overeaters.

Understanding

There is a temptation to individualise eating disorders according to the varying symptoms. However, all the symptoms serve the same purpose and therefore need to be addressed under one umbrella.

Eating disorders are an external way of expressing, covering up and/or controlling inside disease. They are an outward sign that something is wrong and thus serve as a coping mechanism-cum-survival technique for men and women of all ages, from all backgrounds and ethnic groups.

Who has eating disorders?

In reality, most people with an eating disorder would be difficult to identify. Outward appearances, work/school standards and conversation are often to the good, but people do not have to look ill to be ill, even in anorexia nervosa! It is easy to credit only the person exhibiting dramatic weight-loss, for example, with being unwell, but this is a big mistake. Further, it is only for a tiny, though nevertheless significant, proportion of people with an eating disorder that food and eating can become a dangerous and potentially fatal obsession.

Families and Friends

Families and friends are often the first to notice 'something is wrong', but the person with the eating disorder may not be ready to face the problem and may deny it. Because this can leave family and friends feeling responsible yet helpless and puts pressure on relationships, they too need support. Learning more about eating disorders enables them to help more effectively and reduces the feeling that they are responsible.

Dieting

Eating disorders are not about slimming or dieting. Whilst we may hear of them in conjunction with, or following on from, dieting, it is important to see this as only a symptom. The underlying initial need to diet is usually about self-dissatisfaction and low self-worth.

The weight loss and food deprivation lead to a sense of achievement and betterness and an individual who feels life is very difficult to manage may then see this as a viable way of coping. Further, a diet depends on will power and denial so soon becomes broken, hence it becomes important to look at what purpose the food eaten, and otherwise, serves.

When eating patterns become disordered, attitudes to food can become obsessive and people slip out of control and plummet into the lonely and sometimes brutal depths of an eating disorder.

Excercise

Whilst achievement and self-esteem may be sought via weight loss, such denial of food, as well as excessive exercise, purging, vomiting and spitting also serves to control feelings and emotions too painful to talk about. Likewise bingeing and overeating. On the surface the latter is often seen as going out of control. However, the behaviour and obsessions around food serve to similarly depress and/or control emotions.

Fashion

There is temptation to attribute eating disorders to media and fashion. Whilst these outlets do perhaps need to reconsider what they portray as role models, it is important, too, to realise that only those vulnerable in the first place are going to be so influenced. Such people have very low self-esteem and consider themselves useless and hopeless as they are.

Sources of help

Understandably, many people with eating disorders are afraid of the consequence of giving up their illness and of facing up to their difficulties. It is important to know that recovery is possible - even after years of suffering, although the sooner the help is found the better.

Treatments available vary around the country, but the starting point is finding someone to talk to openly and confidentially. Treatments use a range of approaches including talking therapies, self-help groups and organisations and counselling. [5333]

Dieticians

To consult a state registered dietician, contact your GP or for a list of freelance dieticians call the British Dietetic Association on 0121 616 4900. [Jun 200]

Local organisations

First Steps to Freedom

Registered charity which aims to help, in a practical way, people who suffer from phobias, obsessional compulsive disorder, anxiety, panic attacks, anorexia and bulimia, and those who wish to come off tranquilisers, and their carers. For more details, please see main entry in 'Phobias' chapter, page 104.

Face to Face

Face to Face offers general counselling which may include eating disorders. They do not specialise in eating disorders. They offer a free counselling service to young people (16 to 25 years) in the Hastings and Rother area. Only self-referrals are accepted. Referrals to other agencies when appropriate.

Address: Face To Face Counselling Service, 5, Queens Road, Hastings, East Sussex, TN34 1QP. *Tel/Fax*: 01424 466366 (answerphone may be connected). Jun 2000

Eating Disorders Recovery via Self-Help

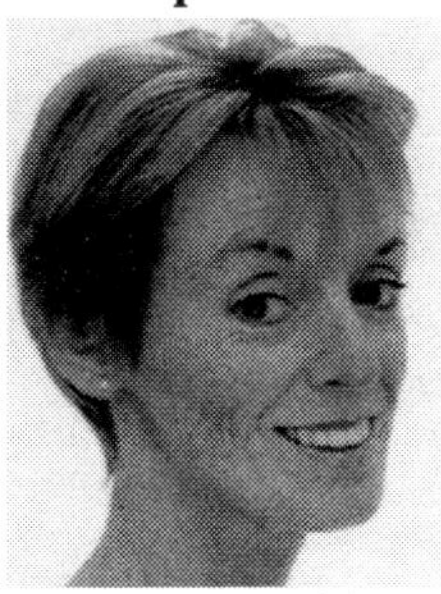

Eating Disorders: Recovery via Self Help (EDRS). "Recovery is possible and for everyone." This is the ethos of EDRS. Ann Cox (photo) was herself ill for 28 years. She made a full recovery in 1989 and decided to pass on her experiences of being unwell, recovering and of (now) being 'normal.' Thus she founded EDRS and sees its role as multi-functional, informative and educational as well as a counselling and help-line service, the latter concentrating on recovery.

Begun in February 1991, this is a benevolent organisation and a voluntary one and help depends on the organisation receiving donations. People are welcome to telephone Ann at any time on the understanding that they may be in contact with the answerphone. If a message is left, Ann undertakes to respond within 24 hours. Self-referrals are the norm and anyone affected by eating disorders, directly or otherwise, is invited to call. She receives calls worldwide.

Contact: Ann Cox. *Tel:* 01424 426880. May 2000

National organisations

Eating Disorders Association

Eating Disorders Assoc-iation is a national charity (formed in 1989 by the amalgamation of three established eating disorders charities) providing information, help and support for people affected by eating disorders and, in particular, anorexia and bulimia nervosa.

Details of local contacts in your area are freely available to callers ringing our National helpline.

EDA offers a range of services which include: national telephone helplines;
a UK-wide network of local self-help and support groups, postal and telephone contacts; a comprehensive range of information, including leaflets for young people; membership which includes a quarterly magazine; lists of treatment available in your area; a helpline and support service for young people; an annual conference for members to learn about the latest developments; a telephone counselling programme for people with bulimia; training for professionals in health, education and social care; a professional journal, European Eating Disorders Review, which provides information and practical help for professionals in all disciplines; service specifications guidelines for the treatment of anorexia and bulimia nervosa.

Chief executive: Mrs Nicky Bryant. Media & information manager: Steve Bloomfield.

Address: Eating Disorders Association, First Floor, Wensum House, 103, Prince of Wales Road, Norwich, NR1 1DW.

Helpline: 01603 621 414, Mondays to Fridays 9.00am to 6.30pm; *Youthline* (up to 18 years of age): 01603 765 050 (Mondays to Fridays, 4 to 6pm). *Recorded Information Service:* 0906 302 0012 (calls cost 50p per minute). *Admin:* 01603 619 090. *Fax:* 01603 664 915 *E-mail:* info@edauk.com *Website:* www.edauk.com

Last year EDA responded to and helped over 40,000 people...16,500 people called our Helpline; 1,300 people called our Youthline; we dealt with 14,000 requests for information; we supported 3000 members; 5,500 people used the Self-Help Network. 5931 Jun 2000

International ED Centre

The International Eating Disorders Centre (IEDC) is a residential centre for adults of 16+ years. It takes people with all eating disorders including compulsive over-eating and binge eating disorders. It is a unit of the Royal Buckinghamshire Hospital, Aylesbury, but is run in a non-institutional environment. The team is headed by a consultant psychiatrist and includes psychologist, psychotherapist, RMN and RGN nurses, a specialist therapist and a dietitian. It also offers day care and out-patient facilities. Unit Co-ordinator: Beryl Foy.

Address: The International Eating Disorders Centre, 119-121, Wendover Road, Aylesbury, Bucks., HP21 9LW. *Tel:* 01296 330557. *Fax:* 01296 339209.
Internet pages: http://www.eatingdis orderscentre.co.uk
E-mail: meating@nildram.co.uk May 2000

Newmarket House

An independent residential clinic dedicated to the treatment of eating disorders. The clinic is set in a spacious house on the outskirts of Norwich. It offers the medical advantages of a hospital within the informed caring environment of a family house.

There is a combination of therapies within a caring, structured atmosphere. Run by Penny & Mark Baily.

Address: Newmarket House Clinic, 153, Newmarket Road, Norwich, Norfolk, NR4 6SY. *Tel:* 01603 452226. *Fax:* 01603 452229. *E-mail:* nhc@clara.net *Website:* www.newmarket-house.co.uk 5210 May 2000

Founder Director: Penelope Baily; Consultant Psychiatrists: Liam Callinan & Justin Gardner; Administrator: Gay Robb; Senior nurse: Amanda Frost. There are almost four staff to each patient, including a clinical director, a consultant psychiatrist, nurses, therapists and a dietician. Newmarket House is a mile from Norwich City Centre.

Further Information

All About Anorexia Nervosa

A booklet for those wanting to know more about anorexia nervosa. Published by the Mental Health Foundation, 1997. *Address:* 20/21 Cornwall Terrace, London NW1 4QL. *Tel:* 020 7535 7474.

All About Bulimia Nervosa

A booklet for those wanting to know more about bulimia nervosa. 18 pages. Published by the Mental Health Foundation. *Tel:* 020 7335 7474. 5004

Autumn Dawn

'Autumn Dawn - Triumph Over Eating Disorders', by Ann Cox. This is an autobiographical account of Ann's struggle and eventual recovery. It is a graphic account that takes the reader through many emotions and whilst it is clearly a horror story, Ann's message of hope triumphs throughout. She believes recovery is possible for anyone. Published by Book Guild Limited. Price £8.50.

Beyond Chaotic Eating

'Beyond Chaotic Eating - A way out of Anorexia, Bulimia & Compulsive Eating', by Helena Wilkinson. The author explores symptoms and the background to eating disorders for people experiencing them, in one way or another. An account is given of the part families play in the build-up to an eating disorder and what they can do to help.

Written from her own experiences of anorexia and as a Christian counsellor, the author also includes guidelines to be found in the Bible. Published by Marshall Pickering. Price £6.99.

Eating Disorders

'Eating Disorders - A Parents' Guide', by Bryant-Waugh & Lask. This is written for parents of children with eating disorders. It describes the different eating disorders and, with sympathy and reassurance, offers guidance on how to decide if your child is unwell and how to get help. Published by Penguin. Price £7.99.

Health Information Service

The HIS is a free and confidential 24-hour service. You can speak to staff during office hours, and you can listen to any of hundreds of tapes at any time, e.g: *Bulimia nervosa* (Tape 276); *Obesity* (Tape 463); *What is a healthy diet?* (Tape 268).

Address: The College of Health, St Margaret's House, 21, Old Ford Road, London, E2 9PL. *Freephone*: 0800 66 5544.

Apl 2000

Helping People

'Helping People with Eating Disorders: A Clinical guide for Assessment and Treatment'. By Bob Palmer, University of Leicester, UK. The author's pragmatic style means that anyone helping people with eating disorders will find this to be a comprehensive, practice based handbook. It incorporates evidence on different treatment methods and guidance on difficult cases. Published by John Wiley and Sons, 2000. ISBN: 0-471 98647-X. 273 pages. Price £17.99. Available from Mind. Tel: 020 8221 9666. 5024

Overcoming Binge Eating

Written by Dr Christopher Fairburn. 'Do you have a binge-eating problem or know someone who does? This authoritative book will show you how to overcome the urge to binge, gain control over your eating behaviour, reduce the risk of relapse, and re-establish stable, healthy eating habits. The advice given has been tested in controlled clinical research'. Published by Guildford Press, 1995. ISBN: 0-89862-179-8. 246 pages. £11.50. Available from Mind Mail Order Service. *Tel*: 020 8221 9666.

Acknlowledgements
Our grateful thanks to Ann Cox of EDRS for editorial assistance with this chapter.

Elderly People

The UK population of people over 65 years has increased fourfold over the last one hundred years and is continuing to grow. An estimated 15% of elderly people have depression and it is reckoned that 5% have some form of dementia. Some of the special help available for elderly people is detailed here. [1571]

Dementia

Dementia is a gradual decline in mental abilities such as memory, thinking, problem solving, concentrating and perception. It is reckoned that one per thousand of the population under 65 have Alzheimer's (a form of dementia), and that most cases develop in later life, affecting one in fifty people over 65, and one in five by the age of 80. [1571]

What is dementia?

'Dementia' is caused by a slowly advancing form of brain damage, although the cause of this is unknown. A person with dementia may become forgetful initially and extremely anxious and confused as the disease progresses. [5224]

Depression

Research has shown that the rate of depression rises in old age. An estimated 15% of people over 65 have depression and an estimated 5% have severe depression. There is a correlation between depression in older people and living alone: an estimated 50% of people over 75 live alone. [1571]

Parkinson's Disease

Parkinson's disease is named after Dr James Parkinson (1755 - 1824) the London doctor whose essay on 'the Shaking Palsy', was published in 1817. James Parkinson established the condition as a clinical entity and his essay continues to be recognised throughout the world as the classic description of the condition. [5615]

Neurological disorder

Parkinson's is a progressive neurological disorder affecting learned voluntary movements such as walking, talking, writing and swallowing. There are three main symptoms: tremor, rigidity and bradykinesia (slowness of movement). However, not everyone will experience all three symptoms. Parkinson's results from the loss of the chemical messenger, dopamine, within the centre of the movement in the midbrain. The cause is as yet unidentified and there is no known cure. Parkinson's is not inherited nor is it contagious. [5615]

Incidence

The incidence of Parkinson's is approximately 1:500 in the general population, rising to 1:100 over the age of 65 and 1:50 over the age of 80. A little recognised fact is that 1:20 people diagnosed are aged under 40. There are more than 120,000 people with Parkinson's in the United Kingdom today and it is common in all parts of the world. [5615]

Treatment

The main treatment for Parkinson's is drug therapy. Because no two people with

Parkinson's are exactly alike, the drug treatment has to be tailored to the individual and the timing of medication is as important as the dosage. With the optimum drug treatment, life expectancy for Parkinson's is normal. Surgical techniques are also being researched. Management plays a very important part in the care of people with Parkinson's and professions such as physiotherapy, speech and language therapy, and occupational therapy have an important role to play. 5615

Local Organisations

Advocacy Service

Do you feel you are not being listened to or not being taken seriously? Are you having difficulty putting your views across? Do you feel you need someone on *your* side? Advocacy is about supporting you to tell your side of the story. Age Concern Advocacy Service is free, confidential and independent. You will be able to speak in confidence to a member of the Age Concern Advocacy Team.

Address: Age Concern East Sussex Advocacy Service, 54, Cliffe High Street, Lewes, Sussex, BN7 2AN. *Tel:* 01273 476704. *Hastings & Rother:* 01424 775766. 6054

Age Concern East Sussex

Information and advice for older people, their families and carers.For home visits in respect of help, an Attendance Allowance application form should be completed. Day care is offered twice a week: Catsfield on Mondays; Hurst Green on Thursdays.

Services

Age Concern offers the following services: Visiting & Befriending Scheme; toenail clipping service; hearing aid battery exchange (Wednesdays from 10am to 12 noon); gardeners' register; Cookery for Men Scheme; Age Concern Insurance; Advocacy Service (also covers Hastings); Home from Hospital Scheme.

Hours: Tuesdays, Wednesdays and Thursdays from 10am to 1pm.
Information Worker: Dorothy Smith; Day Care Organiser: Jackie Dennis; Home from Hospital co-ordinator: Rhiannon Oliver; Advocacy Worker: Jan Jones; Rother co-ordinator: Andrea Talbot;

Address: Age Concern, The Almonry, High Street, Battle, TN33 0EA. *Tel:* 01424 775721. *Fax:* 01424 777050. Jun 2000

Age Concern, Rother

Age Concern, Rother Office, c/o Bexhill Caring Community (affiliated to Age Concern). *Tel*: 01424 215116. May 2000

Age Concern, Hastings

Advice, help and information for older people. Transport services: ambul-ances, voluntary car service and Dial-a-Ride; insurance service. Manager: Angela Colburn. *Hours*: Mondays to Fridays 10.00am to 1.00pm & 2.00 to 4.30pm. Wednesdays 10.00am to 1.00pm only. *Address*: Age Concern, 50, Robertson Street, Hastings, Sussex. TN34 1HL. *Tel*: 01424 426162. May 2000

Age Concern Helpline

Telephone service for older people, their families and people working with them. Call free on 0800 731 4931.
Jun 2000

Alzheimers, Brighton

Address: Alzheimer's Society, 206, Church Road, Hove, Sussex, BN3 2DJ. *Tel:* 01273 726266. *Fax*:01273 749848.
E-mail: alzheimers-brighton@hotmail.com Jun 2000

Alzheimers, Hastings

The Society offers support to the carers of people who are suffering from dementia.

Information Centre is open Mondays to Fridays, 10.00am to 4.00pm. Meetings are held on the first Wednesday in each month in Hastings at 7.00pm at Pinehill, The Ridge, Hastings. Arrangements can be made for transport. *Contact*: Rosemary Iddenden, Co-ordinator. *Hours:* Mondays to Fridays 10am to 4pm.

Address: Alzheimer's Society, Hastings & Rother Branch, 22, Claremont, Hastings, East Sussex TN34 1HA. *Tel:* 01424 720640. May 2000

Bexhill Caring Community

The Caring Community was founded in 1965 to assist the aged and lonely and to offer practical help to those in need. Voluntary helpers visit those requiring our service after an initial visit from the Administrator. For detailed information on services please apply direct. *Contacts:* Mrs Jill Halsall, administrator; Mrs Joan Rudge, deputy administrator.

Address: Bexhill Caring Community, 38, Sackville Road, Bexhill, East sussex, TN39 3JE. *Tel:* 01424 215116. 5867

Care & Repair

For full details of this home improvement agency, please see entry 'Care & Repair' in 'Housing' chapter.

Care Homes

For details of residential and respite care homes in this area please see 'Residential & Respite Care' chapter.

Day Care Centres

Social Services run a number of Day Care Centres. To get a place in one, you need to contact the 'Community Assessment Team'. This is located at Ocean House in St Leonards.

Address: Community Assessment Team, Ocean House, 87, London Road, St Leonards, Sussex, TN37 6BD. *Tel:* 01424 448555. 6064 Aug 2000

Friends of the Old People

FOTOP arranges various functions and minibus outings for members. Referrals by personal recommendation. The annual membership fee is £2.00 per year. Volunteers are required.

Address: Mrs B. Clark, Honorary Secretary c/o 43, Pine Avenue, Hastings, East Sussex, TN34 3PP. *Tel*: 01424 420749. Aug 2000

Hastings Lifeline

Hastings Lifeline aims to enable vulnerable people from all section of the community to remain independent in their own home, secure in the knowledge that help is always available when they need it most.

Address: Hastings Lifeline, 1066 Housing Association, PO Box 1066, Hastings, TN34 1WY. *Tel:* 01424 781234. *Fax:* 01424 781971. *E-mail:* lifeline@connect-free.co.uk

Lucy Wilson, Lifeline business manager. David Nugent, Marketing consultant. Graham Harris, Sheltered Housing manager. Jun 2000

Home from Hospital Service

A volunteer visiting and befriending service for those aged 60+ in the Borough of Hastings area, during the hospital discharge period (2-3 weeks) which offers practical and emotional support.

Anyone may enquire about this scheme, including family, friends or professional staff. A pool of approximately 12 volunteers operate the service at any one time. *Contact:* Mrs Carole Purves. *Hours:* Mondays to Fridays, 10.00am to 4.30pm. Closed Wednesday afternoons.

Address: Hastings Age Concern, 50, Robertson Street, Hastings, East Sussex, TN34 1HL. *Tel*: 01424 440333. Jun 2000

Impact

Home visiting service funded by Social Services and ESCC offering welfare benefits and income maximisation advice for older people. Impact workers will come to visit and help people complete benefit claims form and liaise with outside agencies if they wish. *Tel:* 01323 733374. [5991. Jun 2000]

Parkinson's Disease Society

Bexhill & Hastings Group. Meets on the third Friday in the month at St Michael's Church Hall, Glassenbury Drive, Bexhill, from 2 to 4 pm. *Contact*: Mr E Morley. *Tel*: 01424 712831. See also under 'National Organisations', below. [Jun 2000]

Pinehill Day Centre

Pinehill Day Centre provides a service for older people suffering with mental ill health. The activity programme includes therapeutic memory exercise and ongoing support to the person and their families.

Each individual attending has the opportunity to discuss the activities with a member of staff and will be supported throughout. Referrals can come from anyone in the community and the Assessment Team will complete an assessment of an individual's needs.

Hours: Mondays to Fridays 8.00am to 5.00pm. Saturdays and Sundays 8.30am to 4.30pm. Contact name: Rosemary Gifkins, Resource Officer.

Address: Pinehill Day Centre, 185, The Ridge, Hastings, East Sussex, TN34 2AE. *Tel*: 01424 427818. *Fax*: 01424 421925. [May 2000]

Psychiatry Services

The local NHS Trust provides 'excellent services for individuals over the age of 65.' The consultants in this area are Dr Ramachander and Dr Mutiboko, who work at St Anne's Centre, see below. [5668]

Rother Lifeline

Suppliers of 'community alarms',which provide 24-hour emergency service. Anyone may apply for a unit, - there are no eligibility criteria. The charge for the service is currently £2.25 per week (plus VAT where applicable). The 'units' resemble an ordinary table telephone or are in the form of a pendant which is worn round the neck. Contact: Ray Philby.

Address: Rother Lifeline, Rother Homes, The Watch Oak, Battle, Sussex, TN33 0YA. *Tel:* 01424 776640. *Fax:* 01424 776647. [Jun 2000]

St Anne's Centre

The Department of Mental Health for the Elderly is part of the Hastings & Rother NHS Trust, and is based at St Anne's Centre. The Department provides a psychiatric service for people aged 65 and over. It can also offer help and support to their carers and families.

The service is available to people living in the Hastings, St. Leonards or Rother districts, together with Ninfield and Hooe. The department is headed by two Consultant Psychiatrists, one for the Hastings and St. Leonards district, and one for the Rother district. For those who need it, hospital care can be arranged.

People who are more independent can be helped at the Day Hospital, see below.

A team of 10 Community Psychiatric Nurses (CPNs), are based at St. Anne's Centre and are attached to GP surgeries throughout the district.

The two wards at St. Anne's Centre comprise a total of 48 beds. St. Raphael Ward is a treatment ward, and St. Gabriel Ward is for organically brain damaged patients. Contact Name: Martin Falkner, Senior Clinical Nurse (Ext. 2246). People are referred to St Anne's by their GPs or through hospital consultants. Hours: Mondays to Thursdays 8.30am to 5.00pm. Fridays 8.30am to 4.30pm.

Address: St. Anne's Centre, Department of Mental Health for the Elderly, 729, The Ridge, St. Leonards, Sussex, TN37 7PT. *Tel*: 01424 754889. *Fax*: 01424 755630.

Day Hospital: 01424 754111 (answerphone evenings). *St. Gabriel Ward:* 01424 758099. *St. Raphael Ward:* 01424 758101. May 2000

St Anne's Day Hospital

Patients must be referred by either their GP or by Community Mental Health Nurses. The Day Hospital is restricted to people who can at least walk with sticks. There are 30 places at the St. Anne's Day Hospital used mainly to assess and treat patients who are less dependent.

Address: St. Anne's Centre, 729 The Ridge, St. Leonards, Sussex. *Tel*: 01424 754111. Aug 2000

Social Services

Social Services provide help for people over 65 with a mental health problem. Their services are divided in three areas: Lewes & Wealden, Eastbourne, and Hastings & Rother.

Lewes & Wealden

There are two offices covering this district, one at Seaford and one at Uckfield. *Addresses:* Warwick House, Warwick Road, Seaford, Sussex, BN25 1RG. *Tel:* 01323 895588. *Fax:* 01323 491925; Beechwood Unit, Uckfield Hospital, Uckfield, Sussex, TN22 5AW. *Tel:* 01825 745016. *Fax:* 01825 745013. 5953

Eastbourne

Address: Mental Health Team, Milton Court, Eastbourne, Sussex, TN34 2EW. *Tel:* 01323 434866. 5953

Hastings & Rother

Address: Mental Health Team, St Anne's Centre, 729, The Ridge, Hastings, Sussex, TN37 7PT. *Tel:* 01424 758135 / 01424 754130. 5953

National Organisations

Age Concern

Registered Charity No. 261794. *Address*: Age Concern England, Astral House, 1268, London Road, London, SW16 4ER. *Tel*: 020 8765 7200. Calls are free. *Fax:* 020 8765 7211. *Helpline*: 0800 009966. *E-mail:* ace@ace.org.uk
Website: www.ace.org.uk May 2000

Alzheimer's Society

The Alzheimer's Soc-iety offers a wide range of support, information, advice, literature and local services to those looking after someone with dementia. The Society works through a national network of local branches, support groups and contact people.

These local representatives all have either or professional experience of the disease and are there to help caring relatives and friends of people with dementia in any way they can. The Alzheimer's Society has branches all over the country with one in Hastings and one in Brighton, see above. 6072 Jul 2000

Address: Alzheimer's Society, Gordon House, 10, Greencoat Place, London, SW1P 1PH. *Tel:* 020 7306 0606. *National helpline:* 0845 300 0336 (local rate call, 8.30am to 6.30pm, Mondays to Fridays). Jun 2000

Help the Aged

This agency works to improve the quality of life of elderly people in the UK and internationally, particularly those who are frail, isolated or poor. It does this primarily by supporting groups who provide community services, campaigning on issues which affect older people and by providing free advice and information services.

Address: St James' Walk, London, EC1R 0BE. *Tel*:020 7253 0253. *Fax*: 020 7250 4474. Jun 2000

Parkinson's Disease Society

The Parkinson's Disease Society has over 200 branches all over the UK. They are run by volunteers, often people who have Parkinson's, and their families and carers. Each branch is different in the help which they offer, but generally they provide opportunities for mutual support and social activities through monthly meetings and practical help at a local level.

Helpline

The Society's Helpline offers a 'listening ear' to anyone with Parkinson's, or their families, who need to talk to someone, safe in the knowledge that their call is confidential and the person listening understands Parkinson's. The helpline is available Mondays to Fridays 9.30am to 5.30pm on 0808 800 0303. [Jun 2000] The national office of the Parkinson's Disease Society is in London.

Address: Parkinson's Disease Society of the UK, 215, Vauxhall Bridge Road, London, SW1V 1EJ. Tel: 020 7931 8080. Fax: 020 7233 9908. E-mail: mailbox@pdsuk.demon.co.uk [Jun 2000]

Seniorline

Information service for senior citizens, their relatives, carers and friends. Call free on 0808 800 6565.

Further Information

All About Dementia

A booklet for those wanting to know more about dementia: what is dementia? what is the difference between dementia and Alzheimer's disease? what causes dementia, etc. 28 pages. Published 1997 by the Mental Health Foundation. *Tel:* 020 7335 7474. [5005]

Because You Care

A guide to help carers cope with difficult behaviour in people with dementia. 24 pages. Published 1998 by the Mental Health Foundation. *Tel:* 020 7335 7474. [5006]

Care that Works

Care that works - A relationship approach to persons with dementia. By Jitka M Zgola. A book that shows how caregivers can meet the demanding challenges of their job by building and improving their personal relationships with those in their care.

It pays special attention to communicating with persons who have language deficits and coping with problem behaviours.

Published by John Hopkins University Press. ISBN: 0-8018-6026-1. 258 pages. £14.50. Available from Mind Mail Order Service. *Tel*: 020 8221 9666. [5251]

Factsheet

Factsheet. 'Confusion, Depression or Dementia? The Need for a Comprehensive Assessment'. By Katherine Darton. Published by MIND Information Unit, November 1998. Price 50p. Available from Mind Mail Order Service. *Tel*: 020 8221 9666.

Health Information Service

The HIS is a free and confidential 24-hour service. You can speak to staff during office hours, and you can listen to any of hundreds of tapes at any time, e.g: *Alzheimer's disease* (Tape 175); *Parkinson's disease* (Tape 207); *Caring for a frail or confused older person* (Tape 070); *Living with older people* (Tape 084). *Address:* The College of Health, St Margaret's House, 21, Old Ford Road, London, E2 9PL. *Freephone:* 0800 66 55 44.

The Milk's in the Oven

A booklet explaining dementia to children. Written by Lizi Hann. 36 pages. Published 1998 by the Mental Health Foundation. *Tel:* 020 7335 7474. [5008]

The 36 Hour Day

'The 36 hour day - a family guide to caring

for persons with Alzheimer's disease, related dementing illness and memory loss in later life.' Written by Nancy L Mace and Peter V Rabins. "This book has remained the bible for families who are caring for people with Alzheimer's disease. The practical advice is sympathetic as well as comprehensive, and the book has new sections on the evaluation of persons with dementia and hospice care, and findings on nutrition and new medical research in areas such as drugs, genetics and diagnostic tests."

Published by John Hopkins University Press, 1999, 346 pages, £9.00. ISBN: 08018-6149-7. Available from Mind Mail Order Service. *Tel:* 020 8221 9666. [5088]

Older People & Mental Health

By Kaaren Cruse. Published by MIND Information Unit, May 1993, updated April 1997. £1.36. Available from Mind Mail Order Service. *Tel:* 020 8221 9666. [5367]

Epilepsy

Epilepsy is the most common serious neurological condition affecting at least 300,000 people, of whom 100,000 are children - that is 1 in every 200 of the UK population at any one time. Today, up to 80% of people with epilepsy have their seizures under control with medication and are able to lead a full life. This has been brought about largely by research and a greater understanding of the condition. [5239]

The brain is a highly complex structure composed of millions of nerve cells (neurones). Their activity is usually well organised and they possess mechanisms for self regulation. The neurones in the brain are responsible for a wide range of functions including consciousness, awareness, movement and bodily posture. A sudden temporary interruption in some or all of these functions may be termed a 'seizure' or 'fit'.

Such an event may be caused by some disturbance arising within the brain itself (an intrinsic cause) or, more rarely, by an external factor such as a temporary lack of oxygen or glucose. Many people have a single seizure at some time in their lives, but this does not constitute epilepsy. If an individual has a tendency to experience repeated seizures due to an intrinsic disturbance of neuronal function within the brain, then the term 'epilepsy' may properly be used.

It should be noted, however, that epilepsy is not just one condition, and it is not always easy to give an explanation in each individual case of why seizures begin, or why they continue to occur. The epilepsies, therefore, affect different people in differing ways. When offering explanations of epilepsy, it is important to remember that there are still many misconceptions about this condition.

People may need reassurance that it is not an illness or a disease. [5237]

Causes

Any person's brain has the capacity to produce a seizure if the circumstances are appropriate. But most brains are not likely to do this spontaneously and can therefore be said to have a high 'seizure threshold' or high resistance to seizures. Individuals vary as to their threshold, and it is probably one part of their genetic characteristics. A person with a low threshold might develop epilepsy spontaneously without other factors being involved. Sometimes a predisposition to seizures can be seen in some families where several members are affected.

But the genetics of epilepsy are not straightforward. In some individuals the existing seizure threshold may be lowered if the brain is subjected to unusual stimulation (such as certain frequencies of flickering light and some drugs) or is injured. If the injury is severe, e.g. due to a road traffic accident, infection, birth trauma, stroke or tumour, then epilepsy may develop as a consequence.

Many individuals attribute the onset of their seizures to some relatively minor event such as a blow to the head or an emotional upset. Although these cannot be completely discounted, in such cases it is likely that family predisposition to seizures plays a more important role. [5273]

Research, using Magnetic Resonance Imaging (MRI) has already begun to broaden the understanding of some of the many causes of epilepsy. [5239]

Diagnosis

Unlike most neurological disorders, there may be no physical signs that a person has epilepsy. The diagnosis is, therefore, made on the basis of a history of more than one epileptic seizure. An accurate eyewitness account is crucial to making a correct diagnosis, as the person experiencing the seizure usually has no recollection of what has happened.

A number of investigations may provide additional information, although these tests do not make the diagnosis of epilepsy.

Blood tests - these check the general health of the person and help to exclude a metabolic cause for the attacks.

X-rays of the skull and chest - these help to exclude a structural cause for the seizures. Special studies (CT or MRI scans) of the brain itself may be requested by the physician if there is an indication that the epilepsy has a structural cause. In most people such tests will be normal.

EEG (electroencephalogram) - this test measures the electrical activity of the surface of the brain. Electrodes are placed on the scalp and the signals picked up by the electrodes are then amplified and recorded onto paper. It is a painless procedure lasting about 40 minutes. It should be remembered that the EEG can only give information about the electrical activity of the brain during the period of recording. Only if patterns characteristic of epilepsy are seen during the routine recording, is the EEG of value in the diagnosis of epilepsy. A 'negative' EEG does not exclude a diagnosis of epilepsy. Sometimes ambulatory monitoring (longer term EEG) is used. [5237]

Epilepsy & work

There are about 100,000 people with epilepsy at work in the UK today. Research has shown that, on average, they have fewer accidents than other employees, take less time off work and have good job loyalty records. These facts, together with the right kinds of skills and self-confidence, are positive selling points to an employer.

Remember: An individual with skills and talents is much more employable, despite a few seizures, than someone else with no seizures but no skills. [5238]

Living with epilepsy

If seizures can be completely controlled, and if the person can achieve a high level of confidence and self-esteem, then epilepsy should present no real obstacles to a full life.

However, having seizures for the first time, and being told that the diagnosis is 'epilepsy' (about which there may be many misconceptions in the individual's mind) can be very upsetting.

Careful counselling and health education can do much to alleviate anxiety for the individual and the family.

If the person continues to have seizures, then there may be difficulties in many aspects of daily living. But even in this situation, good psychological health can help minimise physical problems which only occur from time to time. Individuals should be helped not to blame everything on their epilepsy, and there should be an emphasis on abilities rather than the extent of the disability. Details of local self-help groups are available from the Epilepsy Helpline 01494 601400 (Mondays to Fridays 10am to 4pm).

Merely labelling people as 'epileptics' on the basis of a medical diagnosis of epilepsy ignores the rest of their attributes and characteristics both good and bad and should be avoided. [5237]

Treatment

Successful treatment depends on many factors: type of epilepsy, accuracy of diagnosis, accuracy of treatment, compliance, associated handicaps and social problems.

With appropriate drug treatment, seizures can be completely controlled in the majority of people. In some, the tendency to have seizures diminishes with time, but maximum control should still be sought as early as possible. It may be necessary to take anti-epileptic drugs for a period of years even if seizures have stopped.

Some people, however, continue to have seizures despite appropriate treatment. A small proportion of such people may benefit from neurosurgery, but this is only usually recommended in people whose seizures can be shown to arise from activity in one discrete area of the brain. Even if seizures continue it should be possible to adjust the drug regime so that the condition remains stable, to allow the person to function at an optimum level. [5237]

Who has epilepsy?

Epilepsy is the most common serious neurological disorder affecting people of all ages. A prevalence rate of 0.5% (1 in 200) is usually quoted as a minimum prevalence for the UK. This would mean that there are at least 300,000 people with epilepsy in this country. [5237]

Local Organisations

Hares

Hastings & Rother Epilepsy Support (HARES). Advice and information service. *Contact:* Dee Heyfron. *Tel:* 01424 715763. Jun 2000

National Society for Epilepsy

East Sussex office. Sue Willmott gives help and advice over the telephone. *Tel:* 01825 766199. *Mobile:* 07957 714394. See also under 'National Organisations', below. *E-mail:* stmdwillmott@netscapeonline.co.uk Jun 2000

National Organisations

National Society for Epilepsy

The National Society for Epilepsy is striving for a world without epilepsy. In the meantime they will seek to enhance the health and well-being of people with epilepsy by improving clinical treatment and care and by the provision of health information to people with epilepsy, to health professionals and the general public. Founded in 1892. Patron: HM The Queen. May 2000

Clinics

The Society runs, in conjunction with the National Hospital for Neurology & Neurosurgery in London, the largest NHS outpatient epilepsy clinic in the country, with a full range of up to date facilities including an epilepsy surgery programme. Video - EEG telemetry and other EEG facilities are available. The Society also has a private medical service.

Research

The Society owns the only MRI scanner dedicated solely to epilepsy in Europe which helps with research into the causes, effects and treatment of epilepsy. The Society's staff are among the world's leading authorities on epilepsy.

Assessment

The Society has the largest of only three specialist inpatient multi-disciplinary NHS facilities which is used to determine the most appropriate course of medical treatment for each individual. The Assessment Unit has a full complement of medical, nursing, psychological and social work services.

Information & Education
The Society has an Information & Education service that provides a telephone helpline and a comprehensive range of literature and videos for professionals and the public. A wide range of training is offered for professionals, including nurses and doctors.

The Society has an international reputation and provides courses for foreign nationals from many parts of the world.

Address: National Society for Epilepsy, Chesham Lane, Chalfont St Peter, Bucks, SL9 0RJ. *Tel*: 01494 601300. *National helpline:* 01494 601400. *Fax*: 01494 871927. *Website*:
www.epilepsynse.org.uk [5239]

Further Information

Family Health Guide - Epilepsy
By A Hanscomb and L Hughes. Published by Ward Lock, 1995. Available from National Society for Epilepsy. [5237]

Health Information Service
The HIS is a free and confidential 24-hour service. You can speak to staff during office hours and you can listen to any of hundreds of tapes at any time, e.g: *Epilepsy* (Tape 060). Address: The College of Health, St Margaret's House, 21, Old Ford Road, London, E2 9PL. Freephone: 0800 66 55 44. [5367]

Living with epilepsy
By D Chadwick and S Usiskin. Published by Vermillion, 1996. [5237]

Putting you in the picture
An information pack about epilepsy, (video and booklet). Published 1992 by the National Society for Epilepsy. £14.99. [5237]

Acknowledgements
Our grateful thanks to Anna Parikh of the National Society for Epilepsy, for editorial assistance with this chapter.

Abbreviations

EEG. Electroencephalogram.

MRI. Magnetic Resonance Imaging.

Family Problems

Local Organisations

Child & Family Psychiatry

The Department of Child & Family Psychiatry aims to provide assessment and treatment services for children and adolescents up to 16 with emotional and behaviour difficulties and other psychiatric problems. Assessment normally involves parents or carers and may include advice to other professionals working with the child or family. Most referrals are made via GPs, but patients may also be referred by other agencies/professionals. *Hours:* Monday to Friday 9.00am to 5.00pm.

Address: Department of Child & Family Psychiatry, West House, Eversfield Hospital, West Hill Road, St. Leonards-on-Sea, East Sussex, TN38 0NG. *Tel*: 01424 710101. *Fax:* 01424 433870. Jun 2000

Elphinstone Family Centre

A Family Centre working mainly with parents and children under 5; providing support, assessment and treatment for families referred by Social Services. Services include: nursery unit for under 5s (10-15 places); Family Therapy Service (self-referrals); counselling and therapeutic work with adults and children. Contacts: Leslie Hillier and Lotte Risbridger. Hours: Mondays to Fridays 9.00am to 4.45pm.

Address: Elphinstone Family Centre, 211, Elphinstone Road, Hastings, Sussex, TN34 2AX. *Tel*: 01424 440840. *Fax:* 01424 432541. Jun 2000

Family Friends

Address: Hastings & Rother Family Friends, c/o Glyne Gap School, Hastings Road, Bexhill, Sussex, TN40 2PU. *Tel*: 01424 210231. *Contact*: Jean Scotcher. Helping to share the care of a special child.

Family Matters

A charity providing services for parents and young people, including parent support, parenting skills, family counselling, managing challenging behaviour, handling conflict, assertiveness, family work, non-school attendance, relationship difficulties, step-parent conflicts, youth offending, solvent abuse issues. Also, training courses and drop-in sessions.

Address: Family Matters, 128a Battle Road, St Leonards-on-Sea, TN37 7AN.

Contact: Rev'd K. Baird, Director. *Tel*: 01424 851500. *Fax:* 01424 851502. *E-mail:* familymatters@talk21.com or Peter Stevens, administrator. *Tel*: 01424 851502. Jun 2000 5867

Family Support Practioners

'All children are entitled to a safe, loving and stimulating environment to encourage them to achieve their full potential.' A team of specialist health visitors and a school nurse who have developed skills in family dynamics, positive parenting, child management and child protection. Supporting, empowering and encouraging parents in their responsibilities to children; recognising the needs and rights of children.

Team leader: Jenny Willsher. *Other staff:* Mary Dawson, Karen Toohey, Alison Kingwell, Sue Fincham, Elaine Crapper, Maggie Titmas, Vivienne Harrison.

Address: Family Support Practitioners, Hastings & Rother NHS Trust, Eversfield Hospital, West Hill Road, St Leonards-on-Sea, Sussex, TN38 0NG. *Tel:* 01424 710105. 5374

Fernside Family Resource Centre

The aim for the Family Resource Centres is to provide professionally led services that share the principles of the Family Support Strategy; enhance families' quality of life and promote their independence from Social Services Department.

Services include a range of interventions and support strategies to help parents develop their skills to deal with responsibilities and demands of parenthood, healthily and safely. Strategies to assist parents in poverty.

A range of practical, in-home supports. A range of advice, listening, information and support to deal with specific problems, life dilemmas or personal difficulties. Referrals have to be made via Fieldwork team social worker. *Contact:* Phil Riley, unit manager. *Hours*: Mondays to Thursday s9.00am to 5.30pm; Fridays 9.00am to 5.00pm.

Address: Fernside Family Resource Centre, 49, Hollington Park Road, St. Leonards, East Sussex, TN38 0SE. *Tel*: 01424 438417. May 2000

Gingerbread, Bexhill

You may be a lone parent but you are not alone. Our aim is to make life better for lone parents, by assisting with: money problems, child problems and behaviour, bereavement, counselling and social activities. Come and find out how we can help you and we can help each other now. Address: Gingerbread, Bexhill Youth Centre, Station Road, Bexhill, Sussex. Phone Debra on 01424 732814. 5077

Home-Start

Family Support Scheme - a voluntary home-visiting service offering emotional support, friendship and practical help to parents under stress. Volunteers are all parents, who visit for a few hours a week for as long as they are needed.

Referrals can be made by telephone or in writing by a third party, e.g. statutory or voluntary organisations, or by families themselves. The service is available to any family with at least one child under five years. *Contact*: Barbara Mullen or Linda Murry. *Hours:* Mondays to Fridays 9.30am to 12.30pm. *Address:* Home Start, 66, London Road, St. Leonards, TN37 6AF. *Tel*: 01424 443636. Aug 2000

Parents' Helpline

Parents' Helpline is a 24-hour 7 days a week telephone listening service, which is organised by parents for anyone experiencing difficulties with a child, of any age. It is an anonymous, confidential and free service. It is primarily a local service for East Sussex, but calls are accepted from other regions in the UK. *Contact:* Sheila Jones.

Address: Parents' Helpline, Garton House, 22 Stanford Avenue, Brighton, BN1 6AA. *Tel*: 01273 550600. Jun 2000

Parent Link East Sussex

Parents of children with special educational needs often have to contend with complicated systems, forms, meetings, worries, stress and conflict, in order to get their children's needs fully met at school. For further information contact Mike or Helen. *Tel*: 01273 481172. Jun 2000

Playlink Priory
Contacts: Trish Drinkwater and Jan Casson. *Tel:* 01424 448144. Jun 2000

Playlink Hollington
Contact: Carole Adams. *Tel:* 01424 854008. Jun 2000

Playlink Robsack
Contact: Teresa Fuller. *Tel:* 01424 853334. Jun 2000

Sure Start

A programme which will target funding in

areas of greatest need to support the physical, developmental and emotional needs of pre-school children. Sure Start will bring together nursery, child care and playgroup provision with post-natal and other health services. Facilities will be developed to support activities within 'pram pushing' distance of families, backed up by outreach services to offer support in the home. [5090]

Relate South East Sussex

Relate provides a range of services in Seaford, Eastbourne, St Leonards-on-Sea and the Ore Valley, aimed at enhancing relationships. The following services are offered:

Counselling to any couple or individuals who would like help with their relationship; Sexual clinic which can help couples who are having sexual problems in their relationship; Relateen for 11 - 18 year olds who experience family break-up and want to talk to someone; Education & training in many areas of personal development, communication and improved relationships.

Relate will help whether or not you are married, whatever your age, race, personal beliefs, sexual orientation or social background. It costs Relate £30 per hour to provide services and clients are asked to pay what they can realistically afford. As a registered charity Relate relies on the income from clients to keep the service open, but they never refuse a service because of inability to pay.

Contact: Maureen Anstey, manager. Appointments can be made by telephoning the Admin. Centre on 01323 410001 between 9.15am and 1.15pm Mondays to Saturdays; or 5.45pm to 9.15pm Mondays to Fridays. Please telephone for more information or to arrange an appointment.

Address: Relate South East Sussex, 22, Church Street, Eastbourne, East Sussex, BN21 1HS. *Tel/Fax:* 01323 410001. [5488, 5867]

National Organisations

Both Parents Forever

John Bell, Co-director and legal adviser. Margaret Bell, Co-director and medical adviser. Offer help to either of the parents, grandparents and children on their rights to an issue relating to divorce/separation or care proceedings. Help in getting abducted children returned, and overseas contact orders enforced.

The following advice packs are available from the address given below: Married parents' pack (includes grandparents' rights). Price £6.50. Unmarried parents pack (includes grandparents' rights). Price £6.50.Grandparents only pack. Price £2.50.Child abduction and overseas contact pack (please state country). Price £4.50.

Address: Both Parents Forever, 39, Cloonmore Avenue, Orpington, Kent, BR6 9LE. *Tel:* 01689 854343. [May 2000]

Careline

Counselling for children, young people and adults. *Tel:* 020 8514 1177. [Jul 2000]

Contact a Family

Address: Contact a Family. 170, Tottenham Court Road, London, W1P 0HA. *Tel:* 020 7383 3555. *Fax:* 020 738 30259.
E-mail: info@cafamily.org.uk
Website: www.info@cafamily.org.uk [Jun 2000]

Council for One Parent Families

Tel: 0800 018 5026. Lone Parent helpline (calls are free). *Fax:* 020 7482 4851. [Jun 2000]

Exploring Parenthood

This organisation is for any parent who is facing problems with children's behaviour or family relationships. It helps parents look at problems before they become crises and offers advice, education, information and counselling.

Address: Exploring Parenthood, 4, Ivory Place, 20a, Treadgold Street, London, W11 4BP. *Tel:* 020 7221 4471. *Fax*: 020 7221 5501. July 2000

Families Anonymous

Families Anonymous is a fellowship of self-help support groups for friends and families of people abusing drugs. The service is completely confidential and anonymous. Details of meetings, which are held weekly throughout the UK, may be obtained through telephoning the helpline.

Address: Families Anonymous, Doddington & Rollo Community Association, Charlotte Despard Avenue, Battersea, London, SW11 5JE. *Tel. helpline*: 020 7498 4680. *Fax:* 020 7498 1990. *Website:* www.famanon.org.uk May 2000

Families Need Fathers

Jim Parton, Chairman. Keeping children in contact with both parents following divorce or separation. *Address*: Families Need Fathers, 134, Curtain Road, London, EC2A 3AR. *Tel*: 020 7613 5060. *Website:* www.fwf.org.uk Jul 2000

Family Rights Group

Address: Family Rights Group, The Print House, 18, Ashwin Street, London, E8 3DL. *Tel*: 020 7923 2628. *Advice line:* 0800 781 1696 (1.30pm to 3.30pm). Jun 2000

Family Service Units

Contact: H. Evans. Address: Family Service Units, 207, Old Marylebone Road, London, NW1 5QP. *Tel:* 020 7402 5175. *Fax;* 020 7724 1829. Jun 2000

Family Tracing Service

Salvation Army Family Tracing Service, Missing persons helpline. *Tel*: 020 7367 4747. Jun 2000

Family Mediators Association

Address: Family Mediators Association, 46, Grosvenor Gardens, London, SW1W 0EB. *Tel:* 020 7881 9400. *Fax:* 020 7881 9401. *E-mail:* fmassoc@globalnet.co.uk *Website:* www.familymediators.co.uk Jun 2000

Family Welfare Association

Address: Family Welfare Association, 501, Kingsland Road, London, E8 4AU. *Tel*: 020 7254 6251. *Fax:* 020 7249 5443. Jul 2000

Gingerbread, London

A national organisation which has a network of local groups providing lone parents with support, friendship, social activities and a chance to develop skills and grow in confidence.

Address: Gingerbread, 16, Clerkenwell Close, London, EC1R 0AN. *Tel*: 0800 018 4318; *Fax*: 020 7336 8165. *Advice line*: 0800 018 4318. May 2000

Message Home

National Missing Persons Helpline. Left home? Run away? Send a confidential message. *Tel:* 0800 700 740, 24-hour, calls are free. *Tel*: 0500 700 700, calls are free. *All other enquiries:* 020 8392 4545. *Fax:* 020 8878 7752.
E-mail: nmph.casemgrs@virgin.net Jun 2000

Missing Persons Helpline

Tel: 0500 700 700 (calls are free). Jun 2000

National Council for One Parent Families

Lone Parent helpline: Calls are free -
Tel: 0800 018 5026. *Fax:* 020 7482 4851. *E-mail:* info@oneparentfamilies.org.uk *Website:* www.oneparentfamilies.org.uk Jun 2000

National Stepfamily Association

This organisation is now merged into Parentline Plus.

Parentline Plus

Formed following the merger of Parentline, Parent Network and the National Stepfamily Association, to work with families and provide support and information.

Parentline Plus runs a freephone helpline and parenting classes providing information and emotional support to parents under stress.

To talk to someone about any parenting issues or to find out about parenting courses near you call, free, on 0808 8002222. Open Mondays to Fridays 9am to 9pm; Saturdays 9.30 to 5pm. Sundays 10am to 3pm. Alternatively visit their website at: www.parentlineplus.org.uk

Address: Parentline Plus, 520, Highgate Studios, 53-79, Highgate Road, Kentish Town, London, NW5 1TL.
Tel: 020 7284 5500. *Fax:* 020 7284 5501. *Freephone helpline:* 0800 800 2222. *Textphone service:* 0800 7836783. *E-mail:* headoffice@parentlinplus.org.uk *Website:* www.parentlineplus.org.uk 5029 Jul 2000

Parenting Forum

Please see main entry in 'Children & Young People' chapter, page 41. 5037

Parentline

This organisation is now merged into Parentline Plus.

Parent Network

This organisation is now merged into Parentline Plus.

Relate: National Office

Contact: Anne Deas, Information Officer. *Address*: Relate National Marriage Guidance, Herbert Gray College, Little Church Street, Rugby, CV21 3AP. *Tel:* 01788 573241. *Fax:* 01788 535007. May 2000

Young Minds

YoungMinds is the national charity committed to improving the mental health of all children and young people.

Children's Mental Health Matters
When they have it they feel good about themselves, enjoy relationships, learn confidently and overcome their difficulties. When they don't - when they are overwhelmed by misery, anger or fear - all kinds of problems can arise.

Youngminds Parents' Information Service
Tel: 0800 018 2138. Provides information and advice for anyone with concerns about the mental health of a child or young person. Jun 2000

Leaflets & Booklets
YoungMinds literature is provided to help young people, parents and professionals to understand when a young person feels troubled and where to find help. YoungMinds Magazine is a leading source of up-to-date news and features on a wide range of issues affecting children's lives.

Seminars & Training
YoungMinds seminars and training increase professional understanding of children's mental health and improve joint working based on good practice and research.

Consultancy
YoungMinds Consultancy Services works with health, education, social services and the voluntary sector to develop services for children with mental health problems.

People
Director: Peter Wilson; acting chair: Dr Roger Booker; patrons: Dr Anthony Clare, Nick Hornby; president: Prof Fred Stone.

Address: Young Minds, 102, Clerkenwell Road, London, EC1M 5SA. T*el:* 020 7336 8445 (Admin.). *Fax*: 020 7336 8446. *Parents' information service:* 0800 018 2138. *E-mail:*enquiries@youngminds.org.uk
Website: www.youngminds.org.uk 5345 May 2000

Further Information

Children, Feelings & Divorce

'Children, Feelings & Divorce - Finding the best outcome'. Written by Heather Smith. "Why do some children survive the divorce of their parents better than others? What do children of successful divorces have to say about their experience? How can divorcing parents get it right? This book is a distillation of the author's 25 years' experience of working with children whose parents have divorced.

Enlivened throughout by comments made by children and parents themselves, the book is written to increase parents' understanding of their children's feelings and how they express such feelings. In this way it aims to reduce children's distress, giving them a greater chance of growing into happy, successful adults."

April 1999. 200 pp. Paperback ISBN: 1 85343 434 5. Price £15.95. Available from Free Association Books, 57, Warren Street, London, W1P 5PA. *Tel*: 020 7388 3182. *Fax*: 020 7388 3187. *E-mail*: fab@fitzrovia.demon.co.uk 5107

Families And How to Survive Them

By Robin Skinner and John Cleese, published by Mandarin, £5.99; explores routes to a happy, healthy family life.

Adolescence

The survival guide for parents and teenagers, by Elizabeth Fenwick and Dr Tony Smith. Published by Dorling Kindersley. ISBN: 0-7513-0545-6. 5373

See also these chapters...

Children and Young People, page 37.

Acknowledgements

Our grateful thanks to Mary Dawson, family support practitioner, for editorial assistance with this chapter.

Hearing Voices

Local Organisations

Hearing Voices Network

See also under 'Nationsl Organsisations', below. *Contact:* John Milsom, services manager. *Address:* Brighton Community support Services, St Richard's Community Centre, Hove, BN3 7FP. *Tel:* 01273 709060. Jun 2000

National Organisations

Hearing Voices Network

Started in Manchester in 1988. It was inspired by the pioneering work of Marius Romme and Sandra Escher, and a Dutch self-help group, Foundation Resonance.

The aims of the HVN are:

- to support a national network of people who hear voices, as well as mental health workers, family and friends
- to support self-help groups of voice-hearers to share experiences and coping strategies
- to educate society about the meaning of voices
- to develop a range of non-medical ways of assisting people to cope with their voices
- to bring voice-hearers who cope with their voices and so have not been in contact with psychiatric services together with people who are distressed by their voices.

Auditory hallucinations

Psychiatry calls voice-hearing 'auditory hallucinations' and, in many cases, regards it as a symptom of schizophrenia. At HVN we believe voices are similar to dreams - symbols of our unconscious minds. However, it is a basic tenet of HVN that we are open to diverse opinions and we accept the explanation of each individual hearer.

Stigma

HVN aims to destigmatise voice-hearing experiences. This can be achieved in part by promoting more positive explanations of voice-hearing, and giving people a framework for developing their own ways of coping.

There are now over a thousand individual members of HVN and over 80 self-help groups in the UK. Membership is open to anyone interested in voice-hearing, and in raising awareness of voice-hearing experiences. 5968 Jun 2000

Address: Hearing Voices Network, 91, Oldham Street, Manchester, M4 1LW. *Tel/Fax:* 0161 834 5768. *E-Mail:* hearingvoices@care4free.net Jul 2000

Further Information

Accepting Voices

Editors: Professor Marius Romme and Sandra Escher. "*Accepting Voices* illustrates that many people hear voices, and that many cope without recourse to psychiatry, and come to terms with their experience." Published by Mind, 1993. ISBN 1-874690-13-8. 260 pages, £13.99. Mind Mail Order Service. *Tel*: 020 8221 9666.

Hearing Voices

'Hearing voices: A common human experience' by John Watkins. A wealth of information, which will be of great practical value to people who hear voices as well as those who wish to know more. There is a detailed description of a wide variety of voice-hearing experiences, an overview of theories, that attempt to account for voice-hearing, and creative strategies for coping. Published by Hill of Content, 1998. ISBN: 0-85572-288-6. 320 pages, £10.99. Available from Mind. *Tel:* 020 8221 9666. Jun 2000

Making Sense of Voices

'Making Sense of Voices: A guide for mental health professionals working with voice-hearers'. By Prof. Marius Romme and Sandra Escher.

Just under ten years ago Marius Romme and Sandra Escher triggered a seismic shift in the understanding of voice hearing. They put the powerful case for accepting and validating people's own interpretations of their voices, and showed how such interpretations often enabled people to live with them far more effectively than bio-medical approaches.

This new handbook for practitioners builds on this work, combining examples with guidance on the various processes involved in enabling voice-hearers to make sense of their voices and harness them to lead a more fulfilling life. Published by Mind, 2000. ISBN: 1-874690-86-3. 180 pages. Price £25.00. Available from Mind. *Tel:* 020 8221 9666. 5024

The Voice Inside

A practical guide to coping with hearing voices. Written by Paul Baker. Published by Handsell Publishing/Mind, 1997, ISBN 1-874690-71-5, 24 pages, £3.00. "This useful booklet gives an overview of recent research, explains what voices feel like, why they happen and looks at self-management techniques." Available from Mind Mail Order Service. *Tel*: 020 8221 9666.

Working With Voices

Written by Ron Coleman and Mike Smith. "An innovative workbook where the voice-hearer works through a structured course to help them manage their voice or voices." Published by Handsell, 1997, 52 pages, £5.00. Available from Mind Mail Order Service. *Tel*: 020 8221 9666.

Huntington's Disease

Huntington's disease, which is often called HD, is an hereditary disorder of the central nervous system. It used to be known as Huntington's Chorea or HC. Huntington's disease usually develops in adulthood and can cause a very wide range of symptoms. It affects both men and women.[5026]

Causes

Huntington's disease is caused by a faulty gene on chromosome 4. The gene, which produces a protein called Huntingtin, was discovered in 1993. In some way - which is not yet understood - the faulty gene leads to damage of the nerve cells in areas of the brain including the basal ganglia and cerebral cortex. This leads to gradual physical, mental and emotional changes.[5026]

Symptoms

The symptoms of Huntington's disease usually develop when people are between 30-50 years old, although they can start much earlier or much later and can differ from person to person, even in the same family.

The early symptoms include slight, uncontrollable muscular movements; stumbling and clumsiness; lack of concentration and short-term memory lapses; depression and changes of mood, sometimes including aggressive or anti-social behaviour.

Later on in the illness people experience many different symptoms, but these may include involuntary movements, difficulty in speech and swallowing, weight loss, emotional changes resulting in stubbornness, frustration, mood swings and depression.

Sometimes psychological problems, rather than the physical deterioration, cause more difficulties both for the person with Huntington's disease and their carer.[5026]

Treatment

Currently there is no cure for the illness but there are many ways to manage symptoms effectively. Medication can be used to treat symptoms such as involuntary movements, depression and mood swings. Speech therapy can significantly improve speech and swallowing problems. A high calorie diet can prevent weight loss and improve symptoms such as involuntary movements or behavioural problems.[5026]

Organisations

HD Association

The Huntington's Disease Association exists to support people affected by Huntington's disease. The HDA also provides information and advice to professionals whose task it is to support Huntington's disease families.[5025]

Services

- A Central Information, Advice and Support Service which operates from its registered office in London. The administration team consists of paid staff and volunteers. The office is open on weekdays from 9am to 4.30pm.[5025]
- A Regional Care Advisory Service, which consists of a team of Regional Care Advisers who provide information and advice to families.
- Local branches and groups throughout the country.
- A Research Programme which promotes and funds both medical and social research.[5025]

Contact: Eileen Cook, secretary. *Address:* Huntington's Disease Association, 108, Battersea High Street, London, SW11 3HP. *Tel:* 020 7223 7000. *Fax:* 020 7223 9489.[5025]

Learning Difficulties

'Learning difficulties' is a term used to describe a number of difficulties, dyslexia being one of them. [5299]

Dyslexia
Typically, dyslexia is regarded as a learning difficulty and the term is reserved for children who are significantly behind grade level in reading and when there is no evidence of any generally debilitating disorder like a learning disability (previously known as a mental handicap), major brain injury, severe emotional problems or cultural factors such as coming from a home where the language spoken is not the one used in the larger community.

Dyslexia can be overcome through various means and does not stop someone from learning new skills or becoming independent. [5299]

Attention Deficit
Attention Deficit Hyperactive Disorder: please see separate chapter, page 21.

Local Organisations

Hastings College

Courses for Adults with Learning Difficulties. Supportive Education at the School of Health & Social Studies at Hastings College of Arts & Technology. *Contacts*: Peter Suret, head of school; Alison Russell, deputy head of school.

Address: School of Health & Social Studies, Hastings College of Arts & Technology, 80, St Saviours Road, St Leonards, TN38 0AR. *Tel*: 01424 720978. Jul 2000

Hastings Gateway Club

For young adults with learning difficulties. *Contact:* Mr Wilf Elam, vice president. *Hours:* 7 to 9pm Thursday evenings.

Address: Hastings Gateway Club, 13, Linley Drive, Hastings, East Sussex, TN34 2DD. *Tel:* 01424 426444. [5867]

Parent support group

East Sussex Dyslexia support group meetings held every two months at Eastbourne, Hastings, Lewes and Seaford. *Contacts:* Nicky Woodwood, 74, Upper Belgrave Road, Seaford, East Sussex, BN25 3AT. *Tel:* 01323 896542. *E-mail:* nicky@woodward3040.freeserve.co.uk *and* Diane Pearson. *Tel:* 01424 211897. Jun 2000

Parentlink

Information, advice and support to families where there is a child with special educational needs. *Address:* Parentlink, 47, St Anne's Crescent, Lewes, East Sussex, BN7 1SB. *Tel/Fax:* 01273 481172. *E-mail:* parentlink@eastsussexcc.gov.uk Jun 2000

Further Information

Health Information Service
The HIS is a free and confidential 24-hour service. You can speak to staff during office hours, and you can listen to any of hundreds of tapes at any time, e.g. *Dyslexia* Tape 208). *Address:* The College of Health, St Margaret's House, 21, Old Ford Road, London, E2 9PL. *Freephone:* 0800 66 55 44. Apl 2000

Acknowledgements
Our grateful thanks to Trudy Allen and colleagues at Partners in Advocacy, for editorial assistance with this chapter, March 2000.

Learning Disabilities

The term 'learning disability' has been defined as a reduced ability to understand new or complex information and to learn new skills, and a reduced ability to cope independently which started before adulthood with a lasting effect on development. *(Department of Health, 1995).* [1571]

Learning disability has been defined as a reduced ability to understand new or complex information and to learn new skills, and a reduced ability to cope independently which started before adulthood with a lasting effect on development. (*Department of Health, 1995*).

The term 'learning disabilities' is used to describe people who were previously labelled as having a mental handicap, for example someone with Down's syndrome.

The following are points of contact who will be able to respond directly to queries or redirect to an alternative contact.

Down's syndrome
Down's syndrome is a genetic condition caused by the presence of an extra chromosome. People with Down's syndrome have forty-seven chromosomes instead of the usual forty-six. About one baby in every thousand has Down's syndrome. It is the most common form of learning disability (mental handicap).

An increasing number of children with Down's syndrome are now attending mainstream schools and going on to gain employment and lead semi-independent lives as full members of the community.

Please see 'Down's Syndrome Association' below. [5014]

Local Organisations

Community Learning Disability
A service run by Hastings & Rother NHS Trust. A multi-disciplinary specialist support service for adults with learning disabilities in Hastings and Rother. Contact: Peter Baker, head psychologist.

Address: Hastings & Rother NHS Trust, 4, Holmesdale Gardens, Hastings, East Sussex, TN34 1LY. *Tel:* 01424 422238. *Fax:* 01424 465563. [Jun 2000]

Agape Trust
The Agape Trust is a Christian Trust which received charitable status in 1992. The Trust is committed to building purpose-built units in E. Sussex, which encompasses day care, respite and long stay care facilities for young adults with profound disabilities. They are working towards providing two such units - in Hastings and Lewes.

Growing concern

The Trust came into being out of a growing concern for families with children who have profound learning and physical disabilities, and for whom there is a desperate need for appropriate, specialised respite, day care or long-term residential care

Multiple difficulties

The Trust was originally centred around a

young adult with multiple difficulties who has been care for at home by her parents, who are both founder members and current directors of the trust. Emma, the young person in question, requires constant stimulation and 24 hour care from her parents to meet her special needs and, due to a lack of any suitable facilities, her future looks bleak.

Other young people

Unfortunately, there are many other young people in a similar position, whose carers need the assurance of a well-equipped, safe and loving environment for their children, both for immediate respite and for their long-term future. [6089, Aug 2000]

Hastings Project

Contact is the Revd Kenn Baird, Project Development Manager, The Agape Trust, 118, Hastings Road, Battle, East Sussex, TN33 0TQ. *Tel/Fax/Minicom:* 01424 775042. *E-mail:* agape@talk21.com [5036 Jul 2000; 6089,Aug 2000]

Lewes Project

Tel: 01273 400979. [6089, Aug 2000]

Disability Information Line

Children's services. *Contact*: Ann Ling. *Address:* 37, Fellows Road, Hastings, TN34 3TY. *Tel:* 01424 422617 (weekday mornings 9am to noon; answerphone at other times). [Jun 2000]

Learning Disability Forum

The main aim of the forum is to open doors and create opportunities for people who have a learning disability to take part in ordinary activities like education, work and leisure. The forum wants people with a learning disability to be included and accepted as valuable members of the community. Jointly funded by the Catholic Children's Society (Registered Charity No. 233296) and the Diocese of Arundel and Brighton. *Contacts*: John McManus, development worker; Janice Bailey.

Address: Hastings, Rother & Bexhill Learning Disability Forum, 'Osmunda', Fountain Centre, 7, Cranfield Road, Bexhill, Sussex, TN40 1DB. *Tel:* 01424 730536, (John); 430066, (Janice). *E-mail:* fountainscentre@cathchild.org [May 2000]

Mencap

The aim is to provide a service by way of day care for people with a learning disability, which encourages independence and promotes their well-being.

Provision includes further education (based on the arts), residential care, social groups (including disco's, social clubs for adults and children, holidays and outings). Support and friendship is also offered to the families and carers of people with a learning disability.

Chairperson: Mrs Georgina Homes; Treasurer: Mr Chris Dowse; Hon. secretary: Mrs Rosumunde Jordan; Administrator: Mrs Pauline Fletcher; Day care manager: Mrs Veronica Smith; Active arts co-ordinator: Mrs Marilyn Wright.

Address: Hastings & Bexhill Mencap Society, Frimley, 64, London Road, St Leonards-on-Sea, East Sussex, TN37 6AS. *Tel:* 01424 424813. [5450]

My Choice

This is a countywide advocacy service for adults with a learning disability. Formerly known as 'Partners in Advocacy'. Trudy Allen is the county manager and works from the Hastings office. Registered Charity No. 802632. The addresses of the three offices within this service are:

Hastings

Contacts: Trudy Allen, County Manager; Andy Bannister, self-advocacy worker. *Address:* My Choice, The Advocacy Centre, 42, Robertson Street, Hastings, East Sussex, TN34 1HL. *Tel:* 01424 441562. *Fax:*

01424 204687. Jun 2000

Eastbourne

Contact; Stephanie Heng. *Address:* My Choice, EAVS, 8, Saffron Road, Eastbourne, East Sussex, BN21 1DG. *Tel:* 01323 417926. Jun 2000

Lewes

Contact: Shelley Franklin. *Address:* My Choice, South Downs CVS, 66, High Street, Lewes, East Sussex, BN7 1XG. *Tel:* 01273 477700. Jun 2000

Trefoil Guild

The Trefoil Guild is a member of the Girl Guide Organisation and is entirely voluntary. Disabled people who have been members, (18+) of the Scout and Guide movement are welcome. Contact Name: Mrs J. Francis.

They cater for all disabilities including those with learning disabilities and epilepsy or mental health problems. *Secretary*: Mrs Eileen Bolster.

Address: 10, Sheerwater Crescent, Hastings, East Sussex, TN34 2NZ. *Tel:* 01424 424685. May 2000

Social Services

Information Line

Please contact the Social Services Information Line, during office hours, for information about the services provided by the Department and other social care services. *Tel:* 0845 6010664 (calls are charged at local rate). *Fax:* 01424 201946. *E-mail:* information.line@eastsussexcc.gov.uk 5953 Jun 2000

Initial referral points

There are two initial referral points for people with a learning disability, one for Hastings & Rother and one for Lewes & Wealden.

Eastbourne, Hastings & Rother

Address: Learning Disability Assessment Team, Ridgeway, 125, St Helen's Down, Hastings, Sussex, TN34 2AR. *Tel:* 01424 430066. *Fax:* 01424 720338. 5953. Jun 2000

Lewes & Wealden.

Address: Learning Disability Assessment Team, 1, Southview Close, Crowborough, East Sussex, TN6 1HH. *Tel:* 01892 664671. *Fax:* 01892 669928. 5953 Jun 2000

National Organisations

Down's Syndrome Association

The only national charity working exclusively for people with Down's syndrome and their families. The Association has a network of volunteer parent-led branches and groups throughout England, Wales and Northern Ireland.

The National Office of the Association provides information, support and advice on all aspects of the condition and they are always there to help anyone who contacts them. Whenever there is a need for practical guidance, or simply someone to talk to, the Association is there to help.

In addition to the work with families, they work hard to change attitudes towards people with Down's syndrome. Each year they sponsor new research projects which will enhance the lives of all those with the condition.

Address: Down's Syndrome Association, 155, Mitcham Road, London, SW17 9PG. *Tel:* 020 8682 4001. *Fax:* 020 8682 4012. *E-mail:* info@downs-syndrome.org.uk *Website:* www.dsa-uk.com 5014 Jul 2000

Mencap

Address: Mencap, 123, Golden Lane, London EC1 0RT. *Tel*: 020 7454 0454. *Fax:* 020 7608 3254. *E-mail:* mencap@org.uk *Website:* www.mencap.org.uk Jun 2000

Voice UK

Offers information and support to adults and children with learning disabilities who have experienced crime or abuse. *Contact*: Christine Horrocks. Registered Charity No. 2923239.

Address: Voice UK, The College Business Centre, Uttoxeter New Road, Derby, DE22 3WZ. *Tel:* 01332 202555. *Fax* 01332 295888.
E-mail: voiceuk@clara.net *Website:* Website: www.voiceuk.clara.net May 2000

Further Information

Health Information Service
The HIS is a free and confidential 24-hour service. You can speak to staff during office hours, and you can listen to any of hundreds of tapes at any time, e.g: *Down's Syndrome.* (Tape 034).

Address: The College of Health, St Margaret's House, 21, Old Ford Road, London, E2 9PL. *Freephone*: 0800 66 55 44.

Mental Health and Learning Disabilities.
Factsheet by Jackie Golding. Published by MIND Information Unit, May 1999. £1.36. Available from Mind Mail Order Service. *Tel*: 020 8221 9666. 5367

Acknowledgements
Our grateful thanks to Trudy Allen of Partners in Advocacy, Hastings & Rother, and Peter Baker of Community Learning Disability Services for editorial help with this chapter.

Manic Depression

Manic depression - or bipolar affective disorder - is thought to affect about one in every hundred people. In this chapter the illness is described, national and local support groups are listed and there are many recommended books.

Some people experience profound changes in their mood, which can move from depression and lethargy to periods of elation and overactivity. Doctors call this 'manic depression'.

Some people may move from depression to elation and back in a week, while others may go through this cycle once a year or less often.

Highs and lows

Everyone gets mood swings now and then, but for someone who has manic depression, the highs (mania) and lows (depression), can be so severe and out of control that medication and sometimes hospitalisation is needed.

Women are almost twice as likely as men to experience manic depression. Women are particularly vulnerable at adolescence, after having a child, and at the menopause.

Symptoms

Symptoms of mania can include elevated mood, hyperactivity, deluded thinking, irritability, irrational spending of money, inflated self-esteem and poor judgement.
Major depression is characterised by symptoms such as morbid sadness, lowered self-esteem and decreased energy.

Causes

The causes of manic depression are not fully understood, but research is being carried out into genetics, biochemical and environmental factors, each of which can play a role.

Of all psychiatric illnesses, mood disorders are the most responsive to treatment and many cases can be controlled or reduced in severity. On average, it takes five years to be correctly diagnosed for manic depression.

An increasing number of people with manic depression are finding that self-management techniques can help them regain control of their lives. [5222]

Facts about manic depression

The following information is taken from *The Fundamental Facts*, published by the Mental Health Foundation. Hospital admissions: In the UK, there are 370 hospital admissions per ten thousand of the population per year for manic depression; only 3% of these are first time admissions.

This reflects the recurrent nature of manic depression. Repeat episodes: 'an estimated 20% of people who have a first episode of manic depression do not get another.' [1571]

How to help yourself

The following advice is taken from the MDF leaflet "What next? Information for people leaving hospital who have been given a diagnosis of manic depression (bipolar disorder)." [5092]

How to help yourself
You may feel powerless at the moment, but there are ways that you can help yourself. Here are three important things that you can do:

Responsibility
Learn to take responsibility for your own health. Understand what medications you have, how they work and how they are monitored. Make a positive decision to manage yourself and the way you live.

Find out
Find out as much as you can about the condition and help your supporters (your relatives, friends, partner and so on) to do the same.

Support
Start to find people who can support you. Build up relationships of trust with the mental health professionals who work with you - your GP, psychiatrist, CPN, social worker, occupational therapist. Keep them informed and don't be afraid to ask for their help.

Avoiding going into hospital again
There may be occasions when going into hospital is the only appropriate course of action. However there are things that you can do to moderate the severity and impact of mood swings.

Early warning signs
Try to keep to a minimum things that trigger your mood swings - stress, big life changes. Watch for early warning signs. Devise an action/crisis plan. Create strong supportive networks. Don't expect an instant cure.

Avoiding getting low
There may be times when you will become depressed whatever you do. However, there are tried and tested tactics for avoiding the onset and severity of depression.

Structure
Keep a structure or routine to the day. Keep active even if you don't feel like it. Keep up regular exercise and regular eating. Keep a simple journal of your feelings.

Avoiding getting high
There may be times when you will experience an episode of mania despite your best efforts. However, there will often be warning signs and there are preventative measures you can take.
Avoid lots of major life changes all at once. Put a sensible limit on your social or work commitments. Control your intake of stimulants (e.g. coffee, tea, alcohol).

Getting support
It may seem difficult to trust people but it is very important to have at least one friend or family member to confide in. They can also help you to monitor your moods.

Contact a support group for people who have experienced the same thing, e.g. a MDF self-help group. Contact your local mental health organisations and other community groups.

Mood diaries

Mood diaries are a way of recording your moods on a graph so that you can see at a glance how your mood is altering over time. It's useful for seeing when your mood is moving towards being out of control. The following definitions are taken from the Manic Depression Fellowship's *Pendulum,* Spring 1997 issue. Moods are classified into three regions: low, (0-2), normal (3-7) and high (8-10).

Level 0.
Suicidal, numb, scared, trembling, sleeping whenever possible, very low, very anxious, crying, very withdrawn, very slow, mornings very difficult.

Level 1.
Paranoid, unable to make decisions, very negative, lack of co-ordination, slow, memory very poor, poor concentration, almost unable to function.

December

Date	1	2	3	4	5	6	7	8	9	10	11	12	13	14	15	16	17	18	19	20	21	22	23	24	25	26	27	28	29	30	31
Mood 10	10	10	10	10	10	10	10	10	10	10	10	10	10	10	10	10	10	10	10	10	10	10	10	10	10	10	10	10	10	10	10
Mood 9	9	9	9	9	9	9	9	9	9	9	9	9	9	9	9	9	9	9	9	9	9	9	9	9	9	9	9	9	9	9	9
Mood 8	8	8	8	8	8	8	8	8	8	8	8	8	8	8	8	8	8	8	8	8	8	8	8	8	8	8	8	8	8	8	8
Mood 7	7	7	7	7	7	7	7	7	7	7	7	7	7	7	7	7	7	7	7	7	7	7	7	7	7	7	7	7	7	7	■
Mood 6	6	6	6	6	6	6	6	6	6	6	6	6	6	6	6	6	6	6	■	6	6	■	■	6	■	6	■	■	6	■	6
Mood 5	5	5	5	5	5	5	5	5	5	■	5	■	■	■	■	■	■	■	5	■	■	5	5	■	5	■	5	5	■	5	5
Mood 4	4	■	■	■	■	4	■	■	■	4	■	4	4	4	4	4	4	4	4	4	4	4	4	4	4	4	4	4	4	4	4
Mood 3	■	3	3	3	3	■	3	3	3	3	3	3	3	3	3	3	3	3	3	3	3	3	3	3	3	3	3	3	3	3	3
Mood 2	2	2	2	2	2	2	2	2	2	2	2	2	2	2	2	2	2	2	2	2	2	2	2	2	2	2	2	2	2	2	2
Mood 1	1	1	1	1	1	1	1	1	1	1	1	1	1	1	1	1	1	1	1	1	1	1	1	1	1	1	1	1	1	1	1
Mood 0	0	0	0	0	0	0	0	0	0	0	0	0	0	0	0	0	0	0	0	0	0	0	0	0	0	0	0	0	0	0	0

Mood diary - typical entries showing gradual increase in mood level - see text for details

Level 2.
Drowsy, tired, withdrawn, irritable, crying, tense, anxious, hard to get up, hard to take criticism, blaming self, coping with simple tasks.

Level 3.
Apprehensive, pre-occupied, need extra sleep, just coping with everyday tasks.

Level 4.
Needs pushing to do unpleasant tasks, more relaxed, less anxious.

Level 5.
Less sleepy, less tense, coping quite well, more positive, completing daily routines.

Level 6.
Self-confident, enjoying life, thoughtful, balanced viewpoint, realistic, happy, in control.

Level 7.
Quite quick, more talkative, feel just in control of self, feel very well, creative.

Level 8.
Tense, rushing about, irritable of others' slowness, do not listen to advice, poor concentration, not following routine.

Level 9.
Wake up early, need little sleep, craving to spend, 'tipsy' feeling, taking on too much, unrealistic.

Level 10.
Elated, out of control, over spending, sleeping only a few hours, making instant major decisions, aggressive.

Local Organisations

MDF Self-Help Group

FELLOWSHIP

The Hastings & Rother MDF Self-Help Group. The group meets every week on Tuesday mornings between 10.30am and 12.30pm. May 2000

Not only people with manic depression attend these meetings - there are carers, relatives and friends too, who come along to find out more about the illness. A group member says, "We really value a safe space to talk about our experiences and to meet with others who know exactly what it's like, for instance, to have a manic episode."

People often say what a relief it is to just find out that they are not alone. The Self-Help Group is user-led and informally

"We really value a safe space to talk about our experiences and to meet with others who know exactly what it's like, for instance, to have a manic episode"
- group member.
Hastings & Rother
MDF Self-Help Group

structured in a friendly and relaxed atmosphere. Please come along and see if it is for you!

Address: Hastings & Rother Manic Depression Fellowship Self-Help Group, c/o The Advocacy Centre, 42, Robertson Street, Hastings, Sussex. *Tel:* 01424 441597.[5122]

MDFF

The MDFF is the Manic Depression Family & Friends Support Group, started January 1999. It is a support group for relatives and others who live with or care for people with manic depression. The MDFF also tries to bring about improvements to the service received by sufferers.

Contact: John Humphries, secretary, or Maureen Baines, membership secretary. *Address:* MDFF, 33, St Peter's Road, St Leonards, Sussex, TN37 6JQ. *Tel:* 01424 438120 (day); 01424 445540 (evening).

Meetings

All meetings take place at the Moreton Centre, Bethune Court, Boscobel Road, St Leonards, Sussex. Meetings start at 7pm. Schedule of meetings for 2000: Thurs Oct 5; Thurs Nov 2; Thurs Dec 7.

Meetings 2001

The schedule of meetings for 2001: Thurs Jan 4; Thurs Feb 1; Thurs Mar 1; Thurs Mar 29; Thurs Apr 26; Thurs May 24; Thurs Jun 21; Thurs July 19; Thurs Aug 16; Thurs Sep 13; Thurs Oct 11; Thurs Nov 8; Thurs Dec 6.

NSF Carers' Support

The National Schizophrenia Fellow-ship based at Hove offers carers of people with manic depression one to one support. For more details please see entry 'Carers' Support' in the Schizophrenia chapter, page 112.

National Organisations

Manic Depression Fellowship

The Manic Dep-ression Fellowship (MDF) works to enable people affected by manic depression to take control of their lives.

The Fellowship aims to fulfil its mission by supporting and developing its self help groups; publishing information on all aspects of manic depression; developing and providing a range of services for members; providing training in self management techniques; representing the needs of those affected by manic depression to policy making bodies and professional individuals; developing working relationships with other organisations concerned with mental health; combating the stigma and prejudice experienced by those affected by any serious mental health problem.

The MDF was established in 1983 and is today the largest user-led mental health organisation in the UK, with over 130 self-help groups across the United Kingdom.

The aims are to help people with manic depression, their carers, families and friends; to educate the public and the professions about the illness and to encourage research into better methods of treatment. A 24-hour legal advice line and a travel insurance scheme are available to members.[5469]

Patrons: Spike Milligan, Professor Anthony Clare, Dr Miriam Stoppard.

Self-help groups

MDF self-help groups offer the opportunity to meet others who have been through similar experiences. MDF groups can lessen the sense of isolation and provide a safe space. Members understand, from personal experience, the problems and pressures of living with manic depression.

National office staff

Chief exec. . . . . Karen Campbell
Dep chief exec . . . . Michelle Rowett

Employment & development .... Mike Calver
Finance .... Jean Wit
Contact self-manager .... Andy Pattison
Admin .... Brenda Fontain
Fundraising .... Luke Chatterton

Pendulum

Magazine published by the Manic Depression Fellowship. Editor: Polly Mortimer.

Address: The Manic Depression Fellowship, Castle Works, 21, St George's Road, London, SE1 6ES. *Tel:* 020 7793 2600. *E-mail:* pmorti@hotmail.com).

Further Information

A Balancing Act

32-page booklet published by the MDF in August 1997. "Help and coping strategies for those who care for people with manic depression". Price £3. Available from the MDF. *Tel:* 020 7793 2600.

Accepting Voices

Written by Marius Romme and Sandra Escher, published by Mind Publications, 1993.

An Unquiet Mind

A memoir of moods and madness. Written by Kay Redfield Jamison. Published by Picador Publications. Price £9.99. Available from the MDF. *Tel:* 020 7793 2600.

Bipolar Disorder

A guide for patients and their families. Written by Francis Mark Mondimore. Published by John Hopkins Press. Price £9.25.

Cognitive Behavioural Therapy

Cognitive Behavioural Therapy for Bipolar Disorder written by Monica Ramirez Basco and A John Rush. Published by Guildford Press. Price £21.23 (amazon.co.uk).

Carbamazepine & Manic Depression

A guide written by John Greist and published by the Lithium Information Centre, USA. Contents: Carbamazepine and manic depressive disorder; beginning carbamazepine therapy; side effects of carbamazepine; commonly asked questions about carbamazepine. Price £3. Available from the MDF. *Tel:* 020 7793 2600.

Coping with Depression and Elation

Written by Dr Patrick McKeon. Revised edition published by Sheldon Press, 1995. "Dr Patrick McKeon is consultant psychiatrist at St Patrick's Hospital, Dublin. He has a special interest in depression and elation and runs a mood disorder therapeutic programme". Price £6.99. Available from the MDF. *Tel:* 020 7793 2600.

Depression Workbook

A guide for living with depression and manic depression. Written by Mary Ellen Copeland. "Mary Ellen Copeland is a distinguished teacher and lecturer from Vermont, and is herself a manic depressive. In moving language and startling honesty she tells her story here." Published by New Harbinger Publications, 1992. Price £15.99. Available from the MDF. *Tel:* 020 7793 2600.

Drug Treatment of Manic Depression

Written by Anne Cole. Factsheet published by the MDF, 1994. Price £1. Available from the MDF. *Tel:* 020 7793 2600.

Inside out

A guide to self-management of manic depression. Written by David Guinness. 32-page booklet published by the MDF. Price £3. Available from the MDF. *Tel:* 020 7793 2600.

Lithium

Making sense of treatment and drugs. 24-page booklet published jointly by Mind and the MDF, 1994. Contents include: What is lithium? Why is lithium prescribed? Diet guidelines. Adverse effects of lithium. Common questions. Price £2.50. Available from the MDF. *Tel:* 020 7793 2600.

Lithium Treatment

Lithium treatment of manic depressive illness - a practical guide. Written by

Professor Mogens Schou. Fifth edition published by Karger, Basel, 1993. Price £8. Available from the MDF. Tel: 020 7793 2600.

Managing MD Disorders
Edited by Ved Varma. Published by Jessica Kingsley, 1997.

Manic Depression, Bipolar Disorder
Written by Anne Marr and others. A guide to self-help for people with the illness, their relatives and friends. Booklet published by the MDF, 1997. Price £1. Available from the MDF. *Tel:* 020 7793 2600.

Manic Depressive Disorder
Factsheet. Published by the MDF, 1989.

Manic Depressive Illness
Written by Fred K Goodwin and Kay Redfield Jamison. ISBN 0-19-503934-3. (Available as an inter-library loan book from the British Library, reference q90/17257d, through ESCC Library Services, or via publisher at around £70.)

Overcoming Depression
By Dr Richard Gillet. A comprehensive guide to managing depression. Price £8.99. Available from the MDF. *Tel:* 020 7793 2600.

Parenthood
Parenthood and manic depressive illness. The pros and cons of medication during pregnancy. Factsheet published by the MDF, 1992. Price £1. Available from the MDF. *Tel:* 020 7793 2600.

Touched With Fire
Written by Kay Redfield Jamison. Published by Free Press/Simon & Schuster.

Why Did My World Have To Change?
Factsheet published by the MDF which gives support to teenagers whose parents suffer from manic depression. Price £1. Available from the MDF. *Tel:* 020 7793 2600. [5956]

Websites

Have-A-Heart
Mood enhancing exercise, bipolar disorder, tempering the mania of manic depression, understanding suicidal thoughts. Website: www.have-a-heart.com

Society for Manic Depression
This is an American organisation.
Website: www.societymd.org.

Discussion forums
The following three sites are online discussion forums - remember not to give out personal details. *Websites:*
alt.support.depression.manic
soc.support.depression.manic
alt.support.depression.seasonal [5298]

Fact sheets, statistics
Fact sheets, statistics, rapid cycling, creativity, self-care, etc. *Website:*
www.mhsource.com/wb/thow9903.html

Acknowledgements
Our grateful thanks to Alan Mooncie of the MDF Hastings & Rother Self-Help Group for editorial assistance with this chapter. [5925.]

Men

Suicides by men now comprise 75% of all suicides in the UK. Between 1971 and 1996 the suicide rate for women almost halved, while in the same period the rate for men almost doubled.[5032]

Suicide

Suicide rates for men are higher than for women across all age groups. Between the ages of 25 and 44, men are almost four times more likely than women to kill themselves. Men are less likely than women to go to their GP with psychological problems. If men do go to their GP they are more likely to present with physical problems, which may not be recognised as a manifestation of mental distress.[5032]

Alcohol & drugs

The misuse of alcohol and other drugs has long been recognised as a risk factor for suicide. Alcohol and other drugs affect reasoning, and are often depressants; they decrease inhibitions, and so can make someone more likely to attempt suicide.

Men are nine times more likely to abuse alcohol than women, and men diagnosed with alcoholism are six times as likely to commit suicide as men in the general population. Alcohol and drugs are particularly implicated in the suicides of young men. It has been suggested that the increase in drug use by young people in recent years could be a factor in explaining the dramatic rise in young male suicides in Britain in the 1980s and early 1990s.[5032]

Macho

From an early age boys get hurt, abused, ignored, humiliated and called names for showing any vulnerability. Boys are denied access to natural healing processes. This conditioning is often internalised and then acted out in many forms of abuse and self-abuse: minimising or ignoring injuries and illnesses, suppressing and denying feelings of pain and distress, presenting an image of being invulnerable.

Men's fear of talking about their problems can mean they avoid 'difficult' discussions. Many men turn to substance misuse to blot out negative emotions, but this can lead to communication problems, relationship problems and even violence. Young men in distress are more likely to use antisocial behaviour to express themselves than they are to tell someone how they feel.[5032]

Depression

A number of recent studies conclude that depression actually occurs as often in men as in women, even though women get diagnosed and treated twice as often as men. One study, by the Royal College of Psychiatrists, found that men are just as likely to get depressed as women, but frequently feel that it is 'unmanly' and 'weak' to ask for professional help.

Various reasons have been suggested for why depression in men remains hidden or unrecognised. One possible reason concerns the cultural 'norm' - men are simply not supposed to succumb to emotional pain or admit to emotional problems. It has also been suggested that men may manifest depression differently than women; covert depression may be the driving force behind, for example, alcohol and other drug dependencies, domestic violence, or failures in intimacy. [5032]

Patterns of work
During the 1980s and 1990s, dramatic changes in employment affected the numbers of men and women in work. There was a 16 per cent drop in the number of men in employment, while at the same time there was a 12 per cent increase in the number of women in employment. Through the loss of many jobs in manufacturing and heavy industry, and the creation of jobs in service industries, Britain has become the first European country whose workforce is, in the majority, female.

Unemployment

Although there is no such thing as 'gendered' employment in legal terms, in public perceptions there is still a clear division between jobs that are 'men's' and jobs that are 'women's'. Within this new working environment, men are more likely to experience long-term unemployment, and the less well skilled a man is, the more likely he is to be unemployed. Men see work as a man's defining role in the community; unemployment can therefore lead to great alienation. Unemployment is a significant risk factor in suicide; one in seven men who become unemployed will develop a depressive illness within the first six months, while long-term unemployment is associated with a doubling of the male suicide rate. [5032]

Relationships
The breakdown of traditional gender roles have left many men feeling uncertain of what is expected of them, particularly in terms of significant relationships. Stable relationships are a protective factor against suicide in men; men appear to be at a higher risk of suicide if they are single, recently separated, divorced or widowed. It seems that men are less able to cope with relationship breakdown. Most divorces and separations are initiated by women and in 70 per cent of cases the man does not want the family to split up. Where marriages and relationships do break down, men may lose touch with their children as well as their partner and will probably have to find a new home. [5032]

Divorce
A recent British study found that when a man marries and has children, he then has a fifty-fifty chance of divorcing and losing custody of his children. He has a 1 in 3 chance of losing his home and a 1 in 10 chance of losing contact with his children forever. UK courts award custody of children to mothers in 91 per cent of cases.

And there is a cyclical effect. Boys who have little or no contact with their fathers are more likely to become violent, get hurt, get into trouble and do less well at school. Highly involved fathers emerged as a major factor in boys' general well being. A caring, emotionally supportive father seems to be a protective factor against boys experiencing depression and suicidal thoughts.

Mental Health Services

The time is long overdue for men's mental health issues to be recognised and properly addressed. Mental health services need to be more aware of issues of particular relevance to men's mental health, to recognise potential triggers for distress, and risk factors for depression and suicide. It is also important that public health campaigns and strategies begin to address men's health needs. Men's attitudes about themselves, and to other men, need to change if there is going to be any improvements in men's mental health and mental health care. [5032]

Acknowledgement
Taken from 'Machismo & Misery' by George Stewart, with kind permission from *Openmind 104*, July/August 2000. Copyright Mind (National Association for Mental Health). Tel: 020 8221 9661 for subscriptions information.

Migraine

Migraine is probably the most common painful chronic long-term condition which exists, so if you suffer from migraine you are definitely not alone. Any person of any age, class, sex, ethnicity, culture or intelligence level can have migraine. [5247]

If you are a migraine sufferer, then you probably know only too well what migraine is, and just how it affects you. However, let's look at the 'mechanics' of the condition first, as it will be important to your management to know exactly what is going on in your body and to recognise stages and symptoms.

Migraine is a complex condition with a wide variety of symptoms which show that various metabolic, neurophysiological and biochemical changes take place during an attack. For many, the main feature is the headache but for children the headache may be milder, and it is the gastro-intestinal symptoms like stomach ache which tend to be predominant. It is also a disorder which comes and goes, with complete freedom between attacks. [5247]

What is migraine?

'Migraine is a syndrome characterized by extremely severe headaches, usually unilateral and often accompanied by nausea, vomiting and visual disturbances. They show a familiar pattern and are often triggered by stress or by particular foodstuffs.' [5093]

Local Organisations

Migraine Support Group

Contact: June (*tel:* 01424 714285); and Marilyn (*tel:* 01424 221826). *Address:* Withheld. [May 2000]

National Organisations

Migraine Action Association

Address: Migraine Action Association, 178a, High Road, Byfleet, West Byfleet, Surrey, KT14 7ED. *Tel:* 01932 352468. [Feb 2000]

Migraine Trust

Through our Support Services, we help people with migraine manage their condition through accurate, up-to-date, understandable and relevant information; a helpline for advice and regular newsletters. We also help to raise vital awareness of the condition and its significance.

We work to improve the diagnosis and treatment of migraine by helping to set up and fund clinics all over the UK. We provide courses for GPs and other health professionals.

We encourage the new researchers of tomorrow into the field through providing studentships. We hold the only dedicated international migraine symposium as a forum to encourage research.

We hold international workshops as a brainstorming opportunity for leading specialists in migraine and related fields. We fund grants and fellowships into migraine throughout the world, which have brought about some of the major steps forward in research advances.

The Migraine Trust is a registered charity (No. 244250) and relies on voluntary income to maintain its commitments to research, education and support services. You can help us by joining the Trust. The smallest donation will automatically put you on our mailing list. Even if you cannot afford anything at the moment, you can still become a member, just get in touch. The more people we represent, the louder the voice for people with migraine.

Website

Migraine sufferers can now find support through their computer, enabling them to get information on different types of migraine, diagnosis, treatments and support networks.

Address: The Migraine Trust, 45, Great Ormond Street, London, WC1N 3HZ.
Tel: 020 7831 4818. *Fax:* 020 7831 5174.
E-mail: migrainetrust@compuserve.com
Website: www.migrainetrust.org 5247 Jul 2000

Further Information

Headaches & Migraine

Audio cassette. Describes the different types and causes of headaches and migraine. Explains how to treat them, and what self-help techniques can be used to cope with or even avoid them. Includes a 'visualisation' relaxation programme designed specifically for headaches. Published by Talking Life, tel: 0151 632 0662.

Health Information Service

The HIS is a free and confidential 24-hour service. You can speak to staff during office hours, and you can listen to any of hundreds of tapes at any time, e.g: *Headaches* (Tape 087); *Migraine* (Tape 111).

Address: The College of Health, St Margaret's House, 21, Old Ford Road, London, E2 9PL. Freephone: 0800 66 55 44. 5367

Taking Control of Your Migraine

A guide for achieving better migraine control. 16 pages. Published by the Migraine Trust. See above for address and telephone number. 5247

Acknlowledgements
Our grateful thanks to the Migraine Trust for their editorial assistance with this chapter.

Money

Money problems are common when people have mental health problems, and add to their other stresses. Your earning power may be affected; you may lose your job and have to claim state benefits. In this chapter, money, gambling and debt problems are addressed. [5224]

Local Organisations

Bohemia Trust

This Trust is now midway through its fifth year. They have recently moved to new offices in Queens Road, Hastings. They are self-funded and have a retail outlet, also on the Queens Road site. Their staff include a counsellor, RGN, retail/personal consultant and solicitor. Their team is committed to the support and assistance of the extended family and clients who are enduring financial difficulty.

Services

They offer mediation and advisory services between creditors and debtors, use of their free telephones and fax service and they also undertake form completion and budget advice. The Trust runs a home-visiting option for their counsellor/advisor. All their services are free to clients of the Hastings/Bexhill area.

Referrals

The main body of the referrals come from the Conquest Hospital Social Work Office and the Community Assessment Team for Hastings and Bexhill. The Trust is happy to offer its services to anyone in their area and needs no official referral.

Contacts: C. Beaumont, Head Counsellor &Trustee; A.F. Beaumont, W. Nicol Morris, Trustees; Ms S. Young, Nurse/Medical Adviser; M. Clark, Trainee Counsellor.

Address: The Bohemia Trust, 128, Queens Road, Hastings, East Sussex, TN34 1RP. *TelFax:* 01424 722923. [6020 July 2000]

Credit Union

Savings and lending co-operatives for people living and/or working in Hastings and St Leonards. Filling the gap for people outside of traditional banking and providing a community-spirited place to save. Open to the public on Fridays and Saturdays from 10am to 2pm. *Contacts:* Mrs Sam Burt, Credit Union worker; Ms Sandra Pantrey-Mayer, secretary.

Address: Hastings & St Leonards Credit Union Ltd, 41a, Cambridge Road, Hastings, East Sussex, TN34 1DJ. *Tel:* 01424 202651. [5867]

Direct Debt Line

Charity No. 1059127. For advice and information. *Address:* Direct Debt Line, 5b, St Mary's Walk, Hailsham, East Sussex. *Tel:* 0345 626804; 01323 840606. *Fax:* 01323 441422. *E-mail:* info@directdebtline.whd.net [May 2000]

National Organisations

Benefits Enquiry Line
This national freephone DSS helpline gives information on all benefits for sick or disabled people. The lines are open 8.30am to 6.30pm Monday to Friday and 9am to 1pm on Sat. *Tel*: 0800 88 22 00. Jun 2000

Disability Benefits Consortium
For a free copy of a fact sheet on Severe Disablement Allowance, please contact this organisation. *Address:* Disability Benefits Consortium, c/o RNIB, 224, Great Portland Street, London, W1N 6AA. 5425

National Debtline
Tel: 0645 500511. Calls are charged at local rate. Call free on 0808 808 4000. Jul 2000

Gamblers Anonymous
Headquarters: *Address:* Gamblers Anonymous, PO Box 88, London, SW6 3D0. *Gambling Helpline:* 020 7384 3040. Jul 2000

Gamcare
Confidential counselling, advice and information for young people affected by a gambling problem. Local call rate. *Tel:* 0845 6000 133. Jul 2000

Further Information

Disability Living Allowance
Fact-sheet. Factsheet by Kaaren Cruse. Published by MIND Information Unit, December 1999. Price 50p. Available from Mind Mail Order Service. *Tel:* 020 8221 9666.

Incapacity Benefit
Factsheet by Carole Reid-Galloway. Published by MIND Information Unit, August 1998. Price 50p. Available from Mind Mail Order Service. *Tel*: 020 8221 9666.

Managing Your Finances
Mind Rights Guide: Managing your Finances. Factsheet. Price £1.38 + A5 SAE. Available from Mind Mail Order Service. Tel: 020 8221 9666. 5298

Managing Your Finances
Minds Rights Guide 7: Managing your finances. "Answers some of the more common questions about people's rights when their mental health problems affect their ability to manage their financial affairs". Published by Mind. Price £1.00. Available from Mind Mail Order Service. *Tel:* 020 8221 9666. 5106

Social Security Benefits
A-Z of Social Security Benefits for People with Mental Health Problems. With all the latest information on the benefits that can be claimed by people with mental health problems. Published by Mind, 2000. ISBN: 1-874690-62-8. 24 pages. Price £3.00. Available from Mind. *Tel:* 020 8221 9666. 5024

Understanding Problem Gamblers
By Paul Bellringer. 'Gambling in recent years has become a major mainstream leisure activity. For most of us this enjoyable and exciting entertainment remains an occasional social activity, but for an increasing minority it becomes a destructive dependency.

The author describes strategies for breaking through the barrier of denial and explores relapse prevention and the vital role of helping agencies. This book is essential reading for anyone involved with a problem gambler.'

Published by Free Association Books, Oct. 1999. 220 pages, paperback. ISBN: 1 85343 463 9 £15.00. Available from Free Association Books, 57, Warren Street, London, W1P 5PA. *Tel:* 020 7388 3182. *Fax:* 020 7388 3187. *E-mail:* fab@fitzrovia.demon.co.uk 5107

Multiple Sclerosis

Some facts: MS is the most common neurological disorder among young adults and affects around 85,000 people in the UK. People are usually diagnosed between the ages of 20 and 40, but it can be later. It is more common in women than in men - the ratio is three to two. You cannot catch MS. [5082]

Some facts about multiple sclerosis: Anyone can get it, but no two people have exactly the same symptoms. It can strike at any age, but you are most likely to get it in your 20s or 30s. You can't catch MS from another person, and the effects can come and go without warning.

Unpredictable

MS is unpredictable and can play with your emotions. The symptoms can change dramatically from one day to the next - so you may wake to discover you can't see properly, or even walk to your front door to collect the post. You may have trouble remembering things. And then just as suddenly, you may feel incredible relief as your sight or balance returns to normal. For information contact the MS Society. [5044]

Emotions, mind and MS

Directly or indirectly MS can affect your mood, emotions and thought processes. Changes in the way you think and feel may be a response to living with MS or may be a direct result of neurological factors.

Depression

For some people, depression may be a reaction to the stresses that MS places on them. The consquences of living with MS can sometimes be painful, disturbing, fatiguing, intrusive or even embarassing, and it is quite normal for this to affect how you feel and react.

Some MS symptoms, such as fatigue or pain, may be difficult for other people to comprehend, making it hard to make sense of your experience or to know how to offer help. An apparent lack of sympathy or understanding from relatives or friends can cause additonal stress or anxiety. [5078]

Some facts about MS

There are many things we know about MS, some of which still baffle us. We know what forms MS can take and how it can develop, but we are not sure why. We have plenty of clues about the causes, but still cannot quite piece them together.

Neurological disorder

MS is the most common neurological disorder among young adults and affects around 85,000 people in the UK. People are usually diagnosed between the ages of 20 and 40, but it can be later. It is more common in women than in men - the ratio is three to two. You cannot catch MS. MS is a complex condition involving many factors. We know that it affects functions in the central nervous system - the brain and the spinal cord.

Myelin

MS is the result of damage to a substance called myelin. Myelin is a protective sheath surrounding all the nerve fibres in the brain and spinal cord. It works like insulating cable helping to conduct electrical impulses between the brain or spinal cord and the rest of the body, and preventing them from being short-circuited.

When myelin is healthy and functioning properly, electrical impulses get through quickly and efficiently allowing for easy and co-ordinated movement.

When myelin is damaged, messages are slower, distorted, or non-existent and do not get through properly. This causes many of the symptoms of MS. Damaged areas of myelin are known as 'plaques' or 'lesions'.

Symptoms

Symptoms depend on the location of plaques. Myelin damage can affect nerves to the eyes, parts of the brain, the brain stem and the spinal cord. Damage to motor nerves can affect movement. Damage to sensory nerves can result in numbness or tingling. There may be nothing wrong with the actual muscles or organs; it is simply that not all the right messages are getting through. [5082]

MS Awareness week

In 2000, MS Awareness Week was 3rd-7th April.

Local Organisations

Bexhill MS Group

Exists to support all those with multiple sclerosis and their carers. Helpers always welcome. *Contact:* Brenda Cameron, chairman, *tel*: 01424 217117; or Dorothy Jull, welfare officer, *tel*: 01424 845252. [July 2000]

Hastings & District MS Group

Registered Charity No. 207495. The Hastings MS group was started over 40 years ago - in 1958, and is run by a voluntary committee, with Gladys Stewart as its chairman. YAMS is the 'Young & Active with MS' section of the local MS Society. There are about 150 members of whom about 90 have MS. Support is offered to them and their families, their welfare being the main objective, with help available at any time. There are two ambulances so events are able to be arranged throughout the year. Fortnightly classes are held with a qualified physiotherapist for hydrotherapy and physiotherapy. In addition, there are fortnightly remedial Yoga classes.

Gladys Stewart, chairman and regional representative. *Address:* Hastings & District MS Society, 4, Highland Gardens, St Leonards-on-Sea, Sussex, TN38 0HT. *Tel*: 01424 433234.

Mrs B M Carr, honorary welfare secretary. *Address:* Hastings & District MS Society, 16, Capel Court, Albany Road, St Leonards-on-Sea, Sussex, TN38 0LL. *Tel*: 01424 428637.

Anita Brooks, assistant welfare officer. [5867]

National Organisations

Multiple Sclerosis Society

The Multiple Sclerosis Society is a national registered charity dedicated to fighting this unpredictable and frightening disease. There are 350 branches in the UK - a huge network of support. It publishes *MS Matters*, a bi-monthly magazine. There is a national helpline, information booklets, respite care, holiday homes, day centres, regional telephone counselling lines and much more.

Aims

It aims to ensure that everyone affected by MS has equal access to the support and practical help it offers. It is committed to about £8 million of research into the causes and treatment of MS. It answers thousands of calls each year from people with MS, their carers, families and friends through the National MS Helpline and regional telephone counselling lines.

Centres
It also runs eight centres where people with MS can go for respite care, holidays and to give their carers a break. The society publishes a magazine: *MS Matters*. There is an information line manned from 9am to 9pm by professionally trained staff who can answer questions about MS.

Address: Multiple Sclerosis Society of Great Britain and Northern Ireland, 25, Effie Road, London, SW6 1EE. *Contact:* Jackie Bruton. *Tel:* 020 7610 7171. Information line: 0808 800 8000. *E-mail*:info@mssociety.org.uk. *Website*:www.mssociety.org.uk 5044, 5085, 5414 May 2000

Brain & Spine Foundation
British Brain and Spine Foundation. *Tel*: 020 77935 900. *E-mail:* info@brainand-spine.org.uk *Website*: www.brainand-spine.org.uk Jul 2000

Further information

Health Information Service
The HIS is a free and confidential 24-hour service. You can speak to staff during office hours, and you can listen to any of hundreds of tapes at any time, e.g: Multiple Sclerosis (MS) (Tape 173); Multiple Sclerosis: case study (Tape 260).

Address: The College of Health, St Margaret's House, 21, Old Ford Road, London, E2 9PL. *Freephone*: 0800 66 55 44. 5367

Acknowledgements
Our grateful thanks to Gladys Stewart, of the Hastings & District MS Society, for editorial assistance with this chapter.

Obsessions

Obsessive compulsive disorder is a psychological condition characterised by obsessive and persistent thoughts, or repetitive, ritualistic behaviour which the individual feels unable to prevent. [5178]

OCD (obsessive compulsive disorder) is a psychological condition characterised by obsessive and persistent thoughts, or repetitive, ritualistic behaviour which the individual feels unable to prevent. Such obsessions and compulsions are often time consuming, tend to cause the sufferer anxiety and distress and often interfere with daily life. [5178]

Common obsessions

Dirt, germs and contamination; fear of acting on violent or aggressive impulses; unreasonable fear of harming others; abhorrent blasphemous and sexual thoughts; inordinate concern with order, arrangement or symmetry; inability to discard useless or worn out possessions.[5045]

Common compulsions

Excessive washing and cleaning; checking, repetitive actions such as touching, counting, arranging and ordering, hoarding; ritualistic behaviours that lessen the chances of provoking obsessions (e.g. putting all sharp objects out of sight); acts which reduce obsessional fears (e.g. wearing only certain colours).

A person can have a few or many of these symptoms. Most people have one or two rituals and this is entirely normal. Obsessional thoughts and compulsive behaviours only become symptoms of a disorder if they are experienced as 'unwanted' and interfere with social life and/or work. OCD greatly distresses sufferers, despite the fact that they may appear to others to be functioning normally. [5045]

Is OCD a form of madness?

NO. OCD sufferers perform rituals which seem crazy but the person is aware that this behaviour is excessive or irrational. The problem is that the person is unable to control the behaviour. [5177 Mar 98]

Is OCD common?

It is more common that was realised until recently. As many as 1 in 30 of the population may suffer the condition. Sufferers fear that other people will think them mad; they become secretive about their symptoms and reluctant to seek treatment. In addition, they often do not know that their disorder is a recognised condition with recognised treatments. [5177]

What causes OCD?

The cause of the illness is not known for certain although there are probably a number of factors. OCD can run in families and in some cases may be associated with an underlying biochemical disturbance in the brain. Psychological factors such as susceptibility to stress may also be important. [5177]

Can OCD be treated?

Yes. A number of treatments are readily available. There are several drugs which have proved very effective. In addition many sufferers have benefited from psychological treatments such as behaviour therapy. [5177]

Can young people get OCD?
Yes. Children and adolescents' problems are very similar to those of adults, and in fact many adults say that they had their first OCD symptoms as children. Most young children have a phase of ordinary rituals, such as wanting special toys at bedtime, or not treading on cracks in the pavement.

This is not a cause for worry, and is not OCD. If parents are concerned because the rituals upset the child, take up a lot of time and interfere with the child's everyday life (e.g. school, friends etc) it would be worth asking the GP for advice, and if necessary seeing a specialist child psychologist or psychiatrist.

The treatments for childhood OCD are also similar to the treatments used in adults. Therapists will work closely with the child's family to help everyone learn the techniques for fighting OCD.[5177]

Obsessions

Examples of obsessions are fear of shameful behaviour; death and disaster; contamination; perverted sexual thoughts; symmetrical arrangements; intrusive thoughts and images; unsatisfactory body image. [5013]

National Organisations

Obsessive Action

Covering all of the UK, Obsessive Action is a Charity set up by a group of Health Care professionals and sufferers, united by the common objectives of promoting an understanding of Obsessive Compulsive Disorder and educating sufferers, carers, the medical profession and the public about this condition.

Our members receive and are able to contribute to regular newsletters and information bulletins, as well as attend conferences (at a reduced entrance fee) and open days, organised by the Charity.

An OCD Information Pack comprising of factsheets about treatments, a book list, the four most available newsletters, and the list of OCD groups in the UK, is available to anyone wishing to find out more about the condition.

Address: Obsessive Action, Aberdeen Centre, 22-24, Highbury Grove, London, N5 2EA. *Tel:* 020 7226 4000. *Fax:* 020 7288 0828.
E-mail:
admin@obsessiveaction.demon.co.uk
Website: obsessive-action.demon.co.uk [5176]
May 2000

First Steps to Freedom

Registered charity which aims to help, in a practical way, people who suffer from phobias, obsessional compulsive disorder, anxiety, panic attacks, anorexia and bulimia, and those who wish to come off tranquilisers, and their carers. Please see main entry in 'Phobias' chapter, page 103.

No Panic

Work with people experiencing anxiety disorders. Chief Executive: Colin M. Iles. *Address*: No Panic, 93, Brands Farm Way, Telford, Shropshire. *Tel*: 01952 590005 (office); 01952 590545 (helpline). May 2000

See main entry for this organisation on page 98.

Further Information

Obsessive-Compulsive Disorder

'Understanding Obsessive-Compulsive Disorder'. A new booklet specifically on this issue. Published by Mind, 2000. ISBN: 1-874690-98-7. 12 pages. Price £1.00. Available from Mind. *Tel:* 020 8221 9666.
5024

Panic

Panic attacks

A panic attack is a very frightening experience because it seems to come 'out of the blue'. Most people describe a sudden overwhelming sense of anxiety, fast breathing, a racing heart and a feeling that they are about to collapse or faint.

Panic disorders

If you experience repeated panic attacks in different situations this is known as a panic disorder. People who experience panic attacks tend to be unusually aware of change in their bodies, and also tend to assume that these changes are dangerous when they may be quite harmless.

For example, there are lots of reasons for increased heart rate (such as running upstairs or drinking too much coffee) but a person with panic disorder will usually choose the most frightening explanation (such as an imminent heart attack). People with a history of panic attacks also tend to worry about losing control of their bodies and their feelings. [5181]

National Organisations

First Steps to Freedom

Registered charity which aims to help, in a practical way, people who suffer from phobias, obsessional compulsive disorder, anxiety, panic attacks, anorexia and bulimia, and those who wish to come off tranquilisers, and their carers. For more details, please see main entry in 'Phobias' chapter, page 103.

No Panic

No Panic is a voluntary charity which helps people who suffer from panic attacks, phobias, obsessive compulsive disorders and other related anxiety disorders including those people who are trying to give up tranquillisers.

No Panic is based upon self-help through local group meetings and also telephone groups, for those people who don't have a local group or where getting to a group is a problem in itself. The local groups offer regular face to face meetings and, in some cases, home visits, group outings and local helplines.

Services

No Panic provides the following services:

- starts, develops and maintains local self-help groups
- provides a confidential national helpline, 10am to 10pm, every day of the year
- keeps statistics; maintains liaison with statutory services and other interested organisations
- provides a night-time anxiety crisis telephone line (answerphone service only)
- helps to obtain funding, both locally and nationally
- provides telephone recovery groups for those people who are unable to go to a local group
- produces a bi-monthly newsletter and a regularly updated contact booklet for members
- provides advice and support for people trying to come off tranquillisers
- provides literature, books, audio and video cassettes to help overcome anxiety disorders
- provides information and support to families and carers of sufferers
- provides a 'Freephone' Information Pack Line on 0800 783 1531.

Membership

Membership, which costs only £7.00 per year, brings an initial membership information pack which includes a recommended reading list, information on local groups where applicable, a copy of our latest newsletter, access to local helplines where applicable and a contact booklet for those people who have opted to be included in it.

Chief executive: Colin M Iles.

Address: No Panic, 93, Brands Farm way, Telford, Shropshire, TF3 2JQ. *Helpline:* 01952 590545. *Office:* 01952 590005. *Fax:* 01952 270962. *Freephone:* 0800 783 1531 (information line only). *E-mail:* no-panic.co.uk *Website:* www.no-panic.co.uk
5010 Jul 2000

Further Information

Overcoming Panic

Book written by Derrick Silove and Vijaya Manicavasagar. "A step-by-step management programme with monitoring sheets to help you overcome panic and associated agoraphobia." Published by Robinson 1997. ISBN: 1-85487-701-1. 143 pages. Price £6.99. Available from Mind Mail Order Service. *Tel*: 020 8221 9666. 5088

Paranoia

Paranoia is a type of persecutory delusion where someone believes others or organisations are out to harm them. They may then act in accordance with this belief. For example, appearing over-vigilant, listening to police messages over the radio, avoiding situations or trying to protect themselves by wearing an amulet or something of religious significance.

Some people may believe they deserve to be persecuted, others feel very angry and resentful. Feeling threatened and on constant alert can be very frightening, tiring and totally thought consuming. It may be very hard to trust anyone and may interfere with sleep and other daily functions. [5016]

Delusions

A delusion is a strong belief held on insufficient grounds. It is often not in context with the person's cultural and family background. Some delusions appear as if from a vacuum, such as someone suddenly believing they are closely related to the Queen.

Other delusions may derive from some preceding experience or delusion. For example, someone who hears voices may believe they are a gifted psychic, or that the FBI have hidden tape recorders that are triggered to come on whenever they enter a certain room in order to hound them. Someone else who believes they are very rich and powerful may then believe they are controlling the stock markets. [5016]

Further Information

Psychosis

Factsheet written by Kaaren Cruse. Published by Mind. 11 pages. Price £1.36. Available from Mind. *Tel:* 020 8221 9666.

Understanding Paranoia

"Paranoia is a common part of many mental health problems, but is frequently misunderstood. This booklet shows what paranoia is, why people get it, and how best to help them."

Published by Mind, 1999, 20pp. £1 each. Available from Mind. *Tel:* 020 8221 9666.

Personality Disorder

The word 'personality' refers to the enduring pattern of thoughts, feelings and outward behaviour which is characteristic of an individual. We tend to behave in relatively predictable ways, yet our personalities also develop and change in response to changed circumstances. Many people are flexible enough to be able to learn from past experiences and change their behaviour in order to cope more effectively.

Distress

Personality disorders, on the other hand, are characterised by a long-lasting, inflexible and limited range of attitudes and behaviours which are expressed in a wide variety of settings and which deviate markedly from the expectations of the person's culture and cause distress to the person or to others. Personality disorders often begin or become noticeable during adolescence or early adulthood, although they sometimes begin during childhood.

Others

The narrow range of experiences, responses and coping strategies displayed by someone suffering from a personality disorder cause great distress in most circumstances, making it difficult for sufferers to develop friendships, maintain stable partnerships and work co-operatively with others. The suicide risk is reckoned to be three times greater in people suffering from a personality disorder than in the general population.

Depression

Personality disorders differ in the degree to which they disrupt the person's life (or the lives of others) and the extent to which they can be successfully treated. Often a person suffering from a personality disorder suffers additionally from an emotional problem such as depression or phobia. For example, someone suffering from a social phobia or agoraphobia may also be diagnosed as having an avoidant personality disorder. Even if many of the problems associated with the phobia have been resolved, stressful events may trigger an underlying pattern of avoidance and dependency.

For further information, please see Mind's booklet *Understanding Personality Disorder* from which the above is taken. See 'Further Information' page 102. [6080]

National Organisations

PD Network

The PD Network is based at the Henderson Hospital in Sutton. It is a therapeutic community based service, centrally funded for those living in England. It is for people with enduring and complex, emotional, interpersonal and behavioural problems diagnosable as severe personality disorder.

Services

Services available include: provision of intensive residential treatment based on the democratic therapeutic community model; a continuum of care through outreach services; research and integrating findings to improve evidence-based practice; sharing of specialist knowledge and skills through training and education.

Dialogue

Covering all areas of the UK, the Henderson Hospital publishes *Dialogue* which aims to foster communication about the diagnosis of personality disorder. The newsletter contains contributions from people who have been diagnosed with PD, as well as from professionals working in the field. It is hoped that *Dialogue* will reduce the stigma associated with the personality disorder label.

Focus group

The Henderson also plans to set up a focus

group for service users to discuss their experiences of a PD diagnosis and ways to improve existing services.

Contacts

Dr Kingley Norton, Clinical director; Alex Esterhuyzen, consultant psychiatrist. For more information, or to receive a free copy of Dialogue please contact Sue Ryan at the PD Network.

Address: The PD Network, Henderson Hospital, South West London & St George's Mental Health NHS Trust, 2, Homeland Drive, Sutton, Surrey, SM2 5LT. *Tel:* Direct line: 020 8652 2820. *Fax:* 020 8770 3676. *E-mail:* sryan@swlstg-tr.nhs.uk

Website:
www.psyctc.sghms.ac.uk/hendhosp 5258, 5259, 5260, 5452. May 2000

Further Information

Understanding Personality Disorder

Written by Janet Gorman. Published by Mind 1997. 12 page booklet. Available from Mind. *Tel:* 020 8519 2122. 6080

Acknowledgement
Our grateful thanks to Sue Ryan of the PD Network at the Henderson Hospital, Sutton, for editorial assistance with this chapter.

Phobias

Fear of spiders, fear of open spaces, fear of enclosed spaces, fear of bats ... the list of phobias seems endless. And for people suffering, it's no joke. Fortunately there is much that can be done about these debilitating conditions.

A specific phobia is a fear of a particular object or place which is so severe that it affects your way of life. It is possible to develop a phobia for almost anything, but some of the most common phobias are fear of heights, fear of spiders or mice, fear of enclosed spaces (known as claustrophobia) and fear of blood or injections.

Many of us feel some anxiety about these things, perhaps realistically since if we did not fear heights, for example, we might have more accidents! But there is a difference between this ordinary reaction and a phobia, which results in a person going to extreme lengths to avoid the object or situation they fear.

For example, if you have a phobia for injections rather than just a natural dislike of them, you might be unable to go on holiday or travel on business to places where travel injections are required. You might also refuse blood tests even if you knew they were important for your health. [5181]

Facts about phobia

Phobia: 'An estimated 13% of the adult population will develop a specific form of anxiety known as a phobia at some point in their life.' [1571]

Phobias

Here is a list of just some of the things people can have a phobia about:

Bees and wasps; birds; being alone (monophobia); blood; blushing; body defects; cats; daddy long legs; darkness; dentists; dogs; driving; eating; enclosed spaces (claustrophobia); feeling unreal; flying; frogs; heights; hospitals; illness; injections; insects; moths; mice; noise; open spaces (agoraphobia, see below); school; sex; snakes; social (being the centre of attention and/or behaving in an embarrassing or humiliating manner, see below); spiders (arachnophobia, see below); thunder and lightning; vomit; water; wind and weather. [5010, 5015]

Agoraphobia

This is a problem which can lead to people becoming too frightened to leave their home. Agoraphobia is often described as a fear of open spaces, but it is actually more helpful to think of it as a fear of being in places from which it is difficult to escape.

This can include crowds and public places such as shops, cinemas, and public transport. Not surprisingly, if you have severe agoraphobia you can find yourself leading a very restricted life, which is why it is important to get help as soon as possible.

Another aspect of agoraphobia is the fear of 'behaving badly' in public. For example, people worry that because of their anxiety they might faint, panic, rush out or do something embarrassing. For this reason agoraphobia is sometimes described as 'fear of fear'. See also 'Open Door Assn' and 'Pax', both on page 105. [5181]

Arachnophobia

This is a morbid fear of spiders. For help, contact either the Friendly Spider Programme or the Farago Clinic.

Farago clinic

Tel: 0500 002 650. *Fax:* 01753 869447. [Jul 2000]

Friendly Spider Programme

A day course, run at London Zoo, designed to rid chronic arachnophobics of their fear. The programme claims an 82% success rate. Cost is £110 or £55 for concessions. *Tel*: 020 7722 3333. *Contact:* Paul Pearce-Kelly. [Jul 2000]

Social phobia

If you have social phobia this means that you are extremely anxious about what other people will think of you, or how you will be judged by other people. As a result you may have great difficulty in social situations, such as eating or drinking in the presence of other people.

One form of social phobia is severe anxiety about speaking or performing in public. It is quite common to feel rather nervous in these situations, especially when they are unfamiliar, but people with social phobia will find these activities impossible because of the degree of anxiety they experience. At the heart of social phobia is a person's belief that other people will notice their anxiety and that this will make them look foolish or stupid. [5181]

Local Organisations

Dept of Clinical Psychology

Treatment for phobias is available on the NHS. The service offered is based at the Dept. of Clinical Psychology.

Address: Dept. of Clinical Psychology, NHS Trust, Braybrooke House, 9, Holmesdale Gardens, Hastings, East Sussex, TN34 1LY. *Tel*: 01424 435066.

National Organisations

First Steps to Freedom

FSF offers practical help to people suffering from phobias, obsessional compulsive disorders, anxiety, panic attacks, anorexia and bulimia, and those who wish to come off tranquillisers, together with help for their carers.

Patrons

Patrons include: Norman Painting, Robert Robinson, Ken Dodd, Jo Brand, Dr Naomi Fineberg, Dr Mehandra Singh Dayall.

Helpline

First Steps to Freedom offers a confidential helpline available from 10am to 10pm 365 days a year for sufferers and carers, to talk over their anxiety problems with trained volunteers who understand how they are feeling and care about them. They do not use the 1471 number and each call is treated confidentially; practical advice on how to overcome anxiety disorders, or how to overcome withdrawal from tranquillisers.

Telephone self-help groups

FSF has set up telephone self-help groups which are run on a regular basis whereby people get together over the telephone, talk through their anxieties, set themselves goals and steps towards those goals.

Counselling & befriending

FSF provides one-to-one telephone counselling/befriending whereby a sufferer or carer contacts a volunteer on a regular basis, talks over anxieties, sets themselves goals and steps towards those goals.

Books, videos & tapes

Leaflets, self-help booklets, videos, audio tapes and books; relaxation audio tapes - one with relaxation exercises (deep relaxation, quick relaxation, eye exercises, differential relaxation and visualisation), the other with music, the sea, water and bird song.

Advice & training
FSF offers advice and training for those who wish to start their own group or would like to set up their own helpline or become part of the First Steps to Freedom helpline;

Membership

Membership costs £10.00 per year, £25.00 for three years, or there is a concessionary fee of £5.00 for senior citizens, students and those receiving benefit (please provide proof). The hope is that people will join and begin to make the journey which could enable them, a member of their family, or a friend, to lead a more fulfilling life.

Contact: Sheila Harris. *Address*: First Steps to Freedom, 7, Avon Court, School Lane, Kenilworth, Warwickshire, CV8 2GX. *Tel*: 01-926 864473 (office). *Helpline*: 01926 851608 (10am to 10pm every day).
E-mail:
firststepstofreedom@compuserve.com *and* ljh@firststeps.demon.co.uk
Website: firststeps.demon.co.uk 5015 Jul 2000

No Panic
A voluntary charity which helps people who suffer from panic attacks, phobias, obsessive compulsive disorders and other anxiety disorders, including those people who are trying to give up tranquillisers. Please see main entry in 'Panic' chapter, page 98.

Open Door Association
For agoraphobia. They run groups, produce newsletters, books and cassettes. *Address:* 447, Pensby Road, Heswall, Wirral, Merseyside, L61 9PQ. SAE only.

Pax
(Incorporating Agoraphobia Information Service). Information and advisory service for people who experience panic attacks, phobias and anxiety. Books, cassettes and bi-monthly newsletter available. Send SAE for free information pack. *Contact:* Alice Neville, co-ordinator.

Address: 4, Manorbrook, London, SE3 9AW. *Tel*: 020 8318 5026. *Fax:* 020 8852 7048. *Website:* www.panicattacks.co.uk 5032 Jul 2000

National Phobics Society
Living with any form of anxiety is hard work. Fear, avoidance and sheer panic can be a daily experience, making life a constant battle. Many sufferers struggle to cope alone. Yet more than one in ten people in Britain suffer a disabling anxiety disorder at some time in their life.

The national phobics society was set up over 30 years ago by sufferers, to help and support others struggling with anixiety disorders.

The national phobics society has more than 5,000 members, who form an extensive self-help network. Across the country, people with anxiety disorders are learning from each other how to cope and how to live with anxiety.

The society also publishes fact sheets on many different anxiety disorders, some common, some less common. It produces a quarterly newsletter keeping members up to date with developments in therapies and self-help strategies. And it offers advice and support by telephone. So if you're suffering with anxiety, don't panic.

Chief executive: G. Kingsley-Nunes; Chair: K. Lancelot-Taylor; Hon. secretary: N. Lidbetter; Hon. treasurer: P. Taylor. Registered Charity No. 262715.

Address: National Phobics Society, Zion Centre, Royce Road, Hulme, Manchester, M15 5FQ. *Tel:* 0161 227 9898. *Fax:* 0161 227 9862.

E-mail: natphob.soc@good.co.uk

Website: www.phobics-society.org.uk May 2000

Triumph Over Phobia

Triumph Over Phobia was started in 1987 under the auspices of Professor I M Marks, MD, FRCPsych of the Institute of Psychiatry, London, by Celia Bonham Christie MBE, MA, who had overcome her fear of flying by following self-exposure instructions from *Living with Fear*.

The groups are run by lay people and the leaders are generally ex-phobics or ex-OCD sufferers. A structured self-treatment self-exposure programme is followed by group members, using *Living with Fear* as a self-help manual, meeting weekly in a supportive group.

Leaflets available - please send SAE to PO Box 1831, Bath, BA2 4YW. *Tel:* 01225 330353 (admin. line). [5721]

Further Information

Anxiety and Obsession

Written by Dr Brenda Lintner. Booklet published by Sane, 1993.

Health Information Service

The HIS is a free and confidential 24-hour service. You can speak to staff during office hours, and you can listen to any of hundreds of tapes at any time, e.g: *Agoraphobia* (Tape 202); *Fears & phobias* (Tape 246); *Fear of flying* (Tape 247). *Address:* The College of Health, St Margaret's House, 21, Old Ford Road, London, E2 9PL. *Freephone:* 0800 66 55 44. [5367]

Understanding Phobias

A new booklet that looks into the causes and manifestations of phobias. Published by Mind, 2000. ISBN: 1-874690-99-5. 12 pages. Price £1.00. Available from Mind. *Tel:* 020 8221 9666. [5024]

PSP

PSP is short for Progressive Supra-nuclear Palsy. It is described as a 'condition without cure'. It is a neurodegenerative disease affecting the brain stem. It is also known as Steele Richardson Olszewski syndrome, after the three neurologists who identified it as a separate disease in the early sixties. [5117, 5995]

Rare disease

Its progression varies from patient to patient slowly affecting vision, balance, swallowing and speech. This is a formidable, unkind and rare disease which, whilst it has been described as an ugly cousin of Parkinson and Alzheimer, is related only by damaged brain cells, the location of which are different in PSP from these. [5117, 5995]

Brain cells

PSP is often described as being related to Parkinson's because it is caused by damaged brain cells, but the damage is in very different areas. The cause of the degeneration is unknown and there is no cure.

Numbers affected

There are an estimated 20,000 victims in the United States and a similar number in Europe. [5117, 5995]

The comedian Dudley Moore was reported as suffering from this disease, November 1999. PSP affects up to 10,000 people in the UK and has no known cure or treatment, has rarely been researched and has been heard of by so few, despite affecting so many. [5117, 5995]

Local Organisations

PSP Association

Contact: Ian Munro. *Address*: PSP Association, 9 White Hill Drive, Bexhill, TN39 3RN. *Tel*: 01424 842527. [5867]

National Organisations

PSP Association

The PSP Association was established to promote research, to bring together families affected by the disease and to help with rehabilitation. Offering advice, information, support on caring and research into this illness. Contact: Brigadier Michael Coe, Chief Executive.

Address: PSP Europe Association, The Old Rectory, Wappenham, Near Towcester, Northamptonshire, NN12 8SQ. *Fax:* 01327 861007. *E-mail:* psp.eur@virgin.net
Website: www.pspeur.org *Helpline*: 01327 860299 /860342. [Jul 2000]

Race

African Caribbean people
African Caribbean people are twice as likely as white people to be diagnosed with a mental health problem and are 3 to 5 times more likely to be diagnosed and admitted to hospital for schizophrenia. However, most of the research has been based on service use statistics; recent research suggests that the actual prevalence rate of schizophrenia is much lower than originally thought. [1571]

Asian people
Indian men have a high rate of alcohol related problems. Suicide is low among Asian men and older people, but high in young Asian women compared with other ethinic groups. Research has suggested that Western approaches to mental health treatment are often found to be unsuitable and culturally inappropriate to the needs of Asian communities, who tend to view the individual in a holistic way, as a physical, emotional, mental and spiritual being. [1571]

Chinese people
The Chinese community is the third largest minority ethnic group in the UK. A recent study found that the rate of mental illness was particularly low among Chinese people compared with any other ethnic group. This can also be due to the reluctance or inability to recognise mental health problems.

Chinese people are good at somatisation. It has been suggested that the close-knit family structure of the Chinese community provides strong support for its members. While this may be beneficial, it may generate feelings of guilt or shame, resulting in people feeling stigmatised and unable to seek help. [1571, 5360]

Irish people
Hospital admission rates are high for Irish people compared with other ethnic groups, particularly for depression and alcohol problems. [1571]

Local Organisations

Black & Ethnic Support

Provides advice, information and advocacy support for individuals; supports the development of community groups and self-help networks; develops links between individuals and groups; supports the black and ethnic minorities forum, providing a channel of communication between different communities and local service providers.

Available Tuesdays to Fridays 10.30am to 4.30pm. *Contact*: Nadimeh Zeytoun or Lara Desai, community support workers.

Address: Black & Ethnic Minorities Project, 31a, Priory Street, Hastings, East Sussex, TN34 1EA. *Tel*: 01424 204683. *Fax:* 01424 432877.
E-mail: infoworker@hva [May 2000]

Multicultural Forum

This forum meets regularly for all members of the black and ethnic communities in Hastings & Rother. Its purpose is to gather the views of and offer support to these communities. All individuals are welcome.

For further details contact HVA's Black & Ethnic Minority Support Workers, Lara or Nadimeh on 01424 204683 (answerphone available); or 01424 444010. [5325]

National Organisations

ACCI

The African Caribbean Community Initiative (ACCI) provides day care/outreach services to people who have had or have mental health problems. The project offers a culturally sensitive specialist service to its users, particularly for black and ethnic minorities, many of whom experience severe mental health problems, isolation, rejection and marginalisation from society.

Address: Unit 4/5, BDC Building, 21, Temple Street, Wolverhampton, WV2

4AN. *Note:* It has not been possible to contact this group to establish if they still exist. Aug 2000

ACMHA

African Caribbean Mental Health Association. *Address:* African Caribbean Mental Health Association (ACMHA), Suite 37, 49, Effra Road, London, SW2 1BZ. *Tel/Fax:* 020 7737 3603. Jul 2000

Diverse Minds

Diverse Minds is a new programme, set up by Mind with support from the Department of Health, to make mental health services more responsive to the needs of people from black and minority ethnic communities.

In 1993 Mind published a policy statement on black and minority ethnic mental health, which highlighted major concerns in relation to current mental health services, including:

* the impact of racism on people's lives, on their mental health and on the services they receive;

* the inadequate response to the varying needs of people from different cultural, religious and ethnic communities;

* the high numbers of black people picked up by the police under section 136 of the Mental Health Act, compulsorily detained in hospital, diagnosed with schizophrenia and given high doses of medication.

For further information contact Valerie Graham, Outreach Officer *or* Carole Reid-Galloway, Information Officer.

Address: Diverse Minds, 15-19 Broadway, London E15 4BQ. *Tel:* 020 8519 2122. 5277

Horn of Africa

The Horn of Africa Community Group (HACG) offers support and advice to refugees, immigrants, migrants, etc and help with social services, GPs and hospitals. It provides information on issues of concern, does advocacy work, holds workshops and organises events to promote culture and history. It also works with statutory agencies for the benefit of the community.

Address: Horn of Africa Community Group, Lilly Close, St Paul's Court, Gliddon Road, London, W14 9BL. *Tel:* 020 8741 1119.

Jewish Association

The Jewish Association for the Mentally Ill (JAMI) offers guidance, counselling and support to sufferers and their carers. It produces a voluntary newsletter and runs a help and referral line. A day centre is open Sunday to Thursday and Monday evenings throughout the year. Please telephone for details.

Address: JAMI, 16A, North End Road, London, NW11 7PH. *Tel:* 020 8458 2223. *Fax:* 020 8458 1117. *E-mail:* ruth.jami@btclick.com Jul 2000

Language Line

Language Line provides an interpreter on the telephone 24 hours a day. *Tel:* 0800 78 33 503. 5360

NACMHN

We all face difficult times, but it can help to talk to people we trust and can confide in. It can be tempting to keep things in the family, but that's not always best. Everyone needs respect. Experience of racism and other forms of discrimination affects mental health and may create feelings of depression, loneliness and anger. You don't have to cope alone. You can ask for advice and help, including information on complementary therapies.

The National African and Caribbean Mental Health Network (NACMHN) is an umbrella body representing the needs and concerns of the African-Caribbean community with regard to mental health, the provision of appropriate services and the promotion of good practice.

Address: The National African & Caribbean Mental Health Network, Alicia Gordon, c/o African Caribbean Community Initiative, Units 4 & 5, BDC Building, Temple Street, Wolverhampton, WV2 4AN. *Tel*: 01902 715861.

Note: It has not been possible to contact this group to establish if they still exist. [Aug 2000]

Nafsiyat

Nafsiyat Intercultural Therapy Centre. Provides therapy for people from ethnic minorities. Office hours are 9.30 to 5.30, Mondays to Fridays.[Jul 2000]

Address: Nafsiyat, 278, Seven Sisters Road, Finsbury Park, London, N4 2HY. *Tel*: 020 7263 4130. *Fax*: 020 7561 1870. *E-mail:* nafsiyat-therapy@supanet.com *Website:* www.nafsiyat-therapy.supanet.com

Vietnamese Mental Health

The Vietnamese Mental Health Services (VMHS) provide relief for Vietnamese people with mental health difficulties and their families by giving advice, counselling and consultation on mental health issues. It works in partnership with health and social professionals to improve the services delivered to those people in distress. *Contact*: Dr Nx Cam.

Address: VMHS, 49, Effra Road, Units 21 and 23, Brixton, London, SW2 1BZ. *Tel:* 020 7733 7646. *Fax:* 020 7274 1378. *E-mail*: vietnamesemhs@cix.co.uk [Jul 2000]

Further Information

Between Two Cultures

Between Two Cultures: effective counselling for Asian people with mental health and addiction problems. By Zaibby Shaikh with John Reading. Here are fresh, practical ideas from the grass roots on how the specific needs of Asian and other minority ethnic people can be helped through counselling. This book was born out of the work of EACH, an innovation in the provision of counselling for Asian people with an alcohol or mental health problem, which has helped over 2000 people in London. Published by CVS, 2000. ISBN: 0-9019-591-04-2. 80 pages. £6.99. Available from Mind Mail Order Service. *Tel*: 020 8221 9666. [5221]

Ethnicity

Ethnicity: an agenda for mental health. Written by Dinesh Bhugra and Veena Bahl. "This book goes about identifying and meeting the mental health needs of black and other minority ethnic groups. Clinicians, researchers, academics, hospital managers, commissioners and voluntary organisation workers come together to discuss problems in health care delivery. The key emphasis is on involving commissioners and voluntary organisations in meeting the needs of communities."

Published by Gaskell, 1999. ISBN 1-901242-15-13. 262 pages. £25.00 Available from Mind Mail Order Service. *Tel*: 020 8221 9666. [5088]

Getting the Evidence

Getting the evidence - guidelines for ethical mental health research involving issues of 'race', ethnicity and culture. Written by Dr Nimisha Patel. "It will be important for the professional bodies to recognise these guidelines and incorportate them into the training of researchers (Veena Bahl, Adviser, Ethnic Minority Health, Department of Health)." Published by Mind in association with TCPS, 1999. ISBN 187469-79-0. £5.99. Available from Mind Mail Order Service. Tel: 020 8221 9666. 5088

African Caribbean

The Mental Health of the African-Caribbean Community in Britain. Factsheet. By Carole Reid-Galloway. Published by MIND Information Unit, August 1998. £1.36. Available from Mind. Tel: 020 8522 1725. [5270]

Chinese & Vietnamese
'The Mental Health of the Chinese & Vietnamese Communities in Britain.' Factsheet. By Carole Reid-Galloway. Published by MIND Information Unit, August 1998. £1.36. Available from Mind. *Tel*: 020 8522 1725. [5270]

Irish-born
The Mental Health of the Irish-Born People in Britain. Factsheet. By Carole Reid-Galloway. Published by MIND Information Unit, August 1998. £1.36 Available from Mind. Tel: 020 8522 1725. [5270]

South Asian
'The Mental Health of the South Asian Community in Britain'. Factsheet. By Carole Reid-Galloway. Published by MIND Information Unit, August 1998. £1.36 Available from Mind. *Tel*: 020 8522 1725. [5270]

Raised Voices
Written by Melba Wilson and Joy Francis. "A report commissioned by Diverse Minds, the Mind Race and Culture Unit, which examines African-Caribbean and African users' views and experiences of mental health services in England and Wales."

Published by Mind, 1997. ISBN 1-874690-14-6. 34 pages. £5.50. Available from Mind Mail Order Service. *Tel*: 020 8221 9666. [5088]

Resource List
A Resource List of Mental Health Literature in Translation (factsheet). By Carole Reid-Galloway. Published by MIND Information Unit, August 1998. 50p. Available from Mind. *Tel:* 020 8522 1725. [5270 May 2000]

Acknowledgements
Our grateful thanks to Ellen Harley, senior CMHN at Westwood House, for editorial assistance with this chapter.

Schizophrenia

It is estimated that one per cent of the population suffer from this form of mental illness at some time in their life. In this chapter, the illness is described, details of national and local self-help groups are given together with a list of recommended books, helplines and a research project.

Here are three descriptions of schizphrenia taken from different sources:

Schizophrenia
Any of a group of psychotic disorders characterised by a progressive deterioration of the personality, withdrawal from reality, hallucinations, delusions, social apathy and emotional instability.

Schizophrenia
The popular understanding of the term, as describing a Jekyll and Hyde split personality, is not true. Doctors use the term 'schizophrenia' to describe the state of mind in which a person's sense of their own identity, thoughts and perceptions goes beyond the range of normal experience.

People who hear voices, for example, or believe that they are being persecuted by other people, may be disgnosed as suffering from schizophrenia.

Schizophrenia
The term 'schizophrenia' is used to describe a dramatic disturbance in a person's thoughts and feelings. accompanied by behaviour which seems bizarre to others, such as hearing voices, seeing things that aren't there, or believing you are being persecuted by other people. [0534]

Facts about schizophrenia

How many people get schizophrenia? 'An estimated 1% of the population will have schizophrenia at some point in their life'. Another estimate is 'Between 3-4 per 1,000 of the population have schizophrenia at any one time'. Recovery: 'After a first episode, it is expected that approximately a quarter of people with schizophrenia will make a good recovery with some form of treatment within five years'. [1571]

Local Organisations

NSF Hastings & Rother

The NSF Hastings and Rother Group holds its meetings at The Friends Meeting House, 5, South Terrace, Hastings. The Friends Meeting House is in the town centre opposite Priory Meadow Shopping Centre. The group offers support to people with schizophrenia and their carers. *Contact:* Lynne Bingham, secretary.
Address: Lynne Bingham, 2, The Lawn, St. Leonards, Sussex, TN38 OHH. *Tel:* 01424 426833. [5119, 5120, 5867]

NSF Carers' Support

The National Schizophrenia Fellowship provides one to one support for people caring for a relative or friend with schizophrenia. The contact is Suzy Levy, a full-time paid worker, who works from the NSF Hove office. There is "access to respite monies for breaks at Foresters in the New Forest (an NSF managed hotel with staff specifically trained for working with people with mental health difficulties and their carers)".

Address: Suzy Levy, NSF Hove, St Richards Community Centre, Hove, Sussex, BN3 7FP. *Tel:* 01273 709060. [6061 Aug 2000]

National Organisations

NSF

The NSF is the National Schizophrenia Fellowship. It is a national voluntary organisation that helps people with a severe mental illness, their families and carers. NSF campaigns for better services for the mentally ill and runs over 280 projects across the UK along with local carers' and 40 local user support groups. It also provides direct support, advice and services to carers. Training for doctors and other health professionals, social workers, promotion officers, etc is also provided. *Contact*: Cliff Prior, Chief Executive.

Address: 30, Tabernacle Street, London, EC2A 4DD. *Tel*: 020 7330 9100. *Fax*: 020 7330 9102. *E-mail:* info@london.nsf.org.uk

Website: www.nsf.org.uk [Jul 2000]

NSF Mental Healthline

An out of hours free Helpline, run by the NSF, providing information and support to people concerned about their own or others' mental health. Calls are received from users, carers and professionals. People are able to talk in complete confidence. They do not even have to give their name if they prefer not to. Contact name for enquiries: Graham Skinner.

Free Helpline: *Tel:* 0808 808 3333 (6pm until midnight 7 nights a week).

Asian Language Helpline: *Tel:* 0808 800 2073 (Gujrati; Hindi; Punjabi; Urdu;) Hours: Mon & Wed 6 to 9pm; Thu 12 noon to 3pm [12 Jul 2000]

NSF National Helpline

This is run through the NSF national advice centre and offers free, independent advice on a range of mental health issues.

Address: National Schizophrenia Fellowship, 28, Castle Street, Kingston-upon-Thames, KT1 1SS. *Tel. Enquiries:* 020 8547 3937. *Fax*: 020 8547 3862. *E-mail:* info@nsf.org.uk *Website:* www.nsf.org.uk *Helpline:* 020 8974 6814, (10am to 3pm Mondays to Fridays). [Jul 2000]

SANE

SANE: Schizophrenia - A National Emergency. SANE was set up in 1986 as an initiative to tackle schizophrenia, the most widespread and serious mental illness which affects an estimated one in 100 people. Since it was founded SANE has widened its area of interest to include depression and other serious mental illness. The charity has three aims:

Awareness - to campaign for greater awareness and understanding of serious mental illness;

Care - to develop and pioneer care projects, such as SANELINE, and to fund social research into the implementation of the policy of care in the community;

Research - to fund and initiate medical research into the causes, treatment and eventual cure of serious mental illness, through projects such as The Prince of Wales International Centre for Research into Schizophrenia and Depression. [5018]

Address: SANE, 1st Floor, Cityside House, 40, Adler Street, London, E1 1EE. *Tel:* 020 7375 1002. *Fax:* 020 7375 2162. *Saneline (local call rate):* 0845 767 8000, from noon to 2am. [Jul 2000]

Saneline

Saneline is a national telephone helpline offering accurate and up-to-date information to give callers options for action and encourage them to benefit from whatever network of care exists in their own area. It also offers emotional and crisis support to people with mental health problems, their families, friends and information to professionals and organisations working in the mental health field. Trained volunteers answer the telephone, supported by paid co-ordinators. For further infomation contact Michelle O'Brien.

Address: Saneline, 199-205, Old Marylebone Road, London, NW1 5QP. *Tel*: 020 7724 6570. Saneline *Tel*: 0345 67 8000; lo-call number, open 2pm to midnight, every day of the year.

Research

The Maudsley Family Psychosis Study was initiated in 1993 to detect markers of schizophrenia in order to identify predisposing genes and their interaction with environmental factors.

This study is now being extended to manic depression. Participants will have psychological and psychiatric assessments and an MRI brain scan. Professor Robin Murray and colleagues are looking for subjects with manic depression who have a family history of the illness to take part. For further details please contact Muriel Walshe.

Address: Section of General Psychiatry, Division of Psychological Medicine, Institute of Psychiatry, Denmark Hill, London, SE5 8AF. *Tel:* 020 7848 0057. *E-mail:* m.walshe@iop.kcl.ac.uk

Further Information

A Balance of Rights

Edited by Professor Hugh Freeman. A balance of rights - A Report on seminar held on 23rd July 1996. A 44-page, A4 booklet published by Sane, 1996. Reports on speeches made by Marjorie Wallace, Sir Louis Blom-Cooper QC, Professor Hugh Freeman, and others.

Dialectics of Schizophrenia

Written by Philip Thomas. "The author explores the many factors that need to be accounted for if there is to be a significant advancement on our current understanding of what schizophrenia is. He argues that experiences of people with a diagnosis of schizophrenia are not 'understandable' to psychiatrists, as they over-rely on a flawed interpretation of nineteenth century theories."

Publishers by Free Association Books, 1997. ISBN: 1-85343-361-6, 269 pages. Price £9.00. Available from Mind Mail Order Service. *Tel*: 020 8221 9666.

Forgotten Illness, The

Written by Marjorie Wallace and others. A reprint of a series of articles written for The Times by campaigning journalist Marjorie Wallace. A 20-page A3 booklet. Published by Sane, 1994.

Forgotten Illness 2, The

Written by Marjorie Wallace and others. Further series of articles, reprinted from The Times and other newspapers on schizophrenia. A 20-page A3 booklet published by Sane.

Health Information Service

The HIS is a free and confidential 24-hour service. You can speak to staff during office hours, and you can listen to any of hundreds of tapes at any time, e.g: *Schizophrenia* (Tape 091).

Address: The College of Health, St Margaret's House, 21, Old Ford Road, London, E2 9PL. *Freephone:* 0800 66 55 44. Apl 2000

Living with Schizophrenia

Living with schizophrenia - an holistic approach to understanding, preventing and recovering from negative symptoms. Written by John Watkins. "This book combines a review of relevant research findings and the opinions of highly respected researchers in the field with illuminating reports from sufferers. It explains what 'negative' symptoms are, what causes them and how they can be prevented and alleviated without recourse to drug treatments."

Publishers: Hill of Content, 1996. ISBN:0-85572-x. 132 pp. Price £9.00. Available from Mind Mail Order Service. *Tel*: 020 8221 9666. [5088]

Schizophrenia: The Positive Perspective

In search of dignity for schizophrenic people. Written by Peter Chadwick. "People with a diagnosis of schizophrenia are often in the news, usually because of behaviour which alarms the ordinary citizen. Peter Chadwick challenges this cliched view as a user himself, and reveals many areas of enhanced individual functioning and expression." Publishers: Routledge, 1997. ISBN: 0-415-14288-1. 236 pages. Was £15.99 NOW £10.50 + 10% p&p from Mind Mail Order Service, 15-19, Broadway, Stratford, London, E15 4BQ. Tel: 020 8221 9666. Fax: 020 8534 6399. [5106]

Understanding Clozapine Treatment

2nd edition. A 16-page A5 booklet which 'tries to answer some common questions about Clozapine (Clozaril), a medicine used to help people with schizophrenia.' Published by Sane, London, 1997.

Understanding Schizophrenia

A booklet for those wanting to know more about schizophrenia. 20 pages. Published by the Mental Health Foundation 1997. *Tel:* 020 7335 7474. [5007]

Seasonal Affective Disorder

SAD is the abbreviation for Seasonal Affective Disorder, or 'winter depression'. 'Many people find that they sleep and eat slightly more in winter and dislike the dark mornings. For some, however, the symptoms are enough to disrupt their lives and cause considerable stress. These people have SAD. The latest (1998) research indicates that in Britain about half a million people suffer from clinical SAD'. [6070 Jul 2000]

The causes of SAD are thought not to be psychosomatic, but to be connected with the amount of bright light entering the eyes, and its effect on melatonin and seratonin levels. The most effective treatment is thought to be 'light therapy' - exposure to bright light from light boxes for about half an hour per day. [6070 Jul 2000]

Organisations

Outside In

Outside In is a commercial firm producing a range of light boxes and other products for body clock related problems. Free information pack on SAD.

Contact: Steve Hayes. *Address*: Outside In (Cambridge) Ltd, Unit 21, Scotland Road Estate, Dry Drayton, Cambridge, CB3 8AT. *Tel*: 01954 211955. *Fax:* 01954 211956. *E-mail:* 100341.3413@compuserve.com
Website: www.outsidein.co.uk [5191, 6070 Jan, Jul 2000]

SAD Association

This is a voluntary organisation and registered charity which informs the public and health professions about SAD and supports and advises sufferers.

Address: SADA, PO Box 989, Steyning, BN44 3HG. *Tel*: 01903 814942. *Fax*: 01903 879939. *Website:* sada.org.uk [Jul 2000]

Self-harm & Suicide

Rather than being a failure of suicide, self-harm is a positive strategy for survival - a way of coping with and releasing emotional pain which would otherwise be overwhelming - *a service user's view.* [5260]

A personal view

The following view is that of a service-user working for the User & Survivor Network in Wales:

'For many, self-harm is a positive strategy for survival. It is unreasonable to expect people to stop self-harming without putting equally effective strategies in place.

The general view of self-harm is, on the one hand, that it is an issue of failed suicide and, on the other, a deliberate strategy to gain attention. As a result, there is little understanding of self-harm amongst those who are most likely to find themselves dealing with it, i.e. family members, health workers, social workers and teachers.

It has become clear to me that the assumptions made about self-harm are untrue. That rather than being a failure of suicide, self-harm is a positive strategy for survival - a way of coping with and releasing emotional pain which would otherwise be overwhelming. Nor is self-harm a ploy to gain attention but rather a way of acknowledging pain to oneself. In fact is isn't possible to discuss self-harm without talking about pain - not the pain caused by the self-harm but the pain which leads to it. While the causes are varied, it seems general that self-harmers experience extreme emotional distress and it is its expression which results in self-harm.' [5260]

Local Organisations

Samaritans

'Whatever you're going through, we'll go through it with you.' See also under 'Crises & Emergencies', page 206.

Hastings & Rother

Address: The Samaritans, 26, St Andrews Square, Hastings, Sussex. *Tel:* 01424 436666. [Jul 2000]

Eastbourne

Address: The Samaritans, 13, Bolton Road, Eastbourne, Sussex. *Tel*: 01323 735555. [Jul 2000]

Liaison Nurse Service

People who arrive at the Conquest Hospital A & E department who have deliberately harmed themselves by taking an overdose of drugs for example, or cutting themselves, will almost certainly be referred to the Liaison Nurse Service. This is a special facility which aims to provide immediate help, treatment and care to people who are in a mental health crisis.

The vast majority of patients seen by the liaison nurses are not referred to any other mental health professional, as often the patient is suffering a *temporary* mental health crisis, where crisis intervention only, e.g. a one-off counselling type session, is indicated. This involvement can be extended for up to four weeks. The Liaison Nurse

Service is provided 365 days a year and is covered by two nurses. *Contact*: Sarah Tindall.

Address: Liaison Nurse Service, Conquest Hospital, The Ridge, St Leonards-on-Sea, East Sussex, TN37 7RD. *Tel*: 01424 755255.

National Organisations

Befrienders International

Developing volunteer action to prevent suicide. For full details, see under 'Befriending' chapter, page 158.

Bristol Crisis Service

The Bristol Crisis Service for Women is a national helpline for women in distress, particularly those who use self-injury as a way of coping with their problems. The service is open Fridays to Saturdays 9pm to 12.30am. Tel: 0117 925 1119. Aug 2000

National Self-Harm Network

Address: National Self-Harm Network PO Box 16190, London, NW1 3WW.

User & Survivor Network

Address: User & Survivor Network, Office Suite 3, 1, North Parade, Aberystwyth SY23 2JH. *Tel*: 01970 626230. *Fax*: 01970 626233. *Users Freephone:* 0800 216008. *E-mail:* US@usnetworkcymru.demon.co.uk

US Network Policy on Self-Harm, Working Paper No. 5, September 1999. May 2000

Samaritans

The Samaritans

Tel: 0845 7 90 91 92. Jul 2000

Further Information

Cutting: The Risk

Self-harm, self-care and risk reduction. How do I not cut an artery? Talk about my scars? Not harm so badly? This book offers frank answers to questions like these. It is written by survivors and professionals attending the groundbreaking risk reduction conference organised by the National Self- Harm Network last year. Published by National Self-Harm Network, 2000. ISBN: 0-9534027-1-2. 80 pages. Price £10.00. Available from Mind. *Tel:* 020 8221 9666. 5024

Factsheet

Suicide Factsheet. By George Stewart. Published by MIND Information Unit, May 1999. £1.36. Available from Mind Mail Order Service. *Tel*: 020 8221 9666.

Hurt Yourself Less Workbook

"This workbook was written by the National Self-Harm Network, comes in an A4 ringbinder, and looks in detail at the subject. With a practical set of exercises that will help with self-management. It is non-threatening and easy to follow." ISBN: 0-9534027-0-3. 80 pages. Price: £25.00 + 10% p&p. Available from Mind Mail Order Service. *Tel*: 020 8221 9666. Also available from NSHN (National Self-Harm Network) above, 1998. 5088

Night Falls Fast

'Night falls fast - understanding suicide'. Written by Kay Redfield Jamison. "Suicide through literary, historical, anthropological, biochemical, genetic and epidemiological lenses. Suicide rates in the US have tripled in the last 40 years." Published by Knopf. ISBN: 0-375-40145-8. Available through amazon.co.uk. 5069

See also these chapters ...

Crises & Emergencies, page 206.

Sex

For general advice on sex see 'Brook'; for bereavement for lesbian and gay people see 'Bereavement Helpline'; for counselling see 'Pace Project' and the 'Counselling & Therapy' chapter, page 173.

Local Organisations

Blagh

Blagh (Bisexual, Lesbian & Gay Hastings) provides information and support to young people identifying as being lesbian, gay or bisexual. It also provides information and support to those unsure about or questioning their sexuality.The service is available to young people up to 25 years of age.

BLAGH provides a safe space for young people to socialise informally as well as providing information and support with the phone line. *Contact:* Steve.

Address: BLAGH, c/o Bexhill & Hastings Youth Service, 31, Cambridge Road, Hastings, East Sussex, TN34 3DJ. *Tel:* 729292. [5867]

Gay Helpline Hastings

This organisation offers a telephone helpline only. Its first adopted title was 'Hastings Befrienders'. That name was changed to 'Hastings Befrienders Gay Helpline' and more recently to 'Gay Helpline Hastings'. It was founded in the mid-1980s and was then supported by a social group of gay men.

Information & advice

Our remit and purpose is to help any caller in need of information or advice on any aspect of same sex relationships and to give information about any social groups and local venues where same sex relationships are fully accepted.

We have a PO Box address, but no public premises. We have pre-set duty hours currently on one evening per week and an answering machine with message. Out of duty hour calls are answered live whenever possible.

Gay Helpline Hastings is affiliated to National Friend which is itself a registered charity. *Hours:* Wednesdays 7pm to 9pm.

Address: Gay Helpline Hastings, PO Box 6, St Leonards-on-Sea, East Sussex, TN37 6SS. *Tel:* 01424 444777. [5987]

Health Promotion

East Sussex Brighton & Hove Health Authority's Health Promotion department includes a 'Sexual Health Team'.

Positive sexual health

The Sexual Health team comprises of Health Promotion Advisors, administration staff and the Street Outreach Service (SOS) and their key aim is to promote positive sexual health, identity and well-being. In addition, the team aims to reduce HIV infection, unwanted pregnancies, teenage pregnancies and sexually transmitted infections.

Partnership

The team works in partnership with individuals in statutory and non-statutory settings, who have a role in promoting HIV prevention and sexual health. These partners include genito-urinary and family planning clinics, primary health care, education, local authority and voluntary sector agencies.

Address: Health Promotion Department, ESBHHA, Friars Walk, Lewes, Sussex, BN7 2PB. *Tel:* 01273 485300.
E-mail: nhs@esbhhealth.cix.co.uk [5370]

Sexual Health Project

The Hastings & Bexhill Youth Service runs a Sexual Health Project and BLAGH (Bisexual, Lesbian and Gay in Hastings) Group for young people. They are also putting together a sexual health training package which will be available from April

2000.
If interested in any of these initiatives please contact Kerry Smith, Sexual Health Project Manager. *Tel*: 01424 439284 or 430493. *Fax*: 01424 430485.
E-mail: hastingsyouth@aol.com[5246]

Lesbian & Gay Advocacy

Contact: Rose Hall. *Address:* Mind, Lesbian & Gay Advocacy Project, 79, Buckingham Road, Brighton, Sussex, BN1 3RJ. *Tel:* 01273 749600. *Fax:* 01273 771253. [Jul 200]

National Organisations

Brook

Covering the whole of the UK, Brook provides free, confidential sex advice and contraception for young people under the age of 25. Helpline co-ordinator: Paula Currie.

Address: Brook, 421, Highgate Studios, 53-79, Highgate Road, London, NW5 1TL.
Tel/Fax: 020 7284 6093 (direct line). *Freephone*: 0800 0185023. *E-mail:* information@brookcentres.org.uk *Website:* www.brook.org.uk [May 2000]

Bereavement Helpline

Bereavement support for lesbians and gay men, or anyone who is bereaved or preparing to be pereaved by the death of a lesbian or gay person; also support for parents, siblings and other family members, friends, neighbours and colleagues.

The helpline is run by trained lesbian and gay volunteers. The group runs workshops and talks for all people working with death, dying or bereavement. A free 'will pack' is available if an SAE is sent.

Address: Bereavement Helpline, Vaughan M. Williams Centre, Colindale Hospital, Colindale Avenue, London, NW9 5HG. *Tel:* 020 8455 8894 (helpline 7pm to midnight every evening). [Jul 2000]

Family Planning Association

Address: Family Planning Association, 2-12, Pentonville Road, London, NW1 9FP. *Tel:* 020 7837 5432. *Website*: www.fpa.co.uk [Jul 2000]

Contraception Helpline

Contraception Education Service Helpline *Tel*: 020 7837 4044. Mondays to Fridays 9am to 7pm. [Jul 2000]

Pace Project

Project for Advice, Counselling and Education (PACE). Counselling for lesbians and gay men. *Tel*: 020 7700 1323. [Jan 2000]

Employment rights

Lesbian and Gay Employment Rights. Provides support and advice to those experiencing discrimination at work. Lesbians *tel:* (020) 7704 8066. Gay men *tel:* (020) 7704 6066. [Jul 2000]

Project LSD

Information on drugs for lesbians, gay men and bisexuals. *Tel:* 020 7288 1111.

Terence Higgins Trust

For information and advice on HIV/AIDS. *Tel*: 020 7242 1010. [Jul 2000]

Homosexuality Switchboard

For anyone who needs support or information about homosexuality. *Tel*: 020 7704 8066. [Jul 2000]

London Switchboard

A 24-hour service. *Tel*: 020 7837 7324. *Website:* www.llgs.org.uk [Jul 2000]

WellMan Clinic

Private London Clinic dealing with problems of impotence and the male menopause (the andropause). Testosterone replacement therapy is provided. Address: The WellMan Clinic, 32, Weymouth Street, London, W1N EFA. Tel: 020 7637 2018; fax: 020 7637 2019. [Jun 2000]

Further Information

Health Information Service

The HIS is a free and confidential 24-hour service. You can speak to staff during office hours and you can listen to any of hundreds of tapes at any time, e.g: *Masturbation* (Tape 180); *Men's sexual response* (Tape 181); *Homosexuality in men & women* (Tape183); *Impotence* (Tape 218); *Safer sex for drug users worried about AIDS* (Tape 237); *Safer sex for gay men & bisexuals worried about AIDS* (Tape 235); *Safer sex for heterosexuals worried about AIDS* (Tape 234).

Address: The College of Health, St Margaret's House, 21, Old Ford Road, London, E2 9PL. *Freephone*: 0800 66 55 44. 5367

Lesbians, gay men, bisexuals & mental health

By Jackie Golding. Published by Mind Information Unit, June 1996. Price £1.36. Available from Mind Mail Order Service. *Tel*: 020 8221 9666.

See also these chapters ...

Men, page 87.
Women, page 145.

Sleep

Insomnia

The following is reprinted with kind permission from Open Mind 104 *July 2000, (article by David Taylor, The Maudsley, London). Copyright Mind (National Assn for Mental Health). Subscription enquiries to Mind on 020 8221 9661.*

Insomnia is often regarded as more of a nuisance than an illness. However, persistent insomnia can be rather more distressing. While physical harm is thought unlikely to result, people's lives can be blighted by the torture of tiredness and irritability.

Each case of chronic insomnia needs to be carefully examined. Sometimes the cause is readily apparent: painful conditions such as arthritis are very likely to make sleep difficult, and some psychological conditions such as depression and hypomania also disturb sleep. In these cases, the underlying cause of insomnia needs to be treated.

Sleep hygiene

Where no underlying cause can be found, chronic insomnia can often be improved by ensuring good 'sleep hygiene'. This involves establishing a regular sleeping pattern by going to bed at the same time every night and getting up at the same time each morning. It is also important to remove all barriers to sleep - caffeine intake should be restricted, particularly in the evening, and intrusive noises should be avoided. Daytime napping is also discouraged. Exercise and over-stimulation should also be avoided in the hours before retiring.

Alcohol

It is also strongly recommended that nicotine and alcohol intakes are reduced. Both disturb sleep: nicotine by inhibiting the process of getting off to sleep, and alcohol by disturbing sleep during the night. If these sleep hygiene measures are unsuccessful, then relaxation techniques are often very helpful and easy to learn.

Hypnotics

As a last resort, sleeping tablets, also known as hypnotics, can be used. While hypnotics are useful for short-term insomnia - such as that caused by shift-work, jet-lag, or stress - their use in chronic insomnia is very limited. The main reasons for this is that when hypnotics are used regularly for 2 to 4 weeks, their effect tends to wear off. In addition, when taken for long periods (more than a month) and then stopped, so-called 'rebound insomnia' tends to occur.

Temazepam

In the past, benzodiazepines such as temazepam and nitrazepam have been widely used. Benzodiazepines can be addictive if used for long periods. Nowadays, newer drugs such as zopiclone, zolpidem and zaleplon are becoming more popular. These drugs are shorter acting than benzodiazepines, and so do not usually cause morning drowsiness. Their sleep-inducing effects seem to last for up to a month, and rebound insomnia does not seem to be much of a problem with short-term use.

Intermittent use

Nevertheless, the use of these new medications is quite rightly restricted to only a few weeks' regular use. Intermittent use (perhaps every other night or so) is probably better than regular use, but even then, hypnotics are not the answer to chronic insomnia. They should be used only for short periods, and only when all else fails. For the most part, non-drug approaches are best, since they are more likely to work in the long term. 5032. David Taylor, the Maudsley, London.

Sleep Disorder Clinic

Address: Sleep Disorder Clinic, 98, Harley Street, London W1. *Tel*: 020 7629 8304. *Fax:* 020 7409 7854.
E-mail: theprivateclinic.ldn@btinternet.com
*Website: www.*privateclinic.co.uk Jul 2000

Smoking

Deaths from smoking-related causes are estimated to exceed 100,000 a year in this country alone. Do you smoke? Do you want to give up? Maybe you can ... check out this chapter for help in stopping ... and good luck!

Facts about smoking

Addictive 'as hard drugs'.

A report from the Royal College of Physicians describes nicotine as a 'powerfully addictive drug on a par with heroin and cocaine' and calls for cigarettes to be regulated by the Medicine Controls Agency or a new nicotine regulatory authority. Professor Sir George Alberti, president of the Royal College of Physicians says 'At a time when smoking still causes one fifth of all deaths in Britain, measures designed to achieve further reductions in smoking are clearly important.' [5205]

How many people die?

At present, around a third of British people smoke and there are 120,000 smoking-related deaths a year, two-thirds of them from cancer and heart disease. Clive Bates, the director of Action on Smoking and Health, said that the figures showed that a 20-a-day smoker is losing one day of life for every week of smoking. "As if that's not bad enough, smokers are likely to die a more painful death and spend longer being ill while they are alive", he said. [5111]

Did you know?

Smoking 20 cigarettes a day over an average lifetime will cost you about £100,000 (allowing for inflation).[6079]

How many people smoke?

The highest recorded level of smoking among men was 82% in 1948 when surveys started. Latest figures are for 1998 which show that 28% of adult men and 26% of women smoke. However, in East Sussex, Brighton and Hove, 35% of people smoke compared to 27% nationally. [5280, 5090]

Children and smoking

Children who experiment with cigarettes quickly become addicted to the nicotine in tobacco. A Mori survey of children aged 11 to 16 years found that teenagers have similar levels of nicotine dependence as adults, with one third of those who smoke one or more cigarettes a week lighting up their first cigarette within 30 minutes of waking up. [5281]

National Targets

The Government has set the following National targets for smoking reduction. "To reduce the prevalence of smoking in children from 13% to 9% or less by the year 2010; with a fall to 11% by the year 2005.

Reduce the numbers of adult smokers in all social classes so that the overall rate falls from 28% to 24% or less by the year 2010; with a fall to 26% by the year 2005; reduce the percentage of women who smoke during pregnancy from 23% to 15% by the year 2010, with a fall to 18% by the year 2005." [5090]

NHS Trust & smoking

Smoking on Hastings & Rother Trust property will be 'stubbed out' form May 31st 2000. Staff at buildings such as the Conquest and Bexhill hospitals will not be allowed to light up - nor will visitors to the sites, contractors and sub-contractors. But 'further thought' is to be given to patient smoking especially long-stay ones. [5196]

No-Smoking Day

No-Smoking Day is the second Wednesday of March every year, i.e. next year's date will be 14th March, 2001.

Address: No Smoking Day, Unit 203, 16, Baldwins Gardens, London, EC1N 7RJ. Tel: 020 7916 8070. Fax: 020 7916 7556.
E-mail: no.smoking.day@virgin.net
Website: www.no-smoking-day.org Jul 2000

Tabs, patches, gum, etc.

Nicorette

Nicorette Microtabs.These are tablets that help cut the cravings for nocotine. If you are determined to cut out smoking ask your pharmacist for advice or call: *Tel:* 0800 2 GIVE UP (0800 2 448387).
Website: www.nicorette.co.uk [Jul 2000]

Did you know?

Women who smoke 20 cigarettes a day are four times more likely to develop breast cancer.[6079]

Nicotine replacement

Patches, gum, lozenges and inhalers are available. Patches come in 21mg, 14mg and 7mg strengths which allow smokers to wean themselves off nicotine. Gum comes in 4mg and 2mg strengths, and lozenges in 2 mg. Inhalers produce more nicotine the harder you puff. [5194]

Zyban

It was announced in June 2000 that a drug to help smokers quit and which is said to be twice as effective as nicotine patches will be made available on the NHS. The drug is called Zyban and it is claimed it has helped 1.5 million smokers quit in America. Zyban, which is made by Glaxo Welcome, works by changing the brain's sensitivity to nicotine. [Daily Telegraph, 12th June 2000.]

Zyban is a new, prescription only medicine (buproprion hydrochloride) which reduces cravings and withdrawal symptoms. In clinical trials, it helped 30% of smokers to quit for at least one year. It is available on the NHS and is prescribed for 2 months. You start treatment while still smoking and must stop smoking during the second week. The medicine is backed up by a telephone helpline.[6093, Aug 2000]

Local Organisations

Cavendish Clinic, Beckley

Set up early in 2000, by Clive Looker, this clinic runs 'Quit Smoking Workshops'. Cost is £20 for an evening's course, with a follow-up group therapy meeting.

Address: Cavendish Clinic, Main Street, Beckley, Sussex, TN31 6TL. *Tel:* 01797 260557. *E-mail:* clivelook er@cavendish-clinics.com *Website:* www.cavendishclinics.com [5264]

National Organisations

Action on Smoking and Health

ASH ASH is a compaigning and lobbying organisation designed as a health charity. It aims to inform and influence decision makers, the media and the public on topics and related issues on smoking. Publishes a bi-monthly journal, Burning Issue. Director: Clive Bates. Spokesperson: Amanda Sandford. A series of 24 factsheets is available free from the Ash website.

Address: 102, Clifton Street, London, EC2A 4HW. National *Tel:* 020 7739 5902. *Fax:* 020 7613 0531. *E-mail:* action.smoking.health@dial.pipex.com *Website:* www.ash.org.uk [May 2000]

Globalink

An internet discussion forum covering a wide range of smoking topics and news. globalink@globalink.org.[Jan 2000]

Alan Carr Clinics

Alan Carr, anti-smoking guru, used to smoke 100 a day, stopped and wrote a worldwide best selling book on how to stop smoking, available from Penguin. He now has 40 clinics in 18 countries.

Committed Quitters

A study from the University of Pittsburgh found that people trying to give up found it easier when using the Committed Quitters programme, combined with nicotine replacement. (Daily Telegraph, 15 June 2000). *Website:* committedquitters.com

Quitlines & magazines

Don't Give Up on Giving Up
This is a campaign designed to encourage people to stop smoking from 1st January 2000. It is a National Campaign and provides information, support, counselling and general advice for anyone who aims to stop smoking. *National Tel:* 0800 169 0 169. [Jan 2000]

Quit
(UK Smoking Cessation Charity) Counselling line: Tel: 0800 002200. [Jan 2000]

Smokers' helpline
Tel: 0800 169 0169. [Aug 2000]

Stop!
A monthly self-help magazine for those who want to stop smoking. *Address:* Stop, 70c, High Street, Whitstable, Kent, CT5 1BB. *Tel:* 01227 779229. *E-mail:* enquiries@stopmagazine.co.uk *Website:* www.stopmagazine.co.uk [Jul 2000]

Further Information

Health Information Service

The HIS is a free and confidential 24-hour service. You can speak to staff during office hours, and you can listen to any of hundreds of tapes at any time, e.g: *Smoking & heart disease* (Tape 134); *Smoking & how teenagers can stop* (Tape 382); *Smoking & how to give up* (Tape 133); *Smoking & pregnancy* (Tape 135); *Smoking before an operation* (Tape 322); *Dangers of smoking* (Tape 806 in Bengali-Sylheti dialect); *Dangers of smoking* (Tape 906 in Bengali & Sylheti dialect);

Address: The College of Health, St Margaret's House, 21, Old Ford Road, London, E2 9PL. *Freephone:* 0800 66 55 44. [53670]

Acknowledgements
Our grateful thanks to Clive Looker, of the Cavendish Clinic for editorial assistance with this chapter.

Social Exclusion

Organisations

Social Misfit Society

"An important new awareness project, dealing with the public's creation of outcasts." 'Each true personality is formed through the ingredients of opinion, decision, life's experiences and circumstances. Some characters are happy, some are sad, some are sane and some are mad. Others are concealed, whilst others are revealed.' - ('The Big Bruise Show' - 1997). Send SAE for details to 'SMS', PO Box 1, Portsmouth PO2 7YJ. [5201]

Further Information

A Sociology of Mental Illness

By David Pilgrim and Anne Rogers. "Revised issue of a book that gives the background to current drives for social inclusion, and provides a clear introductory overview of the major aspects of the sociology of mental health and illness. An essential read for mental health professionals and students."

Published by Open University Press 1999. ISBN: 0-335-20347-7. 240 pages. Price: £26.99. Available from Mind Mail Order Service. *Tel*: 020 8221 9666. [50880]

Creating Accepting Communities

Report of the Mind inquiry into social exclusion. The Mind Inquiry provides a compelling portrait of the social exclusion of users of mental health services - and also highlights work already being done to promote inclusion. With over 100 recommendations to Government, employers, goods & service providers, local authorities, health authorities, and statutory and voluntary mental health bodies on tackling exclusion.

Published by Mind, 1999. ISBN: 1-874690-87-1. 192 pages. £9.99. Available from Mind Mail Order Service. *Tel*: 020 8221 9666. [5251]

From Psychiatric Patient to Citizen

Overcoming discrimination and social exclusion. Written by Liz Sayce. "In Britain and the USA, people who experience mental distress are amongst the most excluded in society. Liz Sayce's admirable, clear and progressive vision about how to effect the move 'from psychiatric patient to citizen' should be read by all those who care about the quality of life of people who experience mental distress."

Published by Macmillan Press 2000. ISBN: 0-333-69890-8, 280 pages. Price: £13.99. Available from Mind Mail Order Service. *Tel*: 020 8221 9666. [5088]

Outsiders Coming In?

Achieving social inclusion for people with mental health problems. Written by Liz Sayce and David Morris. "Local work to improve social exclusion for people with mental health problems, from employment projects to supported education, can bring demonstrable health gain. This report outlines key evidence and makes a practical proposal for action which could be pursued by mental health primary care services with a number of partners."

Published by Mind 1999. ISBN: 1-8784690-90, 42 pages. Price: £4.00. Available from Mind Mail Order Service. *Tel*: 020 8221 9666. [5088]

Stammering

Stammering can be a devastating social barrier which many people endure for decades before seeking help or finding a remedy.

Stammering is characterised by involuntary disruptions in fluent speech, and may take the form of repetitions and prolongations of sounds, syllables or words.

Speech may sound forced, tense or jerky. People who stammer may avoid both words and situations which they know will cause them difficulty.

Communication problem

Stammering is not simply a speech difficulty, but a serious communication problem. It can undermine a person's confidence and self-esteem; affect their interaction with others; impede their education and seriously hamper employment prospects.

The causes of stammering are not known, but research suggests that a combination of factors is involved. Men are four times more likely to be affected than women.

Children

Five per cent of pre-school children stammer. This means that, at any one time, about 188,000 children under five are affected in the UK. Around a quarter of these children are at risk of developing a chronic stammer in adult life unless they receive speech and language therapy during the pre-school years. Approximately 109,000 school-age children and 450,000 adults in the UK stammer (i.e. one per cent of their respective age group).

For further information please contact The British Stammering Association. 5834

National Organisations

British Stammering Association

Address: The British Stammering Association, 15, Old Ford Road, London, E2, 9PJ. *Tel:* 020 8983 1003. *Helpline:* 0845 603 2001. *Fax:* 020 8983 3591. *E-mail:* mail@stammer.demon.co.uk *Website:* www.stammer.demon.co.uk 5834

McGuire Programme

The McGuire Programme holds four-day intensive courses throughout the UK. The main goal is to help stammerers become eloquent speakers rather than simply non-stammerers. To do this there are four objectives -

Physical objective

The objective is to speak powerfully from the thorax by training to use your costal diaphragm.

Mental objectives

The mental objectives are - (a) to understand the dynamics of stuttering; (b) to counteract the tendency to 'hold back' and use avoidance mechanisms; (c) to deal with the fear through concentration and non-avoidance techniques. To understand and reduce the fear thereby preventing severe relapses;(d) to accept yourself as a recovering stutterer until you have proven yourself a fluent speaker with occasional reminders of past affliction; (e) to develop an assertive attitude to attack your remaining feared situations.

Emotional objective
Once you have dealt with the fear, the objective is to let go and have fun speaking.

Spiritual objective
The objective is self-actualization. Once your verbal self is set free, who will be doing the talking? Are you the person you want to be? This positive internal change - beliefs, intentions, perceptions, etc. - is necessary to hold on to your fluency.

Follow-up
The success of the programme is also due to the follow-up support and guidance from coaches, as they can understand and relate to the feelings of isolation and loss of dignity that a stammerer feels; along with support group meetings, telephone list and e-mail discussion linked to the other world centres of the programme.

Costs
The programme is very much a programme for stammerers run by stammerers. Initial fee is £600 and is due on the second day of your first intensive course. If you decide after the first day that the programme is not for you there is no charge. Subsequent courses are £10.00 a day, maximum of £30.00 for the four day course (plus accommodation charge). An information pack on the McGuire Programme, Intensive Fluency Courses is available.

Personnel
David McGuire, Founder. Bernadette Bailey, Regional Director (UK North). Heidi Bristow, Regional Director (UK South); Maree Sweeney, Regional Director (Ireland); Scott Mackintosh, Regional Director (Australia); Rob Young, Regional Director (USA). 5933, 6009 Jul 2000

Address: The McGuire Programme, Freedoms Road, Box 54, 266, Banbury Road, Summertown, Oxford, OX2 7DL. *Tel:* 0800 9176579. *E-mail:* heidipg@bristow30.freeserve.co.uk

Stress

The word 'stress' has become part of our modern vocabulary. While the term is often used casually for those whose ability to cope with day-to-day matters is at crisis point, stress can have serious debilitating consequences... *Professor Cary Cooper, President ISMA (UK).*[5885]

'The word 'stress' has become part of our modern vocabulary. While the term is often used casually for those whose ability to cope with day-to-day matters is at crisis point, stress can have serious debilitating consequences for the individual, the family and the work organisation.

The costs to the UK economy in sickness absence, in premature medical retirements, in labour turnover, in lack of added value to products and services, in the disruptions to family life and in the cost to the health service to repair the damage are enormous...' *Professor Cary Cooper, President ISMA (UK).* May 2000

National Organisations

Centre for Stress Management

The Centre specialises in training professionals in stress management, the cognitive behaviour therapies and allied therapies. In-house training in stress management is provided to industrial and commercial organisations. Professional and self-help books are also for sale.

Professor Stephen Palmer, director; Peter Ruddell, clinical director. Professor Stephen Palmer is an expert on stress and stress management. His recent book with Cary L Cooper is *Conquer your Stress* and is published by the Institute of Personnel and Development at £5.95.

Address: Centre for Stress Management, 156, Westcombe Hill, London, SE3 7DH. *Tel/Fax*: 020 8293 4114 (24 hours); 020 8853 1122 (general enquiries); 020 8318 4448 (course reservations). *Website*: www.managingstress.com [5922]

Stress Management Association

The ISMA is the International Stress Management Association Founded in 1984, ISMA (UK) is the largest of 12 national branches worldwide. Registered Charity No. 294743.

A key role of ISMA (UK) is to establish professional standards for trainers and coaches in the stress management field, as well as encouraging continuing professional development. The UK needs trained and competent professionals to work with individuals and organisations in helping to manage, humanely, the increasing pressures of modern life.

Chair: David Newth; Secretary: David Slight; Treasurer: Lucie Slight; Administrator: David Moore. *Address*: International Stress Management

Association (UK), 18, Albury Ride, Cheshunt, Waltham Cross, EN8 8XF, Hertfordshire. *Tel*: 07000 780430. *Fax*: 01992 426673. *E-mail*: stress@isma.org.uk *Website*: www.isma.org.uk May 2000

Training Institute

Stress Management Training Institute. The honorary director of this charity is Mike Atherton.

Address: Stress Management Training Institute, Isle of Wight, Hampshire. *Tel*: 01983 868166. Aug 2000

Unwind

Information and advice about pain and stress management. Contact Marie Langley. Address: Melrose, 3, Alderlea Close, Gilesgate, Durham, DH1 1DS. Tel: 0191 384 2056. Jul 2000

Further Information

Coping With Stress at Work

Audio cassette. 'Presented by broadcaster and psychiatrist Professor Anthony Clare. Learn how to recognise stress symptoms; cope with brain overload; avoid burn-out; manage your time effectively; improve relationships at work; recognise stress in colleagues; avoid stress entirely! Includes a relaxation exercise.' Published by Talking Life, tel: 0151 632 0662.

BMA Family Doctor Guide to Stress

"A practical, full-colour guide to the symptoms, recognition, treatments, defences and lifestyle choices that may help you prevent stress." Published by Dorling Kindersley, 1999, 96 pages £4.99. Available from Mind Mail Order Service, 15, Broadway, Stratford, London, E15 4BQ. Tel: 020 8221 9666.

Coping With Stress

Written by Dr Tom Trauer. Published by Salamander Books, £3.95.

Health Information Service

The HIS is a free and confidential 24-hour service. You can speak to staff during office hours, and you can listen to any of hundreds of tapes at any time, e.g: *Stress* (Tape 081); *Stress: work related stress* (Tape 467).

Address: The College of Health, St Margaret's House, 21, Old Ford Road, London, E2 9PL. *Freephone*: 0800 66 55 44. 5367

Instant Calm

Written by Paul Wilson. Over 100 techniques for dealing with stress. Includes a variety of self-help techniques. Published by Plume-Penguin Books. Price £9.99.

Stress Busters

16-page, A5 booklet published by the Hastings & Rother Health Promotion Unit. A very brief look at recognising and coping with stress.

Stress at Work Factsheet

By George Stewart. Published by MIND Information Unit, August 1998. £1.36. Available from Mind Mail Order Service. *Tel*: 020 8221 9666.

Ultimate Stress Buster

By Dr Sarah Brewer. Published by Ebury Press. Price £14.99.

Substance Misuse

Drug and alcohol abuse is a major problem and represents a very serious challenge to health. It places a strain on communities and exposes them to the risk of drug-related crime. Substance misuse and dependence do not occur in isolation and are often related to other social problems. [5090]

About drugs

'Drug and alcohol abuse is a major problem and represents a very serious challenge to health. It places a strain on communities and exposes them to the risk of drug-related crime. Substance misuse and dependence do not occur in isolation and are often related to other social problems. The issue is complex and there are no easy answers to it. Our goals aim to contribute to the creation of healthy and confident communities.' [5090]

Drug dependence

An individual is said to have developed dependence on a drug or other substance when there is a strong, compelling desire to continue taking it. Note that this 'desire' may derive from a wish either (a) to experience its effects or (b) to avoid or escape the aversive experiences produced by its absence. Dependence on a drug may in origin be largely psychological or physiological.

Drug tolerance

A condition of diminished responsiveness to a particular drug resulting from repeated exposure to it. Once tolerance has developed, increased doses are required to produce the effects achieved earlier with small doses.[5093]

Targets

Local targets

Toni Wilkinson, head of the Hastings & St Leonards Primary Care Group and chair of a local action group has set out the following aims:

- Cut drug-related crime by 25% by 2005 and 50% by 2008.
- Cut the number of drug related deaths.
- Provide more help outside hospitals.
- Provide treatment services for under 18s.
- Increase the uptake of immunisation programmes.
- Ensure swift and clear access to treatment.
- Prevent people starting to take illicit drugs.
- Reduce local access to prescribed and illicit drugs. [5048]

National target

'To help young people resist drug misuse in order to achieve their full potential in society, protect communities from drug-related anti-social and criminal behaviour, enable people with drug problems to overcome them and live healthy and crime-free lives and stifle the availablity of illegal substances.' [5090]

Illicit drugs in hospital
The following advice is given by Hastings & Rother NHS Trust to all patients who have a mental health problem.

"If you take an unprescribed drug or are under the influence of alcohol you are effectively untreatable, since it is impossible for the clinical team to assess and treat your mental health problems when your thinking and feelings are altered by these non-prescribed substances. Such use may in itself cause dramatic worsening of your mental health. We are, therefore, required to take certain steps to eliminate this very serious problem.

1. You may be asked on admission to provide a breath test or urine sample for detecting the presence of illicit drugs or alcohol. The levels detected will be recorded.

2. Random testing for illicit drugs and alcohol may occur during your stay in hospital, at the nurses' discretion.

3. If you are too ill or disturbed to be discharged as a result of taking non-prescribed drugs or alcohol, you will be closely supervised until fit for discharge.

4. The clinical staff will inform the police in any case where you, other patients or visitors are suspected of possessing or are known to be supplying drugs to any other person." [5172]

Substances
The various substances which can be misused are listed below in alphabetical order. Some, like 'Alcohol' have their own chapters.

Alcohol
Please see 'Alcohol' chapter, page 12.

Amphetamines
Also known as 'speed', 'uppers', 'whiz', etc. Widely used. The effects include increased breathing and heart rates, widening of the pupils and a lessening of appetite. The user feels more energetic, confident and cheerful. There is a risk of psychological dependence. Regular users of high doses may develop delusions, hallucinations and feelings of persecution. [6062, Dept of Health]

Barbiturates
Also known as 'downers'. Used medically to calm people down and as sleeping pills. Barbiturates depress the central nervous system in the same way as alcohol. Large doses can produce unconsciousness and eventual breathing failure and death. Long term use can result in mental and physical dependence. [6062, Dept of Health]

Cannabis
Cannabis is the name of a genus of plants. The sativa variety is the most common and is cultivated legally for the hemp and illegally for its various psychoactive products which are known by a wide variety of names including hashish, marihuana, marijuana, charas, bhang, ganja, dagga and just plain cannabis - in addition to an ever increasing number of slang terms.

The active ingredients are tetrahydrocannabinols, the primary one being an isomer, delta-9-tetrahydrocannabinol, which has been synthesized and is known to produce central-nervous-system effects. The range of effects of the drug is quite large and is dependent on dosage, the setting in which it is taken, the psychological and physical make-up of the individual and other substances such as alcohol taken at the same time.

There is currently considerable debate over the short- and long-range effects of cannabis. The 'social degeneration' occasionally seen with extensive use may be cause as much as effect. [5093]

Cocaine
An alkaloid obtained from the coca leaf. It has anaesthetic properties when applied locally and stimulating and mood-elevating effects when taken internally by ingestion,

injection or inhalation. Both drug dependence and drug tolerance develop with continued use. Cocaine acts by blocking the reuptake of dopamine. Long-term abuse is associated with a toxic psychosis similar to that seen with amphetamines. [5093]

Ecstasy

Also known as E, XTC, Doves, Disco Biscuits, Adam, Eve, Fantasy, Cities, Essence, Burgers, M & Ms, Rhubarb & Custard, Flatliners, New Yorkers, M25s, Shamrock, Dennis the Menace, Phase 4s. Can lead to forgetting safe sex (e.g. use of condoms). Risks are: fainting, death, brain damage and dependence. Ecstasy can get mixed with talc, flour, baking powder, rat poison and Angel Delight. Users can experience dehydration, energy rush, loss of appetite, mild hallucinations, calmness, happiness. Sometimes the tablets aren't ecstasy at all - they're just worming tablets. Don't mix with alcohol - ever. Ecstasy is illegal. You risk heavy fines if caught in possession. Effects begin after 20-60 minutes and last for 3-4 hours or more. Swallowed as tablets or capsules. [5022]

GHB

The following information is taken from 'ashesonthesea' website, May 2000.

Names

GHB: Gamma hydroxy butyrate or Gamma hydroxybutyric acid, Sodium Oxybate. *Street names* for GHB: GHB, 'G' (most common), Gamma-OH, Liquid E. *Description:* A clear liquid. Looks just like water.

Effects

Intoxication, increased energy, happiness, talking, desire to socialize, feeling affectionate and playful, mild disinhibition, sensuality, enhanced sexual experience, muscle relaxation, loss of coordination due to loss of muscle tone, possible nausea, difficulty concentrating, loss of gag reflex. Many people have bad reactions. These can include nausea, headaches, drowsiness, dizziness, amnesia, vomiting, loss of muscle control, respiratory problems, loss of consciousness, being conscious but unable to move, and death - especially when combined with alcohol or other drugs.

Effects of large doses

Disinhibition, sedation, desire to sleep, rambling incoherent speech, giddiness, silliness, difficulty thinking, slurred speech, passing out, and death. WARNING: If your friend passes out, always seek medical attention immediately, no matter what anyone else tells you.

Website: www.ashesonthesea.com [5797]

Heroin

An opiate derived from morphine with analgesic, euphoric and sedative effects. Like all the opiates, repeated dosages lead to development of tolerance and a marked drug dependence. The effectiveness of heroin to alter mood, relieve tension, fears and anxieties and produce a gentle drowsy euphoria has made it the most abused of the narcotics. [5093]

LSD

Lysergic acid diethylamide (LSD). Also known as 'Acid', 'Tabs', 'Trips'. One of the chemical substances derived from lysergic acid, LSD is an exceedingly powerful psychoactive drug capable of producing extreme alterations in consciousness, hallucinations, dramatic distortions in perception and unpredictable mood swings. It is difficult to predict what a person's reactions to LSD (or, for that matter, any psychoactive drug) will be.

The effects are dependent on a number of factors other than dosage such as the expectations of the user, the setting in which the experience takes place and the individual's general psychological state of mind at the time. There was, for a time, hope that it might have some therapeutic role to play and a few researchers reported some success in treating various disorders from schizophrenia to alcoholism. Follow-up work failed to confirm these early reports and today the drug is regarded as having essentially no clinical value. As a 'recreational' drug it harbours a number of very real psychological dangers. [5093]

LSD is a 'Class A' drug and supplying the drug can mean life imprisonment. LSD "distorts your mind and therefore makes you hallucinate and believe you're seeing images. It can also make you think you can do things that you cannot - for example, FLY!" [6062 Dept of Health]

Magic Mushrooms
Several species of mushrooms, including Liberty Caps, can produce hallucinations when eaten. The active ingredient is psilocybin or psilocin. The effects are similar to a mild LSD experience, but come on quicker and do not last as long. As with LSD, tolerance rapidly develops. The greatest danger is the possibility of picking a poisonous mushroom by mistake. Some mushrooms, e.g. Amanita species, can cause death in even tiny amounts. [6063, Health Promotion.]

Nicotine
Please see separate chapter, 'Smoking', page 123.

Solvents
This includes 'glue sniffing', when someone deliberately breathes the fumes from everyday products in order to become intoxicated or 'high'. For example, cigarette lighter refills, adhesives, aerosols and even petrol. The greatest number of victims are aged between 14 and 17. [5998 Oct 1999]

Please see 'Resolv' under 'National Organisations' in this chapter.

There are over a hundred deaths each year from solvent sniffing and most of those who die are teenagers. Some youngsters who sniff have accidents while intoxicated and some suffer damage to their health. [5023]

Tranquilisers
Minor tranquilisers are used to control anxiety and tension, to sedate and to induce sleep, and include Valium, Librium, Ativan and Temazepam. Tranquilisers depress mental activity and alertness. Long term use can result in dependence and the withdrawal effects can be very unpleasant. Please see 'Battle Against Tranquilisers' and 'CITA' under 'National Organisations' in this chapter. See also 'Coming off Tranquilisers' in the 'Further Information' section. [6002 Dept of Health]

Local Organisations

ADCESBH
The Alcohol & Drugs Council for East Sussex and Brighton & Hove (ADCESBH) is based in Eastbourne and runs training courses for those working in this field.

Address: ADCESBH, Centenary House, The Avenue, Eastbourne, Sussex, BN21 3XY. *Tel*: 01323 430003. *Fax*: 01323 644687. [5019]

Training Courses
Further information from one of the following offices, Brighton: 01273 703100; Eastbourne: 01323 430003; Hastings: 01424 441933. [Jul 2000]

Addaction Criminal Justice Project
The aims of the 5A Day Programme is to enable drug misusers to make positive changes in their life.

The organisation has proved over a number of years through working with substance misusers that this will be via a process of replacement activities, which aim to bridge the gap between problematic drug use, stability and a drug-free lifestyle. The aim of this is to stabilise any chaotic substance misuse and associated lifestyle and to thereby reduce any drug-related offending behaviour. Each person will have a treatment plan drawn up for them by their key-worker, identifying which groups each client will attend, to ensure that all individuals' needs are being addressed.

Groups are also an integral part of the 5A Day Programme, covering offending behaviour, relapse prevention, computer courses, new direction 'back to work plans', as well as open discussion groups. *Contacts:* Mrs Nadia Clarke, Team leader; Gerard Horobin, Project worker.

Address: Addaction Criminal Justice Project, 5a, Trinity Street, Hastings, East Sussex, TN34 1HG. *Tel:* 01424 441548. *Fax:* 01424 429803. [5093]

Aftercare Services

Aftercare Services Co-ordination (ASC) provides emotional and practical support to people who have a prior history of drug and/or alcohol misuse and are currently substance free. The service is also open to people who may have lapsed who wish to become substance free again. ASC covers people who have been through rehabilitation programmes, hospital, community or self-detox.

Services

The catchment area is Hastings and Rother. Service includes befriending/support on an individual level; access to other appropriate services; lapse prevention and management; an opportunity to focus and develop ideas; involvement in, and access to, community-based activities, groups and networks; supporting client/group led activities; access to training/support and voluntary work for people who wish to contribute to ongoing or potential projects.

Access to ASC is through a referring agency, e.g. Substance Misuse, Housing Association, Probation. ASC can meet the client at the referring agency. After an initial assessment it then becomes possible to consider seeing the client in their own home. If this is not appropriate, an alternative venue, as agreed between the client and ASC, can be arranged.

Hours: Mondays to Thursdays 9.30am to 5.30pm. The aim is to organise a support group in the near future. *Contact:* Nick Muriel.

Address: ASC, 85, Mount Pleasant Road, Hastings, East Sussex, TN34 3SL. *Tel:* 01424 729022. *Fax:* 01424 200842. [5867 Jun 2000] C

DAIS

DAIS is a local charity working in the community and used by an increasing number of people dependent on prescribed medication, illegal drugs or alcohol. It is accessible to users and their families seeking counselling or advice on our Helpline: 01424 220788.

DAIS offers information, advice on harm minimisation and nutrition, one-to-one counselling, crisis intervention and aftercare. It also runs self-help groups for those reducing their dependencies, who benefit by sharing their problems and successes in a safe setting and who can use the support network.

Complete confidentiality within the organisation is assured. However, if a client wishes, DAIS can liaise with a wide range of agencies including legal, medical, mental health, probation, prison, hospital and rehabilitation services, enabling them to assist with other related problems.

If a volunteer is not available to answer the telephone any message left will get a quick response.

Visits by trained volunteer counsellors can be arranged to any mutually agreed location. [5997]

Drug Dependency Unit

Please now see under 'Substance Misuse Service', page 137.

Families Anonymous

For details of local groups, please contact the head office, listed under 'National Organisations', page 138.

Get It While You Can

The GIWYC (Get It While You Can) project was established in Hastings in April 1996. It was started in Brighton two years earlier and is now claimed to be 'the most effective arrest referral scheme in the country.' What is offered is 'a pro-active approach to the repetitive cycle of drug and alcohol related crime.'

Access

People who misuse alcohol or drugs all have points in their lives when they have flashes of wanting to stop. The GIWYC project offers appropriate help to individuals at a time of vulnerability, when they are more likely to consider change. Anyone involved in the criminal justice system who has substance misuse or related problems may apply to GIWYC.

They are available to see anyone who finds themselves in police custody, on probation, released from prison or appearing before magistrates. GIWYC is often approached by family and friends or partners who themselves might need support and advice.

GIWYC discusses the difficulties experienced by the client, looks at priorities and explores the options open to him or her.

'A great deal of our work is concerned with giving up to date and accurate information, filling in gaps in clients' awareness and dispelling myths about drug use. We advocate a harm reduction approach and recommend the use of counselling and other services in the town.'

Hastings office

Address: CRI, Get It While You Can Project, Hastings & Rother Law Courts, Bohemia Road, Hastings, Sussex, TN3 1ND. *Tel:* 01424 432000. Drop in hours: Mondays to Fridays 10am to 1pm. Office hours: 9.15am to 5pm. *Contact:* Robyn Rimmell, project worker. May 2000

Eastbourne office

Address: The Law Courts, Eastbourne Magistrates Court, Old Orchard Road, Eastbourne, Sussex, BN21 4UN. *Tel/Fax:* 01323 725765. Drop in hours: Mondays to Fridays 10am to 1pm. Office Hours: 9.15am to 5pm. *Contact:* John Malone. Aug 2000

Brighton

Address: Brighton Magistrates Court, 2nd Floor, Edward Street, Brighton, Sussex, BN3 3JD. *Tel:* 01273 676246. *Drop in hours:* Mondays to Fridays 10am to 1pm. Office *Hours:* 9.15am to 5pm. *Contact:* Norma Buss or Mike Byrne. 5147, 5148 May 2000

Health Promotion

The Substance Misuse Team works as part of a co-ordinated multi-agency approach to implement the National Drugs Strategy in accordance with the local Drug Action Team's plan of action, which also includes issues related to the misuse of alcohol. The strategy has four aims: to reduce drug use amongst young people; to protect communities from the consequences of drug use and related crime; to improve access to treatment for drug users; and to reduce the availability of drugs. See page 321. 5370

Narcotics Anonymous

There are weekly local meetings held in Brighton (on every day of the week); Eastbourne (Thursdays); and Tunbridge Wells (Fridays). Please telephone the UK Service office for further details, see below.

Phoenix House

Phoenix House is the largest national provider of residential care and rehabilitation services to substance misusers.

The Bexhill project provides a safe and supportive environment where clients use groups and individual counselling to explore their problems with drugs and learn new skills aimed to help them develop independent lives free from problematic substance misuse.

The main house has accommodation for up to 30 men and women. A smaller house in Hastings provides semi-independent accommodation for up to a further five people.

The rehabilitation programme concentrates on promoting change by challenging individual attitudes and behaviour, encouraging self worth and personal responsibility and the development of social and life skills.

Contact: Christine Reddington, project manager; Ben Fitzpatrick, business manager.

Address: Phoenix House, Colwall Court, 1, Pages Avenue, Bexhill-on-Sea, East Sussex, TN39 3AP. *Tel:* 01424 732171. *Fax:* 01424 733480. Jun 2000

Social Services

The countywide Service Manager for Substance Misuse is James Johnson.

Address: East Sussex Social Services, Substance Misuse Service, 1a, Shepherd Street, St Leonards, Sussex, TN38 0ET. *Tel:* 01424 443893. *Fax:* 01424 465822. 5081

Young people

Two drug and alcohol abuse specialists are working with young people as part of a countywide initiative. For information on where to find help, contact Social Services' Vicky Finnemore on 01273 517038. *Fax:* 01273 514367. July 2000

Substance Misuse Service

Formerly known as the Drug Dependency Unit, it is a department of Hastings & Rother Trust. It caters primarily for people addicted to opiates. People with other addictions, e.g. amphetamines, are referred to other places, e.g. the Trinity Project. 'We adopt a holistic approach to client care - focusing on individuals' psychological, physical and social needs.'

Anyone may attend by simply turning up, or by making an appointment first. The service is free.

The SMS is a prescribing clinic providing information, advice, support, health education, counselling, in-patient detoxification, community detoxification, medical and psychiatric assessment. Clients may apply in person direct to the SMS or they may be referred by their GP or other professional. Total confidentiality is observed.

Community nursing sisters: Kate Barry & Maggie Jones; Charge nurse: Ray Harrison; Charge nurse: Ian Stewart (temp.); Support worker: Debbie Fraser; Social worker: Richard Arnison.

Address: Substance Misuse Service, 9a, Holmesdale Gardens, Hastings, Sussex, TN34 1LY. *Tel:* 01424 720088. *Fax:* 01424 438111. Jul 2000

Trinity Project

Helping individuals and communities to manage the effects of drug and alcohol misuse. A confidential service which offers: advice and information for anyone concerned about substance misuse; needle exchange, health advice, HIV and Hep. B and C testing; support and counselling; rural outreach programme; peer education training; shared care scheme. Clients may be referred via family, friends or GPs, or may make direct contact themselves.

Manager: Frank Clarke; Administrator: Karen Brooker; GP liaison worker: Bill Dyer Wright; Project worker: Vivien Anderson; Outreach worker: John Stiles; Nurse/project worker: Gill Fields.

Hours: Mondays to Fridays 9.15am to 12.30pm (appointments only); Mondays to Fridays 1.00pm to 4.45pm (open access). Needle exchange available: 9.15am to 12.30pm and 1.00 to 4.45pm.

Address: Trinity Project, 6, Trinity Street, Hastings, East Sussex, TN34 1HG. *Tel:* 01424 426375. *Fax:* 01424 72207.
E-Mail: trinity@addaction.org.uk May 2000

National Organisations

Battle Against Tranquilisers

'To lessen the harm caused by benzodiazepine tranquilisers and sleeping pills'.

We support people to withdraw as comfortably as possible. We do this through groups, individual visits and telephone helpline. We support people who are addicted through prescription. We work with the statutory sector and other voluntary sector organisations with BZ/alcohol/illicit drug problems. We do training (post-graduate and other) for professional workers, voluntary sector organisations and community groups, tailoring presentations to specific requirements. Registered Charity No. 1056508

Chair: Tom Turvey; Vice-Chair: Edith Milne; Company Secretary: Hilary Furnivall. Secretary: Sonia Garland. *Contact*: Una Corbett, Co-ordinator.

Address: Battle Against Tranquilliers, PO Box 658, Bristol, BS99 1XP. *Tel:* 0117 9663629 or 9653463 or 9620249. *Fax:* 07970 090483. 5472

CITA

Providing help, advice, counselling, support and information for those addicted to their prescribed mind-altering medication, especially tranquilliers and anti-depressants; and for their friends, relatives, doctors and health professionals. Help and counselling offered regarding anxiety and stress management. Literature, tapes, books all available. The service is available throughout the UK and abroad. Registered Charity No.519334.

Administrator, scientific adviser & company secretary: Paul Entwistle; Consultant trainer: Pam Armstrong; Treasurer: Peter Tallent.

Address: CITA, Cavendish House, Rooms 15 and 17, Brighton Road, Waterloo, Liverpool, L22 5NG. *Tel:* 0151 474 9626. *Fax:* 0151 284 8324. *Helpline:* 0151 949 0102. *Website:* www.liv.ac.uk/~csunit/community/cita.htm 5483

DrugScope

DrugScope has been created through the merger of the UK's foremost drug information and policy organisations: the Institute for the Study of Drug Dependence (ISDD) and the Standing Conference on Drug Abuse (SCODA) - two charities with a total of sixty years in the national and international drugs field.

DrugScope is today one of the UK's leading centres of expertise on drugs. Our aim is to inform policy development and reduce drug-related risk. We provide quality drug information, promote effective responses to drug taking, undertake research at local, national and international levels, advise on policy-making, encourage informed debate and provide a voice for our member bodies working on the ground.

Address: DrugScope, 32-36, Loman Street, London, SE1 0EE. *Tel:* 020 7928 1211. *Fax:* 020 7928 1771.
E-mail: services@drugscope.org.uk
Website: www.drugscope.org.uk 6075 Jul 2000

Families Anonymous

Families Anonymous is a completely independent, non-professional organisation set up for all families and friends of anyone with a former, suspected or current drug problem.

"When drug addiction enters a family via one of its members, the effect can be devastating. If you have reason to believe or even a vague suspicion that someone close to you may have a drug problem, we know how you feel. We know what is is like to be alone with this problem. We remember the feelings of panic and frustration that resulted from this discovery. We in Families Anonymous have experienced this too.

Families Anonymous is a fellowship of self-help groups for those concerned about drug abuse, or related behavioural problems of a relative or friend. It is based on the 'Twelve Steps' of Alcoholics Anonymous, and was started in this country in 1980. About 50 groups now meet every week in various parts of the country." [5886]

For details of local meetings as well a mail order literature service, please telephone the head office of Families Anonymous.

Hours: Mondays to Fridays, with volunteers who man the helpline between 6 and 11pm each evening and all day on Saturdays and Sundays.

Address: Families Anonymous UK Office, Doddington & Rollo Community Association, Charlotte Despart Avenue, London, SW11 5JE. *Tel:* 020 7498 4680. *Fax:* 020 7498 1990. *Website:* www.famanon.org.uk [5886]

First Steps to Freedom

Registered charity which aims to help, in a practical way, people who suffer from phobias, obsessional compulsive disorder, anxiety, panic attacks, anorexia and bulimia, and those who wish to come off tranquilisers, and their carers. For more details, please see main entry in 'Phobias' chapter, page 104.

Narcotics Anonymous

Narcotics Anonymous is an international, community-based, non-profit fellowship of men and women for whom drugs have become a major problem - recovering addicts who meet regularly to help each other stay clean. Membership is open to anyone irrespective of age, sex, religion, race, creed or class and the only requirement for membership is a desire to stop using drugs.

Meetings

Narcotics Anonymous started in the USA in 1953 and is one of the oldest and largest organisations of its type in the world. More than 20,000 meetings take place in 90 countries *each week.*

The first NA meeting in the United Kingdom took place in London in 1980. There are currently more than 340 weekly meetings throughout England, Scotland and Wales. Narcotics Anonymous is a completely voluntary organisation. Membership is open to anyone with a drug problem seeking help, regardless of what drug or combination of drugs have been used.

Twelve steps

The core of the Narcotics Anonymous programme is a series of twelve steps, adapted from the recovery programme of Alcoholics Anonymous. These steps include admitting to a drug problem, seeking help, self-appraisal, confidential self-disclosure, making amends where possible where harm has been done, achieving a spiritual awakening and supporting other drug addicts who want to recover.

Achieving recovery

Narcotics Anonymous is a non-religious fellowship, encouraging each member to cultivate an individual understanding, religious or not, of a 'spiritual awakening'. Narcotics

Anonymous believes one of the cornerstones of its success is the therapeutic value of addicts working with each other to achieve recovery.

In meetings members regularly share their personal experiences with each other, not as professionals but as ordinary people who have discovered that sharing brings about solutions to their problems.

Narcotics Anonymous encourages its members to abstain completely from all drugs including alcohol because NA members have discovered that complete and continuous abstinence provides the best foundation for recovery and personal growth.

Clean Times
"If you have not seen a copy of the new Clean Times, you don't know what you're missing". One copy costs £1.50, a subscription costs £6.00 (4 issues). Send cheques (payable to *Clean Times*) or postal orders to *Clean Times*, address below [5865]

Address: 202, City Road, London, EC1V 2PH. *Tel:* 020 7251 4007. *Fax:* 020 7251 4006. UK Helpline: *Tel:* 020 7730 0009. UK Service Office: *Tel:* 020 7251 4007. *E-mail:* ukso@ukna.org [5864]

National Drugs Helpline
Helpline for drug users, their families, friends and carers. *Tel:* 0800 776600. [Jul 2000]

Release
Information and advice around drugs and legal issues. 24 hour helpline. *Tel:* London 020 7603 8654. [Jul 2000]

Project LSD
Information on drugs for lesbians, gay men and bisexuals. *Tel:* 020 7288 1111. *Note:* Telephone number not verified at August 2000.

Re-Solv
Re-Solv is The Society for the Prevention of solvent and Volatile Substance Misuse and offers advice and support to parents of children involved with solvent abuse, as well as individuals caught up in solvent abuse themselves.

Address: Re-Solv, 30a, High Street, Stone, Staffordshire, ST15 8AW. *Tel:* 01785 817885. *Fax:* 01785 813205. *Freephone Helpline* 0808 800 2345. *Website:* www.re-solv.org [May 2000]

SCODA
SCODA is the Standing Committee On Drug Abuse. It is now part of 'DrugScope', please see above.

SHARP
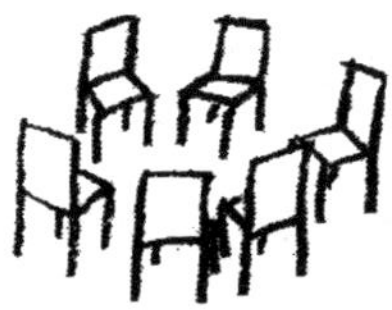

Self Help Addiction Recovery Programme (SHARP) is an out-patient treatment programme managed by The Chemical Dependency Centre which aims to improve the lives of people affected by alcohol or drug dependency by providing high quality, abstinence-based treatment options which integrate 12-step recovery programmes and other appropriate therapies.

SHARP provides a structured day programme over 48 days for men and women with severe drug and alcohol problems. Clients must be involved for at least 24 hours.

Chief executive: Tristan Millington-Drake; Manager, day and out-patient services: Sue Mercer; Team leader: Dave Mullaney; Referrals worker: Christina Pocapaglia.

Address: SHARP, 11, Redcliffe Gardens, London, SW10 9BG. *Tel:* 020 7352 2552. *Fax:* 020 7351 4498. [May 2000]

Turning Point

Turning Point is the UK's largest charity helping people with drink, drug and mental health problems, with more than 100 service centres across the country.

Turning Point provides residential and rehabilitation day care and street level advice and support for those seeking help and treats people as individuals - they believe there is no one type of person who develops drink, drug or mental health problems, no single reason why, and no set cure or treatment. Because of this no single project is run in the same way as any other. However, they all have one thing in common - they offer free, confidential and non-judgemental help to people whom society often regards as difficult to care for or sees as undeserving of help. Registered Charity No. 234887.

Chief executive: Ted Unworth; *executive director, north:* David Edwards; *executive director, south:* Rosanna O'Connor; *head of communications:* Ron Alexander.

Address: Turning Point, New Loom House, 101, Backchurch Lane, London, E1 1LU. *Tel:* 020 7702 2300. South regional office: 020 7702 1458. *Fax:* 020 7702 1456. *E-mail:* tpmail@turning-point.co.uk *Website:* www.turning-point.co.uk May 2000

Further Information

Alcohol, Drugs and Mental Illness.
Written by Dr Brenda Lintner. Booklet published by Sane, 1993.

Coping with tranquiliser addiction.
'Addicted to tranquilisers or sleeping pills? Thousands have been helped to withdraw from their pills by this tape. How to kick the habit safely, avoid panic attacks and cope on a daily basis with your addiction. Useful breathing exercises.' Published by Talking Life, *tel:* 0151 632 0662.

Coming off Tranquillisers
'Coming off Tranquillisers, Sleeping Pills and Anti-depressants: A Safe and Effective Withdrawal Plan'. Written by Shirley Trickett. "Withdrawing from tranquillisers, if not managed properly, can bring on other distressing symptoms: panic attacks, hallucinations and insomnia. This highly acclaimed guide to safe withdrawal is widely recommended by doctors, therapists and nurses."

Published by Thorsons, 1998, 176 pages, ISBN: 0-7225-3611-9, £7.99. Available from Mind Mail Order Service. *Tel:* 020 8221 9666. *Fax:* 020 8534 6399. *E-mail:* publications@mind.org.uk 5088

Forbidden Drugs
By Philip Robson. 'I urge anyone interested in the issues surrounding illegal drugs to read this book' - Will Self. This book avoids generalisation and delivers realistic, unemotive information about the effects (positive as well as negative) of all types of drugs including alcohol and nicotine. It concludes with suggestions for limiting the damage to individuals and society.

Published by Oxford University Press, 1999. ISBN: 0-19-262955-7. 302 pages. Price £12.99. Available from Mind. *Tel:* 020 8221 9666.

Street Drugs
Understanding the Psychological Effects of Street Drugs. 12-page booklet written and edited by Terry Brown & Sara Dunn. Published by Mind 1998. Available from Mind. *Tel:* 020 8519 8122. 5021

Health Information Service
The HIS is a free and confidential 24-hour service. You can speak to staff during office hours, and you can listen to any of hundreds of tapes at any time, e.g: *Heroin* (Tape 360); *Ecstasy* (Tape 356); *Marijuana* (Tape

305); *LSD and magic mushrooms* (Tape 359); *Solvent abuse & glue sniffing* (Tape 092); *Crack: the long & short-term effects* (Tape 306).

Address: The College of Health, St Margaret's House, 21, Old Ford Road, London, E2 9PL. *Freephone:* 0800 66 55 44. [5367]

See also these chapters ...

Alcohol, page 12.

Acknowledgements
Our grateful thanks to Nick Casey of ESBHHA Health Promotion for editorial assistance with this chapter.

Tinnitus

Tinnitus is defined as 'a subjective sensation of a ringing or tinkling in the ears experienced in the absence of any external acoustic stimulus. It can be produced by a number of causes including diseases of the outer, middle or inner ear, nerve damage or as a reaction to some drugs such as quinine and aspirin'. [5093, Reber]

There is no cure for tinnitus and those newly diagnosed will be devastated by the news and may well benefit from contact with a support group. Tinnitus is not a 'mental illness' in that it probably has a physical cause. It can affect young and old alike; in fact some children are born with it and think everyone has it. Even totally deaf people may have tinnitus. Many famous people are sufferers and manage to lead normal lives, e.g. William Shatner, Barbra Streisand, Leonard Nimoy. [Constable, Aug 2000]

Local Organisation

Sussex Tinnitus Association

Offering newsletters, information, research and meetings including contact with audiology departments and liaison with ENT consultants and GPs. 24 hour answerphone - helpline. *Contact:* Mrs Mavis Constable, secretary & treasurer. There are six groups in Sussex, including Hastings, Bexhill and Eastbourne.

Address: Sussex Tinnitus Association, 6, Shortbrow Close, Lower Willingdon, Eastbourne, East Sussex, BN22 0QX. Tel: 01323 503751. [5867 Jun 2000]

National Organisation

British Tinnitus Association

Address: British Tinnitus Association, 4th Floor, White Building, Fitzalan Square, Sheffield, S1 2AZ. Helpline: 0800 018 0527. Fax: 0114 279 6222.

E-mail: bta@tinnitus.org.uk

Website: www.tinnitus.org.uk [Jul 2000]

Acknowledgements

Our grateful thanks to Mavis Constable of the Sussex Tinnitus Association for editorial help with this chapter.

Trauma

Post Traumatic Stress Disorder

Post-traumatic stress disorder (PTSD)is the name given to the after-effects of an unusually frightening or horrifying experience; for example, seeing someone killed, surviving an accident or losing your home or family.

If you have PTSD you will tend to re-live your traumatic experience by dreaming about it, thinking about it, and becoming upset if you see similar events or scenes. You may find yourself avoiding places or activities which remind you of that experience, and you may also find it difficult to be positive and plan for the future.

Obviously it is quite normal to feel upset immediately after a painful or distressing experience, so the term PTSD is only applicable if the feelings persist. It is also important not to confuse PTSD with grief following the death of a loved one. [5181]

Organisations

Trauma Aftercare Trust

Address: Trauma Aftercare Trust HQ, Buttfields, The Farthings, Withington, Gloucester, GL54 4DF. *Helpline:* (24 hour *Tel*: 01242 890306. *E-mail:* tacta@tacthq.demon.co.uk
Website: www.tacthq.demon.co.uk [May 2000]

Traumatic Stress Clinic

Address: Traumatic Stress Clinic, 73, Charlotte Street, London, W1P 1LB. *Tel*: 020 7530 3666. [May 2000]

Further Information

Overcoming Traumatic Stress.

Overcoming Traumatic Stress: a self-help guide using cognitive-behavioural techniques. By Claudia Herbert and Ann Wetmore. Terrible events cause many people to become permanently changed. This book provides practical advice and exercises to help people overcome this.

Published by Robinson, 1999. ISBN: 1-84119-016-0. 208 pages. £7.99. Available from Mind Mail Order Service. *Tel*: 020 8221 9666.

Post Traumatic Stress

Post Traumatic Stress - the Basics. 20 page booklet available from the Trauma Aftercare Trust. For address and telephone number please see this chapter. [5011]

Women

For advice about sex and contraception see 'Brook', page 146; for advice about violence see 'Refuge', page 146, 'Hastings Women's Refuge' and 'St Jude's', this page. For advice about self-injury, see Bristol Crisis Service, page 146.

Local Organisations

National Childbirth Trust

"We offer antenatal classes for pregnant mothers and their partners and breastfeeding help and information. Also postnatal support for newly delivered mothers and mothers with young children." Anyone may apply for help. *Hours:* antenatal classes are held in the evenings only.

Breastfeeding counsellors and postnatal supporters are mothers with young families, and can be contacted at any reasonable time. Breastfeeding counselling and postnatal support are provided free of charge. *Contact:* Ros Vinall.

Address: National Childbirth Trust Hastings & Rother, Tinkersden Cottage, Lower Northlands, Bodiam, East Sussex, TN32 5UN. *Tel:* 01580 850997. *E-mail:* vinall@tinkersden.fsnet.co.uk Jul 2000

St Jude's Women's Refuge

Tel: 01424 732060. *Fax:* 01424 730060.

Temporary refuge for women (Rother district & Hastings) who are afraid or have suffered violence themselves or to their children. Also: Outreach service, support and advice manned 24 hr. *Tel:* 01424 732060. Jul 2000

Hastings Women's Refuge

A local refuge in Hastings providing accommodation for local women experiencing violent relationships, and their children. Besides accommodation, the refuge provides support and information for women and a dedicated play-worker for the children. *Contact:* Ms Jacqui Ballard, development worker for domestic abuse across East Sussex.

Address: Hastings Women's Refuge, Ocean House, Hastings, East Sussex, TN37 6LW.

Contact information: A 24hr a day, 365 days a year national crisis line (4 lines) for women experiencing violent/abusive relationships. They link with Language Line, to provide a service for women whose first language is not English. They also provide refuge accommodation all over England. 5867 Jul 2000

Women's Network

Hastings & Rother Women's Network. Enables women to exchange information, ideas and experiences through networking with other groups. Giving a voice to women's views on important issues such as housing, GPs, hospitals, social and council services.

Encourages the development of new services and changes/developments in existing services to ensure that women's needs are understood and met. Offering a monthly drop-in for all women and providing network and information exchange.

Meet on the first Friday of each month from 12 to 2pm (bring your own lunch). *Contact:* Mrs Susan Lyle, co-ordinator.

Address: Hastings & Rother Women's Network, c/o Pinehurst Centre, 3, Avondale Road, St Leonards-on-Sea, East Sussex, TN38 0SA. *Tel:* 01424 423686. 5867

Pilgrim House Trust

Drop-in centre with group work. Offering support and information to women aged 16 plus regarding relationships, housing, benefits, education, training, parenting skills etc. Also, teenage pregnancy support group (14 to 18 years). The service also includes a Rapid Response Crisis Intervention Team which will provide both an immediate and outreach service to women experiencing violent relationships; as well as a specialist alcohol worker. *Contact:* Ms Mandy Martin, project leader.

Address: Pilgrim House Trust, 45, Cambridge Road, Hastings, East Sussex, TN34 1DT. *Tel:* 01424 716629. 5867 Jul 2000

Police

Any woman who is at risk of physical violence is advised to contact the Police. They, in partnership with Hastings Borough Council, can offer assistance and a safe environment either in a refuge or elsewhere.

Address: Sussex Police, Bohemia Road, St Leonards, Sussex. *Tel*: 0845 60 70 999. Aug 2000

Brighton Rape Crisis

Address: PO Box 323, Brighton, BN2 2TY. *Tel*: 01273 203773 (24-hr answphone). Open Mondays and Fridays 6 to 9 pm. Or for immediate help ring London Rape Crisis on *tel:* 020 7837 1600. Confidential service, answered by women, telephone counselling and advice service. Jul 2000

Threshold

Women's Mental Health Initiative. Registered Charity No. 1000835.

Address: Threshold, 14, St George's Place, Brighton, BN1 4GB, Sussex. *Tel:* 01273 626444. *Fax:* 01273 626444. *E-mail:* thrwomen@globalnet.co.uk May 2000

Victim Support

Practical and emotional help for the victims of crime, by unannounced visits to the victim's home, by a volunteer, where possible. Deals with minor and major crime including sexual assault and rape. Offers assistance to families of victims of murder and road traffic accidents. Also support for court witnesses.

Anyone may apply for help. The organisation does not become involved with victims under the age of 17, unless they are victims of crime.

Hours: Mondays to Fridays 10.30am to 2.00pm. Emergencies between 8am to 8pm outside office hours: via Hastings Police. Specific services are provided to women for rape and sexual assault who are visited only with their agreement. Our rape volunteer visitors receive special training and offer long-term support. This differs from 'one-off' calls for other crimes. *Contacts:* Shirley Porte, Phil Craig, Valerie Bailey.

Address: Hastings & Rother Victim Support, First Floor Suite, 6, Cambridge Road, Hastings, East Sussex, TN34 1DJ. *Tel:* 01424 424393. Emotional support and practical advice for victims of crime. *Fax:* 01424 721100. *Victim Support Line: Tel:* 0845 303 0900 (local call rate). Jul 2000

National Organisations

Brook

Covering the whole of the UK, Brook provides free, confidential sex advice and contraception for young people under the age of 25. Helpline co-ordinator: Paula Currie.

Address: Brook, 421, Highgate Studios, 53-79, Highgate Road, London, NW5 1TL. *Tel/Fax*: 020 7284 6093 (direct line). *Freephone*: 0800 0185023. *E-mail:* information@brookcentres.org.uk *Website:* www.brook.org.uk May 2000

Refuge

24-hour crisis line providing practical advice and emotional support for women experiencing domestic violence. *Tel:* 0870 599 5443. Jul 2000

Bristol Crisis Service

Bristol Crisis Service for Women. National helpline for women in distress, particularly those who use self-injury as a way of coping with their problems. The service is open

Fridays to Saturdays 9pm to 12.30am. *Tel:* 0117 925 1119. *Website:* www.users.zetnet.co.uk/bcsw/ Jul 2000

Miscarriage Association

Can provide written information and put you in touch with a local support group. *Tel:* 01924 200799. *Fax:* 01924 298834. Jul 2000

Association for Postnatal Illness

Covering the whole of the UK, the Association offers advice, information and support to mothers suffering from post-natal depression, and their families. Support is given by letter, telephone or e-mail. All volunteers are ex-sufferers.

Address: Association for Postnatal Illness, 25, Jerdan Place, Fulham, London, SW6 1BE. *Tel:* 0207 386 0868. *Fax:* 0207 386 8885. *E-mail:* info@apni.org *Website:* www.apni.org May 2000

Premenstrual Society

Covering the whole of the UK, the Society provides information and support to sufferers from premenstrual syndrome (PMS) and period pains, and those who care for them. They also support local support groups and run courses (most for nurses) as the need arises. They have recently started a Research Fund.

Chairman: Dr Michael Brush; Local Groups Co-ordinator: Mrs Zoe Manning; Hon. Medical Adviser: Dr Marta Perry.

Address: Premenstrual Society, PO Box 429, Addlestone, Surrey, KT15 1DZ. *Tel:* 01932 872560 (professional & admin. only); other enquiries by letter with SAE. May 2000

Premenstrual Syndrome

The National Association for Premenstrual Syndrome (NAPS) offers positive and energetic support to sufferers and their partners by giving personal advice and support when asked. NAPS supplies information on a continuous basis to members, and works with the medical profession to alleviate suffering and to promote the interests of sufferers where appropriate. Registered Charity No. 289901. Chief executive officer: Mrs S Allen; Network development officer: Mrs C Baker.

Address: National Association for Premenstrual Syndrome, 7, Swift's Court, High Street, Seal, Kent, TN15 0EG. *Tel/Fax:* 01732 760011. *Helpline:* 01732 760012. *E-mail:* naps@charity.vfree.com *Website:* www.pms.org.uk May 2000

Rape Crisis Centre

Helpline for women and girls who have been raped or sexually assaulted. London Office: *Tel:* 020 7916 5466. *Helpline:* 020 7837 1600. Jul 2000

Women In Special Hospitals

Women in Special Hospitals (WISH). *Tel:* 020 7329 2415. *E-mail:* wish@wishlondon.freeserve.co.uk Jul 2000

Women's Aid Federation

The aims of the Women's Aid National Helpline are to provide support, information and a listening ear to women experiencing domestic violence and to those seeking help on a woman's behalf; to discuss the available options and, if appropriate, to refer callers on to refuges and other sources of help and information.

The WANH currently responds to some 25,000 calls a year. Everyone taking calls has been trained in telephone counselling skills and domestic violence issues. A caller experiencing domestic violence may be referred to a registered family law solicitor or a local face to face support group or to emergency refuge accommodation. (There are over 200 throughout the UK affiliated to the Women's Aid Federation).

Address: Women's Aid Federation of England, PO Box 391, Bristol, BS99 7WS.

Tel: 0345 023 468 (National Helpline); 0117 944 4411 (Admin); 0117 942 1396 (Training Team). *Fax:* 0117 924 1703.

E-mail: wafe@wafe.co.uk
Website: www.womensaid.org.uk 6066 Jul 2000

Women's Therapy Centre

Provides individual and group psychotherapy for women, particularly those who do not usually have easy access to psychotherapy. Also, nationwide advice and information on counselling and psychotherapy services contained on a database.

Address: Women's Therapy Centre, 10, Manor Gardens, London, N7 6JS. *Tel:* 020 7263 6200. *Fax:* 0207281 7879. *E-mail:* info@womenstherapycentre.co.uk *Website:* www.womenstherapycentre.co.uk May 2000

Further Information

Guide to Postnatal Depression.

Written by Erika Harvey. 'A clear and practical guide to all levels of postnatal depression which outlines the causes and symptoms, and how to deal with special circumstances including ill or disabled babies or multiple births. It contains self help techniques and information on natural remedies.'

Published by Element 1999. ISBN: 1-86204-330-2, 118 pages. Price £5.99. Available from Mind Mail Order, *tel:* 020 8221 9666. 5251

Health Information Service

The HIS is a free and confidential 24-hour service. You can speak to staff during office hours, and you can listen to any of hundreds of tapes at any time, e.g: *Post-natal depression* (Tape 124). *Address*: The College of Health, St Margaret's House, 21, Old Ford Road, London, E2 9PL. *Freephone*: 0800 66 55 44. 5367

Women and Mental Health

Editor: Dora Kohen. Why are women more vulnerable to mental health problems than men? This is a comprehensive and clear tour through the issues relating to women and mental health, including perinatal psychiatric disorders, depression, eating disorders, schizophrenia and alcohol and drug abuse. Written from a female perspective, *Women and Mental Health* is an invaluable tool. Published by Routledge, 2000. ISBN: 0-415-18885-7. 230 pages. Price £16.99. Available from Mind. *Tel:* 020 8221 9666. 5024

Acknowledgements
Our grateful thanks to Anne Guildford of Threshold & Women's Mental Health Initiative, Brighton for editorial assistance with this chapter

HASTINGS MIND

good health guide

help

This second part of the *Guide* gives information about local and national organisations which can provide help. For a quick overview of this section, please see the Contents on page 6

Advice

Obtaining peace of mind about the right way of dealing with the day to day concerns that can arise as a result of being mentally ill is a vital part of coping with the illness. Housing difficulties, debt problems and a variety of legal issues can be resolved far more easily once you know who can help and where to find them.

This section contains information about those who can help you the most, should the need arise. So if, for example, mental illness has caused you or someone you care for to be out of work with mounting debts and possible homelessness, a good place to start looking for help is at your nearest Citizens' Advice Bureau.

Your local CAB centre, together with HARC (Hastings and Rother Representation Centre) specialise in providing practical help and advice to people who simply can't deal with these matters on their own. Their services will cost you nothing and anyone is welcome to ask for their help.

Money problems
CABs can help you to deal with debt problems including housing repossession and eviction. You will receive any necessary advice or help with Court proceedings, administration orders or bankruptcy, preparation of financial statements and negotiations with creditors. [5214] Please see also 'Money' chapter, page 91.

Citizens' Advice Bureaux

Citizens' Advice Bureaux (CABs) offer free, independent, impartial and confidential information and advice service, covering a wide range of subjects including benefits advice, housing problems, employment difficulties, racial issues and personal matters both individual and family related.

Their advice is given professionally by fully trained voluntary and paid staff, using a national information system.

They also offer a specialist money advice service to clients in debt, those involved with social security appeals and industrial tribunals. This is a free service that can be used by anyone. The various local offices are listed below. [5214]

Advocacy
If necessary the CAB may (if you agree) be able to take up your case on your behalf - for example, make telephone calls, write letters or attend a court hearing with you. [5214]

Counselling
Counselling is different from advice. It may help just to talk about your problem. People often need this kind of help with bereavement, relationship problems, work problems or career changes.

Clients are seen at the Bureau by trained counsellors for up to five sessions. The sessions last one hour and are free. [5214]

Free advice
CAB advice workers can give you free advice and information on a wide range of subjects including social security benefits, consumer rights, taxation, debt problems, credit, housing, work problems, family and relationship problems, the legal system, local services and groups, health and disability, neighbourhood problems, immigration and nationality, human rights, education, travel and much more.

Their advice is completely free and impartial and whatever you tell them is treated in the strictest confidence. [5214]

Legal problems
If you have a legal problem the CAB may refer you to a solicitor on duty at the Bureau for a 15 minute advice session, by previous appointment only. You will first need to discuss the matter with one of our advisers to see if this is appropriate. [5214]

Battle CAB

Hours: 'Outreach' sessions. Open Mondays

only from 10am until 12 noon. *Address:* Citizens' Advice Bureau, Battle Memorial Hall, High Street, Battle, Sussex. *Tel:* 01424 215055. [Jul 2000]

Bexhill & Rother CAB

Hours: Mondays, Wednesdays & Fridays 10.00am to 12 noon & 2.00 to 4.00pm; Tuesdays & Thursdays 10.00am to 4.00pm. (Thursday: telephone enquiries only 12 noon to 2.00pm). There is disabled access. *Contact*: Mrs Jill Loader, manager.

Address: Citizens' Advice Bureau, 38, Sackville Road, Bexhill, East Sussex, TN39 3JE. *Tel*: 01424 734549. *Fax:* 01424 734513. [Jun 2000]

Friends of Bexhill & Rother CAB
Contact: Clive Loader. *Address*: Friends of Bexhill & Rother CAB, 10, Broadoak Lane, Bexhill, TN39 4HE. *Tel*: 01424 218165. [Jul 2000]

Bexhill Hospital CAB

'Outreach' sessions.Every Tuesday from 10 to 12 noon. Held in the relatives' room. *Address:* Bexhill Hospital, Holliers Hill, Bexhill, Sussex. *Tel:* 01424 215055. [Jul 2000]

Burwash CAB

Hours: 'Outreach' sessions. Open on Mondays only between 2.30 and 4.30pm. *Address*: Citizens' Advice Bureau, Fairfield Doctors Surgery, Burwash, Sussex. *Tel*: 01424 215055. [Jul 2000]

Camber CAB

'Outreach' sessions. *Hours:* Tuesdays, 10am-12noon. *Address:* GP Surgery, Camber. *Contact:* Sandra Garner, manager. *Tel:* 01424 430400. [Jul 2000]

Hastings & Rother CAB

Clients may call at the office during normal hours or they can make an appointment by telephone. The CAB is located in the town centre a few minutes walk from British Rail Station.

Hours: Mondays to Fridays 10.00am to 1.00pm when clients may simply walk in without an appointment; and from 2.00 to 4.00pm with an appointment. On Wednesday the office is open from 5 to 7pm for appointments only. There is disabled access.

Facts about Hastings CAB: The Bureau dealt with 17,500 enquiries in 1999. All of the generalist advisers are volunteers. 80% of the admin. workers are volunteers. The volunteers give over 10,000 hours per year to the community by working in this Bureau.

Contacts: Sandra Garner, manager; Jan Waller, deputy manager.

Address: Hastings and Rother Citizens Advice Bureau, 24, Cornwallis Terrace, Hastings, East Sussex, TN34 1EB. *Tel*: 01424 430400. *Appointments:* 01424 718882. *Fax:* 01424 442253. [5214]

Herstmonceux CAB

'Outreach' sessions. *Tel*: 01424 215055 and 734549. [Jul 2000]

Robertsbridge CAB

Hours: 'Outreach' sessions. Friday only between 10.00am and 12 noon. *Address*: Citizens' Advice Bureau, c/o Robertsbridge Community Hall, Robertsbridge, East Sussex. *Tel*: 01424 215055. [Jul 2000]

Rye CAB

Hours: Mondays 10am to 12.15pm and Wednesdays from 2.00 to 4pm. Appointments may be made via the Hastings office.

Address: Citizens' Advice Bureau, 1st floor, 48, Cinque Ports Street, Rye, TN31 7AN. *Tel*: 01797 223746, during opening times only. At other times please call the Hastings office. *Tel*: 01424 430400. [5214]

Sedlescombe CAB

'Outreach' sessions. Wednesdays only from 2 to 4pm. *Address:* The Village Hall, Sedlescombe, Sussex. *Tel*: 01424 215055 and 734549. [Jul 2000]

Ticehurst CAB

'Outreach' sessions. *Tel*: 01424 215055 and 734549. Wednesdays only from 10 to 12 noon. *Address:* The Annexe, High Street, Sussex. May 2000

Local Organisations

HARC

HARC is the Hastings Advice & Representation Centre. Their mission is 'To relieve local poverty and improve the quality of life for people on a low income.

Our aims

To ensure the correct benefit is received by those on a low income; to protect the rights of employees; to facilitate a return to employment; to assist disabled people to live independently; to provide free educational courses and to give practical help to the homeless.

Our objectives

To provide comprehensive information on all welfare benefits and employment law; to provide impartial confidential advice by telephone, drop-in service, appointments and home visits. To represent clients at: Social Security Appeal Tribunals, Disability Appeal Tribunals, Medical Appeal Tribunals, Employment Tribunals and Commissioners.

Rural Outreach

In addition to our Advice Centre services we offer a Rural Outreach Service in Rother seeing clients at home or in rural surgeries in various locations. This service is intended for people with physical disabilities or mental health problems who are unable to visit the Centre. Home visits in Hastings are also available on request, but these are limited to staff availability.

Patron: Michael Mansfield QC. Manager: Jacky Everard. Devolpment worker: Sandra Lewis. Advice workers: Clive Edwards, Donna Jenkinson, Sue Paquette, Debbie Hunt, Beverly Banks. Rural Outreach adviser: Teresa Andrews. Reception/Admin: Ian Harries & Geoff Elliot.

HARC Advice Centre

Address: HARC, 8, Cambridge Road, Hastings, East Sussex, TN34 1DJ. *Tel:* 01424 428375. *Fax:* 01424 423266. *E-mail:* harc@bt.internet.com 5031

HARC Shops

HARC also operates two charity shops in Queens Road, Hastings, and London Road, St Leonards-on-Sea, which help raise funds for our work. Both shops welcome donations of clothing, books and bric-a-brac as well as offers of voluntary help.

Opportunities exist for shop staff, 'back room' staff and volunteer drivers. Expenses are available if required. For further information contact Sandra Lewis on 01424 718056.

Address: HARC, 186, Queens Road, Hastings, East Sussex, TN34 1RG; and London Road, St Leonards-on-Sea, East Sussex, TN37 6AN. *Tel*: 01424 722164 or 01424 720500. 5867

Oasis

Ore Advice Support Information Service. For all residents of the Ore Valley. Legal and benefit help, information, library, education and careers guidance, health advice. *Contact*: Clare Croft, co-ordinator.

Address: Oasis, 46/48, Chiltern Drive, Hastings, Sussex, TN34 3PZ. *Tel*: 01424 448141. *E-mail*: claremarion@aol.com 5273 May 2000

Trinity Project

If you wish to talk about the problems you are experiencing with substances, or as a family member or friend you would like advice, then the Trinity Project may be able to help. For full details of the Trinity Project see 'Substance Misuse' chapter, page 137.

National Organisations

Citizens' Advice Bureaux

For information on the CAB Service nationally. *Address:* National Association of Citizens' Advice Bureaux, Myddelton House, 115, Pentonville Road, London N1 9LZ. *Tel:* 020 7833 2181. *Fax:* 020 7833 4371. *Website:* www.adviceguide.org.uk - for 24 hour online CAB information and advice. May 2000

See also these chapters ...

Money, page 91.
Information, page 220.
Legal Matters, page 223.

Acknowledgements
Our grateful thanks to the staff of Hastings & Rother Citizens Advice Bureau for providing editorial assistance with this chapter.

Advocacy

An advocate is someone who can represent and defend the views, needs, wishes, worries and rights of individuals who do not feel able to do this themselves. [5251]

"Within mental health services, an advocate is someone who can represent and defend the views, needs, wishes, worries and rights of individuals who do not feel able to do this themselves.

Advocacy can also support service users to participate in and make decisions. Advocates are wholly independent; they represent their client's without taking a view on their best interests." [5091]

What an advocate can do

The emphasis is on the pursuit of the individual's rights which, if necessary, will be pursued in an adversarial context. In particular, mental health advocates:

- assist clients to express their views and needs, e.g. at a ward round in relation to their care and treatment;
- can provide support for patients detained under the Mental Health Act at a Hospital Manager's Review or Mental Health Review Tribunal;
- support clients to make comments or complaints about the services they receive;
- ensure clients can access specialist legal advice where appropriate;
- support clients to access health/social care professionals and other relevant agencies, e.g. welfare rights and Citizens, Advice Bureaux;
- gather information to allow clients to make an informed choice;
- do not provide counselling, therapy or other forms of care and treatment. [5091]

Patients' Charter 2001

The NHS National Plan, announced by the government in July 2000, says that by 2002 there will be an NHS-wide Patients' Advocacy & Liaison Service in every major hospital. [6042 Jul 2000]

Local Organisations

Advocacy Centre

This is now known as South East Advocacy Projects. Please see separate paragraph.

Children & young people

For advocacy services for children and young people see under 'Xpress', page 155.

Mental Health Advocacy

Mental Health Advocacy is a project of South East Advocacy Projects. It exists to represent the views of users of mental health services, or to help them to express their views themselves. The current service is confined to Hastings and Rother, but it is hoped to extend mental health advocacy throughout East Sussex.

The Mental Health Advocacy Project (MHAP) is staffed by Anne Dawson and Geoff Barnes. Anne says, "We provide advocacy support to people aged 16 to 65 who are currently receiving service from the Hastings & Rother NHS Trust." Anne explains that 'currently' would include anyone who has received service over the last two years.

The sort of support given by the MHAP includes: accompanying clients on appointments with psychiatrists, supporting clients at ward rounds, managers' hearings, and so on. Allison Peterson is county co-ordinator.

Address: Mental Health Advocacy Project, 42, Robertson Street, Hastings, East Sussex, TN34 1HL. *Tel*: 01424 441597. *Fax:* 01424 204687. [5923]

South East Advocacy Projects

South East Advocacy Projects started as the Advocacy Centre which was set up in 1992 as part of Hastings Voluntary Action. In April 2000 the various projects came together as one charity, South East Advocacy Projects. There are seven paid workers spread between three departments:

- Xpress Advocacy Service,
- My Choice,
- Mental Health Advocacy Project. Please see separate entries for each of these departments. [5935]

My Choice

My Choice is part of South East Advocacy Projects and is for people with learning disabilities. My Choice joins together the former projects Speak Out, Lewes; Speak Out, Eastbourne; Our Voice, Wealden and Partners in Advocacy, Hastings. County manager is Trudy Allen. *Contact:* Trudy Allen, county manager, My Choice. *Address:* The Advocacy Centre, 42, Robertson Street, Hastings, East Sussex, TN34 1HL. *Tel:* 01424 441597. [5100 Jul 2000]

My Choice, Eastbourne
Address: My Choice, 8, Saffrons Road, Eastbourne, Sussex, BN21 1DG. *Tel*: 01323 417926. [5100]

My Choice, Hastings
My Choice, The Advocacy Centre, 42, Robertson Street, Hastings, East Sussex, TN34 1HL. *Tel:* 01424 441562. [Jul 2000]

My Choice, Lewes
Address: My Choice, 66, High Street, Lewes, Sussex, BN7 1XG. *Tel*: 01273 477700. [5100]

My Choice, Wealden
Address: My Choice, 1st Floor, 2 The Broadway, Crowborough, East Sussex, TN6 1DF. *Tel:* 01892 668830. [Jul 2000]

Xpress

A free, independent and confidential ad-vocacy and information service for children and young people aged up to 21 living in Hastings and Rother especially those in foster care or who 'present complex and/or multiple issues and needs'. Advocates support for young people in having a voice in the way they are cared for, in decisions that are made about their lives and in accessing complaints procedures.

Xpress, Eastbourne.
Address: Xpress Eastbourne, EAVS, 8, Saffrons Road, Eastbourne, East Sussex, BN21 1DG. *Tel:* 01323 733111. [5923]

Xpress, Hastings.
Hours: Office: Mondays to Fridays 8.30am to 5.00pm. *Freephone Helpline*: Mondays & Wednesdays 6.30pm to 9.00pm. *Contact*: Jill Miles, project manager; Sallie Thomsett, deputy manager.

Address: Xpress Advocacy Service, 42, Robertson Street, Hastings, East Sussex, TN34 1HL. *Tel:* 01424 441597; 01424 440118. *Helpline:* 0800 454424. [Jul 2000]

HARC

Hastings Advice and Representation Centre. Please see under Advice chapter, page 152. [Jun 2000]

National Organisations

CAIT

CAIT (Citizen Advocacy Information & Training). Citizen advocacy is the offer of sustained, individual and freely given support and representation by one citizen to another. The person seeking a citizen advocate may be someone who is excluded from or marginalised within their own community and is unable or unwilling to voice their views and wishes.

Address: CAIT, Unit 64, Lee Valley Technopark, Ashley Road, Tottenham Hale, London, N17 9LN. *Tel:* 020 8880 4545. *Fax:* 020 8880 4113. E-mail: cait@teleregion.co.uk Website: www.citizenadvocacy.org.uk June 2000

Director: Sally Carr. National Development Team (South): Allison McClean. National Development Team (North): Joe Monaghan. Volunteers: Juanita Michael & Robin Lomas.

Survivors Speak Out

Provides a contact point for people who are survivors of the mental health services. Contact: Rob Ford, *tel:* 0116 255 2309. *Address:* Survivors Speak Out, 34, Osnaburgh Street, London, NW1 3ND. Aug 2000

UK Advocacy Network

UKAN is a network of user-led groups involved in advocacy, patient councils, service planning etc. It exists as a two-way process, supporting user groups with advice and examples of good practice, and also acts at a national level to pass on views from grass-roots to the highest levels of the mental health system. The UKAN helped develop 'Advocacy - a code of practice', published by NHS Executive Mental Health Task Force User Group in February 2000, written by Edna Conlan and others. Edna Conlan is founder chair of UKAN. "A civilization is measured by its treatment of its most vulnerable groups. We must remember that citizens in care are no less citizens and their voices should be heard, their views respected and their interests defended." Edna Conlan. 6049 Feb 2000

Address: United Kingdom Advocacy Network, Volserve House, 14-18, West Bar Green, Sheffield, S1 2DA. *Tel/Fax:* 0114 272 8171.

E-mail: ukan@can-online.org.uk *Website:* www.comcom.org/ukan Jul 2000

Further Information

Guidelines

'Guidelines on Advocacy for Mental Health Workers'. By Jim Read and Jan Wallcraft. Published by Mind/Unison, 1995. 28 pages. Price £2.50. This book explains why advocacy in mental health is necessary, clarifies the distinction between service providers and independent advocates and gives guidance on how they can work together. Mind Mail Order Service. *Tel:* 020 8221 9666.

Factsheet

'Key facts about advocacy'. By Katherine Dunton. Published by Mind, Nov. 1998. Price £0.50. Available from Mind Mail Order Service. *Tel:* 020 8221 9666.

Acknowledgements

Our grateful thanks to Anne Dawson, Trudy Allen and Jill Miles of South East Advocacy Projects for editorial assistance with this chapter.

Befriending

Befriending is the provision of quality support of a friendly nature intended to lessen a person's sense of personal or social isolation.

Local Organisations

Befriending Scheme, Hastings

This is run by the APCMI (Assn for the Pastoral Care of the Mentally Ill which provides a one-to-one befriending service to people in the community who have bec-ome isolated as a result of mental health problems.

The organisation recruits and trains volunteers who are prepared to befriend someone for 1 to 2 hours a week. APCMI seek to promote a better understanding of mental illness among the general public. They co-operate fully with other statutory and non-statutory organisations working in the field of mental health.

Address: Association for the Pastoral Care of the Mentally Ill, 49, Cambridge Gardens, Hastings, Sussex, TN34 1EN. *Tel:* 01424 424152. *E-mail*: apcmi@beeb.net

Office hours are Mondays to Thursdays, 9.30 to 12.30 pm; there is an answerphone service outside these hours. Chairman: Rev. B Trill; Secretary: Mrs M Moss; Treasurer: Mr D Harding; Co-ordinator: Ms C Jowitt. Contact: Lynn Jenkins: Administrator. [6055]
May 2000

Befrienders needed!

The APCMI (Association for the Pastoral Care of the Mentally Ill) needs volunteers. Volunteers undertake a commitment to visit their friend for 1-2 hours a week and attend monthly group meetings and regular supervision sessions with the co-ordinator (for an initial period of 1 year). All expenses incurred are covered by APCMI. Recruitment takes place twice a year. A seven week part-time induction training programme must be attended prior to selection, (see below). In the first instance please contact Lynn Jenkins. [5189]

Training programme

The aims of the training programme run by the APCMI are to:

- Provide an account of the origins and background of the befriending scheme.
- Encourage participants to explore the values of human relationships and learn more about mental health issues, providing an opportunity to consider their commitment to volunteering. At the end of this foundation programme candidates will be asked to attend a selection interview prior to being accepted as a befriender. The training programme is free to all who wish to attend and participants will not be committing themselves to volunteering by attending the course. Anyone interested should please ring Lynn Jenkins on 01424 424152, and leave your name and address on the answerphone. [5189]

Hastings Befrienders

This organisation is not a 'befriending group' as the term is usually understood. It has changed its name to 'Gay Helpline Hastings'. Please see 'Sex' chapter, page 119.[5987]

National Organisations

Befrienders International

Befrienders International is a network of over 300 befriending centres world-wide. Trained volunteers are used and the service offered is free, confidential and non-judgmental. People are befriended by telephone and in meetings face-to-face and by letter and e-mail. Founded 1974 by Chad Varah, CBE.

Address: Befrienders International, 26/27, Market Place, Kingston-upon-Thames, Surrey, KT1 1JH. *Tel:* 020 8541 4949. *Fax:* 020 8549 1544. *Website:* www.befrienders.org [6059 Aug 2000]

Acknowledgements
Our grateful thanks to Lynn Jenkins of APCMI for editorial assistance with this chapter. [Jan & Mar 2000]

Carers

Caring can mean giving emotional, practical or physical support to a relative, a friend or neighbour. It can be difficult and painful, but it can also be very rewarding. Carers need all the help they can get, and information, support and acknowledgement can make a great difference. [0534]

Carers' rights & expectations

The National Service Framework for Mental Health, 1999 states, under standard 6 (Caring about Carers), all individuals who provide regular and substantial care for a person on CPA should:

- Have an assessment of their caring, physical and mental health needs, repeated on at least an annual basis.
- Have their *own written care plan* whichi is given to them and implemented in discussion with them.

What carers should expect

The following is taken from *Information for carers of people with mental health problems,* published by the Basingstoke & Alton Mental Health Carers Empowerment Forum in June 1996:

- A prompt and positive response when you ask for help or an assessment.
- Information and help as soon as it becomes clear that you are providing care for someone with mental health problems.
- Help in understanding the nature of the mental illness that the person you care for has and how it affects them and the people they come into contact with.
- An explanation of the treatments available, how they work and any likely side-effects.
- Details of what services are available (including services provided by voluntary organisations) and how to get them.
- Advice on how best to cope with the effects of mental illness on the person you care for.
- Information about your rights and those of the person you care for, particularly under the Mental Health and Social Security Acts.
- Involvement in the assessment of the person you care for, unless he or she has asked that you should not be involved.
- To be dealt with courteously and with respect and to have your point of view listened to.
- To choose to have someone to help you put your point of view across in discussions with Health and Social Services staff.
- To be told how the information you give will be used by the people who provide services.

Please see also 'Your Rights' chapter, page 269. [5291]

Local Organisations

Association of Carers

A relief sitting service in Hastings, St Leonards, Bex-hill and surrounding area, on a regular basis in the client's home. Volunteers are willing to sit with someone who is unable to be left on their own through illness or disability, offering companionship and friendly support, and enabling the carer some free time. Volunteers are not asked to carry out tasks or nursing duties.

Assessments

Other help and support is offered to our carers internally. Anyone may apply direct to the organisation by telephone or in person. Assessments are carried out in the carer's home There is no charge for the service provided. *Contacts*: David Southerden, Fundraiser/PR Manager; Yvonne Hartnoll, Services Manager. 5417

Address: Association of Carers, Theaklin Drive, St Leonards-on-Sea, East Sussex, TN38 9AZ. *Tel*: 01424 722309. *Fax:* 01424 422522. Registered Charity No. 1004055. 5432 May 2000

Care for the Carers

Care for the Carers is a registered charitable company set up in 1989. We work right across East Sussex, Brighton and Hove. Our head office is in Lewes and we have four area offices, addresses below. Registered Charity No. 1074906.

What we do

We work to support all those people who look after sick or disabled relatives, friends, neighbours, partners or children in their own homes. There are an estimated 47,000 carers in East Sussex and 25,000 in Brighton & Hove aged over 16.

How we do it

We work closely with social services and the health authority to ensure that, as far as possible, the services these organisations provide satisfies carers' real needs.

Carers' forums

These are regular informal meetings where carers and the health professionals come together to exchange news and views, needs, comments and criticisms. This ensures carers' needs and views get fed directly into the service planning process.

Information

Information on a wide variety of topics including getting help at home, social security benefits, arranging a break from caring, support groups, counselling, legal matters and much more. There is a free magazine, Careline.

Hastings & Rother Office

Address: Care for the Carers Ltd, 49, Cambridge Gardens, Hastings, Sussex, TN34 1EN. *Tel*: 01424 717931. *Fax:* 01424 439179. *E-mail:* jan@hastingscarers-freeserve.co.uk Jul 2000

Lewes District Office

Address: Care for the Carers, Chandlers Wharf, Railway Lane, Lewes, Sussex, BN7 2AQ. *Tel*: 01273 486625/486641. *Fax*: 01273 486554. *E-mail:* liz@cfclewes.freeserve.co.uk Jul 2000

Brighton & Hove Office

Address: Care for the Carers, Community Base, 113-117, Queens Road, Brighton, Sussex, BN1 3XG. *Tel*: 01273 234758. *Fax*: 01273 234757. *E-mail:* cfcbton@freenet.co.uk Jul 2000

Eastbourne, Seaford & Wealden Office

Contact: Anna Geall. *Address*: Care for the Carers, Heffle Court Annexe, 1, Station Road, Heathfield, Sussex, TN21 8DR. *TelFax*: 01435 862376. *E-mail:* anna@hefflecarers.fsnet.co.uk 5064 Jul 2000

Bexhill Caring Community

The Caring Community offers visits to the lonely and housebound; shopping, collecting pensions and odd jobs depending on the need; a library service for the housebound; occasional outings, usually in the summer; assistance with heating and other expenses at the discretion of the Administrator; wheelchair outing for shopping once a month; taped music and book library; bath service.; dial-a-ride service (small charge made). Registered Charity No. 250517.

Contact: Mrs Jill Halsall, Administrator. *Hours:* Mondays to Thursdays 10 to 12 noon and 2 to 4pm; Fridays 10 to 12 noon. *Address*: Bexhill Caring Community, 38, Sackville Road, Bexhill, TN39 3JE. *Tel*: 01424 215116. 5506 Jul 2000

Careline

To provide confidential telephone counselling throughout the UK for children, young people and adults. Chairman: Angela Sharp; Administrator: Sarah Moore.

Address: Careline, Cardinal Heenan Centre, 326, High Road, Ilford, Essex, IG1 1QP. *Tel*: 020 8514 5444. *Fax:* 020 8478 7943. *Helpline*: 020 8514 1177. May 2000

MDFF

Manic Depression Friends & Family Support Group. For full details of this support group, please see in 'Manic Depression' chapter, page 84.

Crossroads

This is a major registered charity which provides practical support and care for carers. Its objective is to relieve the stresses of carers - people who care for relatives or friends who have disability or illness. Carers are of all ages and have differing needs. Crossroads provides the service based on carers' needs. It has regional centres throughout the UK. *Contacts*: Mrs Janet Cackett, manager; Ken Saunders, development worker; Jen Batchelor, assessor; Graham Barnell, chairman/trustee; Barry Turnwell, company secretary/trustee.

Address: Hastings & Rother Crossroads Care Attendant Scheme Limited, 135, Hughenden Road, Hastings, Sussex, TN34 3TF. *Tel*: 01424 444964. *Fax:* 01424 435972. *E-mail:* crossroads@hastingsrother.freeserve.co.uk Registered Charity No. 1060552. May 2000

Young Carers' Project

This is a special service which supports young people up to 18 who look after family members. *Contact:* Wendy McGowan-Griffin, project co-ordinator.

Address: Ground Floor, Glebe House, Rotten Row, Lewes, Sussex, BN7 1TN. *Tel*: 01273 487723 & 01424 446663. *Fax:* 01273 480397. *E-mail:* wendy@esussexyoungcarers.fsbusiness.co.uk Jul 2000

National Organisations

Carers' National Association

The CNA has a telephone helpline for carers of elderly, ill or disabled relatives and friends. CNA works to improve recognition and services for carers by drawing carers' issues to the attention of government and other policy makers. The CNA publishes many excellent free booklets. Please telephone for a list.

Address: Carers' National Association, 20, Glasshouse Yard, London, EC1A 4JT. *Tel*: 020 7490 8818. *Fax*: 020 7490 8824. *Free helpline*: 0808 808 7777 (10 am to 12 noon & 2 pm to 4pm Mondays to Fridays).
E-mail: internet@ukcarers.org
Website: www.carersnorth.demon.co.uk Jul 2000

Carers' Line

Carers' Line. Advice and information for all carers. Call free on 0808 808 7777. Aug 2000

Crossroads

For details of the work of this charity, please see under 'Local Organisations', above.

Address: Crossroads Association. *Contact*: Carolyn Robb. *Address*: Crossroads Association, 10, Regent Place, Rugby, CV21 2PN. *Tel*: 01788 573653. May 2000

NARMI

The National Alliance of the Relatives of the Mentally Ill, (NARMI) offers support and advocacy to those with mental health problems and their carers. It specialises in welfare benefit, mental health legislation and acts as a campaigning organisation.

Contacts: Pamela Jenkinson, chairman; Ray Missell, treasurer; Mrs Pearl Baker, secretary/director.

Address: 'Tydehams Oaks', Tydehams, Newbury, Berkshire, RG14 6JT. *Tel*: 01635 551923. *Fax*: 01635 550229. *E-mail:* pearl-baker@talk21.com May 2000

NSF

The National Schizophrenia Fellow-ship employs Suzy Levy full-time, based at Hove, with responsibility for all of East Sussex. She provides support for carers of people with manic depression and schizophrenia. For further details please see 'Carers' Support' in the Schizophrenia chapter, page 113. Jul 2000

Princess Royal Trust for Carers

The Princess Royal Trust for Carers (PRTC) is establishing a network of carers' centres across the UK providing information, advice and support to all carers, irrespective of the illness or disability of the cared-for. There are currently (July 2000) 96 such centres in the UK. *Contact*: Jean Collingwood.

Address: The Princess Royal Trust for Carers, 142, Minories, London, EC3N 1LB. *Tel*: 020 7480 7788. *Fax*: 020 7481 4729. *E-mail:* info@carers.org *Website:* www.carers.org Jul 2000

Further Information

Benefits

What's available and how to get them. 16 page booklet. Published by the Carers National Association. Free. *Tel:* 020 7490 8810. 6044

Carers' Resource List

By Louise Flory. Published by MIND Information Unit, March 1999. £1. Available from Mind Mail Order Service. *Tel*: 020 8221 9666.

Comfort for Carers

MDF Factsheet. Leaflet published by the MDF.

How do I get help?

A carer's guide to assessments. 24 page booklet. Published by the Carers National Association. Free. *Tel:* 020 9490 8818. 6045

Living with Mental Illness

Written by Liz Kuipers & Paul Bebbington. Published by Souvenir Press. A book for relatives and friends. Price £9.99; available from the MDF. *Tel:* 020 7793 2600.

Taking a break

Everyone needs a change and some time off occasionally, whether it's for an hour, a day or a week. This 20 page, free booklet shows how you *can* get a break. Published by the Carers National Association. *Tel:* 020 9490 8818. 6046

Acknowledgements
Our grateful thanks to Sandy Lazarus of Care for the Carers for editorial assistance with this chapter.

Chemists

Pharmacies

Pharmacy: the practice or art of preparing or dispensing drugs; from Greek pharmakon, drug. 0526

Pharmacists (or chemists), are experts in medicines. They dispense prescriptions given to you by your GP. They can advise you about these medicines, how to take them and possible side effects. You can also ask your pharmacist for advice about medicines sold 'over the counter' and for advice about health problems and minor illnesses. A pharmacist will refer you to a GP if a prescription is needed or a serious illness is suspected. 5047

Prescription charges

The current NHS prescription charge is £6.00 for each medicine. NHS prescriptions are free for patients under 16 years of age; patients under 19 years of age and in full time education; men and women aged 60 years and over; patients with a current exemption certificate (FP92); patients or their partners currently receiving Income Support; patients or their partners currently receiving Full Working Families Tax Credit or Credit reduced by £70 or less; patients or their partners currently receiving Full Disabled Persons Tax Credit or Credit reduced by £70 or less; patients or their partners who hold a current NHS charges certificate for full help (AG2); patients who are War/Service Pensioners with an exemption certificate. 5041

Free prescriptions?

From April 1999, people between 16 and 60 who claim free prescriptions will be asked to provide proof that they are entitled to do so.

Not sure if you qualify for free prescriptions? Call the Adviceline for advice and guidance. Adviceline - *Tel:* 0800 91 77 711. Jul 2000

Prepayment Certificates

The 'season ticket' for prescriptions. You can save time and money by using these 'season tickets'. A four month one costs £31.40 and a 12 month one costs £86.20. Anyone who has to pay for their NHS prescriptions can buy one. Simply get a form from the post office or pharmacist, fill it in and return it to the pharmacist with payment. You will get your prepayment certificate straightaway. You can also order them direct from East Sussex Brighton & Hove Health Authority at 36-38 Friars Walk, Lewes, Sussex, BN27 2PB. Make cheques payable to 'HM Paymaster General'. 6084 ESB-HHA

Prescription collection service

A new service offered by Boots. If you take prescribed medication regularly you will know how long it can take to order a prescription, collect it from your doctor's surgery, visit your local pharmacy and wait for it to be dispensed.

Boots can collect prescriptions from the surgery on your behalf and have your medication ready for you to pick up at an agreed time.

To arrange for your repeat prescription to be collected, fill in your details on the registration form provided and give the completed form to the pharmacist who will explain how the prescription collection service works in your area.

Next time you require a prescription, simply order it from your doctor's surgery as usual and follow the guidelines given to you or by your local store.

Your medication will be ready for you to collect at your Boots store at an agreed time. 5040

Medilink

A scheme run by all branches of Boots. If you join their patient medication record scheme - Medilink - they can keep a confidential record of your dispensed medicines for you at your request, no matter which of their pharmacies you call into. [5042]

Local Chemists

This section of the directory lists all the chemists where prescriptions may be fulfilled, including those in supermarkets. Details given include times of opening, names of resident pharmacists, with qualifications, telephone numbers, e-mail addresses, website addresses and any other useful information. The list is arranged alphabetically by town for easy reference.

Battle

Boots The Chemists

The pharmacist is Miss S M Wright, MRPharmS. Shop opening hours are 9am to 5.30pm Mondays to Saturdays. Closed Sundays. There is wheelchair access.

Address: Boots The Chemists, 8, High Street, Battle, Sussex, TN33 0AE. *Tel*: 01424 772010. [Jun 2000]

Moss Chemists

The pharmacist presently is a locum only.

Hours:

Mon	9am to 7.00pm
Tue.	9am to 7.00pm
Wed	9am to 6.30pm
Thur.	9am to 7.00pm
Fri	9am to 7.00pm
Sat	9am to 5.00pm
Sun	Closed

Address: Moss Chemists, 21-22, High Street, Battle, Sussex, TN33 OAE. *Tel*: 01424 772069. *Fax:* 01424 775047. [Jul 2000]

Bexhill

Boots The Chemists

The pharmacist is Ms Janet Crawford, MRPharmS. Opening hours are Monday to Saturdays 9am to 5.30pm. Closed on Sundays. There is wheelchair access via lift to the first floor. Special services include advice to Residential Homes and Nursing Homes and monitored dosage system. *Address*: Boots The Chemists, 14-16, Devonshire Road, Bexhill, Sussex, TN40 1AS. *Tel*: 01424 734788. Website: www.boots.co.uk. [5143]

Collington Pharmacy

The pharmacist is Mr Patel, MRPharmS. Opening hours are Monday to Friday 9am to 6.30pm and 9am to 1pm on Saturdays. Closed on Sundays.

Address: Collington Pharmacy, 4, Collington Mansions, Bexhill, Sussex, TN39 3PU. *Tel/Fax*: 01424 220232. [Jul 2000]

Collis, L J.

The pharmacist is Mrs Sara Cook, B.Sc, MRPharmsS. The hours of opening are Mondays to Saturdays 8.45am to 5.30pm and are closed on Sundays. There is a free delivery service. There is wheelchair access.

Address: L J Collis (Paydens Ltd), 9-11, St Leonards Road, Bexhill, Sussex, TN40 1HJ. *Tel:* 01424 211341. [5153 May 2000]

Little Common Pharmacy

Opening times are Mondays to Fridays 9am to 6pm. Saturdays are 9am to 5pm and closed on Sundays.

Address: Little Common Pharmacy, 77, Cooden Sea Road, Little Common, Bexhill, Sussex, TN39 4SL. *Tel/Fax*: 01424 843080. [Jul 2000]

Lloyds Pharmacy

Opening hours are Mondays to Fridays 9am to 6.30pm. Saturdays are 9am to 12 noon. Closed on Sundays. There is wheelchair access.

Address: Lloyds Pharmacy, 15, De La Warr Road, Bexhill, Sussex, TN40 2HG. *Tel/Fax*: 01424 730309. [Jul 2000]

Lloyds Pharmacy

The pharmacist is a locum at present. The Manager is Sarah Goring, MRPharmS.

Shop opening times are Mondays to Fridays, 9am to 6pm; Saturdays 9am to 5.30pm and closed on Sundays. There is wheelchair access (ramp in front of shop).

Address: Lloyds Pharmacy, 60, Ninfield Road, Sidley, Bexhill, Sussex, TN39 5AB. *Tel/Fax*: 01424 220424. Jul 2000

Marsh Pharmacy

The pharmacist is Mr N H M Jiwani, B.Sc, MIPharmM, MRPharmS, Dip.Com.-Pharm. Hours of opening are Mondays to Fridays 9am to 7pm. Saturdays 9am to 5pm. Closed Sundays. There is wheelchair access.

Address: Marsh Pharmacy, Bexhill Mobility and Healthcare Centre, 30, St Leonards Road, Bexhill, Sussex, TN40 1HT. *Tel*: 01424 219516. *Fax*: 01424 732240.*E-mail*:marsh@healthcarespecialists.co.uk 5152

N Neate Chemists

The pharmacist is Mr N Neate MRPharmS. Shop opening hours are Mondays to Saturdays 9am to 5.30 pm. Closed Wednesday afternoons & Sundays.

Address: N Neate, 1b, Western Road, Bexhill, Sussex, TN40 1DU. *Tel*: 01424 219422. Jul 2000

Crowborough

Boots The Chemists

The pharmacist is Mr Jerry Brookman, MRPharmS. The opening hours are Mondays to Saturdays 9am to 5.30pm and closed on Sundays, but with a rota service every fourth Sunday. (See local press for details). There is wheelchair access.

Address: Boots The Chemists, 3, London House, High Street, Crowborough, Sussex, TN6 2QA. *Tel*: 01892 652714. *Fax:* 01892 667832. Jul 2000

Chappell Pharmacy

The pharmacist is Mr M Sharma, MRPharmS. Shop opening hours are Mondays to Fridays 8.30am to 7pm, Saturdays 9am to 5pm and closed on Sundays but with rota duty. (See local publication of details). Special services include oxygen collection and delivery and wheelchair access.

Address: Chappell Pharmacy & Chemist, 1-3, Croft Road, Crowborough, Sussex, TN6 1DL. *Tel/Fax:* 01892 652012. Jul 2000

St Denys Pharmacy

The pharmacist is Mrs Jane Ward, BSc.Ph., MRPharmS. Shop opening hours are Mondays to Thursdays from 9am to 5.30pm and Fridays to Saturdays 9am to 1pm. Lunch is taken from 1pm to 2.15pm.

Address: St Denys Pharmacy, Brook Health Centre, Crowborough Hill, Crowborough, Sussex, TN6 2ED. *Tel*: 01892 667284. Jul 2000

Hastings & St Leonards

Andersen's Pharmacy

The pharmacist is Mr Barry Power, B.Pharm., M.Sc., M.Pharm.S. Opening hours are Mondays to Fridays 9am to 5.30pm; closed 12.30pm to 2pm. Closed all day Saturdays and Sundays.

Address: J Andersen's Pharmacy, 164, Harold Road, Hastings, Sussex, TN35 5NH. *Tel*: 01424 721390. 5150 May 2000

Andersen's Pharmacy

Address: J Andersen's Pharmacy, 87, Mount Road, Hastings, Sussex. The pharmacist is Mr J Andersen, MRPharmS. Shop opening hours are:

Mon	9am to 5.30pm
Tue	9am to 5.30pm
Wed	9am to 1.00pm
Thur & Fri	9am to 5.30pm
Sat	9am to 1.00pm
Sun	Closed

Address: J Andersen's Pharmacy, 87, Mount Road, Hastings, Sussex, TN35 5LA. *Tel*: 01424 421191. 5150 May 2000

Bloom Pharmacy (Vantage)

The pharmacist is Mr Bloom MRPharmS. Shop opening hours are Mondays to Fridays 9.00am to 5.30pm and Saturdays 9.00am to 4.30pm. Closed on Sundays. A special range of items is offered on bath aids and walking aids. The shop has wheel-chair access.

Address: Bloom Pharmacy, 55-57, Bohemia Road, St Leonards, Sussex, TN37 6RE. *Tel/Fax*: 01424 421072. Jul 2000

Boots The Chemists

The pharmacist is Miss Jane Richards MRPharmS. The shop is open on Mondays to Saturdays 9.00am to 5.30pm and is closed on Sundays. Domicilliary Oxygen service offered during open hours.

Address: Boots The Chemists, 35-37, London Road, St Leonards, Sussex, TN37 6AJ. *Tel*: 01424 420769. *Fax:* 01424 712848. Jul 2000

Boots The Chemists

The pharmacist is Ann Cherry, (MRPharmS). Opening hours are Mondays to Saturdays 9am to 5.30pm, and Sundays 11am to 4.30pm. There is wheelchair access and other special services include a disabled toilet and mother and baby room.

Address: Boots The Chemists, Kings Walk, Priory Meadow Shopping Centre, Hastings, Sussex, TN34 1QP. *Tel*: 01424 718334. May 2000

Boots The Chemists

Opening hours are Mondays to Saturdays 9am to 5.30pm. Closed on Sundays. The shop is accessible for wheelchairs.

Address: Boots The Chemists, 17-19, Robertson Street, Hastings, Sussex,TN34 1HL. *Tel*: 01424 436111. May 2000

Day Lewis Porter's Chemist

Pharmacist is a locum; no manager has been appointed at present. Opening hours are Mondays to Fridays 9am to 6.15pm, with lunch from 1.00 to 2.15pm. Saturdays opening hours are 9am to 1pm.

Address: Day Lewis Porter's Chemist, 25, Mount Pleasant Rd, Hastings, TN34 3SB. *Tel/Fax*: 01424 422891. Jul 2000

Hirst, J L

The pharmacist is Mr G Delves, MRPharmS. Opening hours are:

Mon	9am to 6.00pm
Tue.	9am to 6.00pm
Wed	9am to 5.30pm
Thur & Fri	9am to 6.00pm
Sat	9am to 1.00pm
Sun	Closed

Closed for lunch from 1pm to 2.15pm on Mondays to Fridays.

Address: J L Hirst, 3, Parkstone Parade, Hastings, TN34 2PS. *Tel/Fax*: 01424 433541. Jul 2000

Laycock Chemists

Opening hours: Mondays to Fridays 9am to 6pm; Wednesdays 9am to 5.30pm; Saturdays 9am to 1pm; closed Sundays.

Address: Laycock Chemists, 30, Little Ridge Avenue, St Leonards, Sussex, TN37 6AJ. *Tel/Fax*: 01424 755395. Jul 2000

Lloyds Pharmacy

Opening hours: Mondays to Saturdays 9am to 5.30pm; closed Sundays.

Address: Lloyds Pharmacy, 128, Battle Road, Hollington, St Leonards, Sussex, TN37 7AN. *Tel/Fax:* 01424 851050. Jul 2000

Lloyds Pharmacy

Opening hours: Mondays to Fridays 8.45am to 6pm; Saturdays 9am to 5.30pm; closed Sundays.

Address: Lloyds Pharmacy, 39-41, Sedles-combe Road North, St Leonards, Sussex, TN37 7DA. *Tel/Fax*: 01424 421132. Jul 2000

Lloyds Pharmacy

This is a small pharmacy serving the local area. There is a locum serving this chemist with no manager appointed at present. Opening times are Mondays to Fridays

8.30am to 6.30pm. Closed for lunch from 1-2pm. Open on Saturdays from 9am to 1pm. Closed on Sundays.

Address: Lloyds Pharmacy, 25, The High Street, Hastings, Sussex, TN34 3EY. *Tel/Fax*: 01424 420944. May 2000

Safeway Supermarket

Hours of opening are: Mondays to Saturdays 9am to 9pm; Sundays 10am to 4pm; Closed 1.30 to 2.30pm. There is wheelchair access.

Address: Instore Pharmacy, Safeway Supermarket, Queens Road, Hastings, Sussex, TN34 1RN. *Tel*: 01424 445505. 5155 May 2000

Silchester Pharmacy

Opening hours: Mondays to Fridays 9am to 6pm; Saturdays 9am to 1pm; closed Sundays.

Address: Silchester Pharmacy, 4, Silchester Road, St Leonards, Sussex, TN38 0JB. *Tel/Fax*: 01424 436663. Jul 2000

Tesco

TESCO The pharmacist is Mr Brian Hunt, MR PharmS.

Address: Instore Pharmacy, Tesco Superstore, Churchwood Drive, St Leonards, Sussex, TN38 9RB. *Tel*: 01424 786449. May 2000

Theaker Chemists

Opening hours: Mondays to Saturdays 9am to 5.30pm; closed Sundays.

Address: Theaker Chemists, 8, York Buildings, Hastings, Sussex, TN34 1NN. *Tel/Fax*: 01424 428523. Jul 2000

Warrior Pharmacy

The pharmacist is Mr Brent Auld MRPharmS. Shop opening times are Mondays to Fridays 9am to 8pm, Saturdays 9am to 1pm and Sundays 10am to 12noon.

Address: Warrior Pharmacy, 27, Grand Parade, St Leonards, Sussex, TN37 7DN. *Tel/Fax*: 01424 446611. Jul 2000

West St Leonards Pharmacy

'Computerisation, recording of patient medication records, advising and visiting patients and helping nursing homes are our new roles.' Established 1889. Pharmacist: Brian Sullivan, B Pharm, MRPharmS.

Opening hours: Mondays to Fridays 9am to 1pm and 2 to 5.30pm; Saturdays 9am to 1pm; closed Sundays.

Address: West St Leonards Pharmacy, 7, Bexhill Road, St Leonards, Sussex, TN38 0AH. *Tel*: 01424 422020. *Fax*: 01424 442525. Jul 2000

Hawkhurst

Hawkhurst Pharmacy

Opening hours: Mondays to Fridays 9am to 7pm; Saturdays 9am to 5.30pm; closed Sundays and bank holidays.

Address: Hawkhurst Pharmacy, 1, The Colonnade, Hawkhurst, Kent, TN18 4ES. *Tel/Fax*: 01580 753222. Jul 2000

Heathfield

Proctor, A

Opening hours: Mondays to Fridays 9am to 1pm & 2 to 5.30pm; Wednesdays 9am to 1pm & 2 to 6.30pm; Saturdays 9am to 1pm & 2 to 5pm; closed Sundays.

Address: A Proctor & Son Ltd, 63, High Street, Heathfield, Sussex, TN21 8HU. *Tel*: 01435 862064. *Fax:* 01435 868038. Jul 2000

Proctor, A

Opening hours (alternate weeks): Mondays to Fridays 9am to 5.30pm & 9am to 6.30pm; Saturdays 9am to 5pm; alternate Sundays 11am to 12 noon.

Address: A Proctor & Son Ltd, Station Road, Heathfield, Sussex, TN21 8LD. *Tel*: 01435 862067. *Fax:* 01435 868039. Jul 2000

Ore

Ore Village Pharmacy

The pharmacy is able to provide oxygen therapy. There is wheelchair access. Hours:

Mon . . . . 9am to 5.30pm
Tue . . . . 9am to 5.30pm
Wed . . . . 9am to 1.00pm
Thur . . . . 9am to 5.30pm
Fri . . . . 9am to 5.30pm
Sat . . . . 9am to 5.30pm
Sun . . . . Closed

Address: Ore Village Pharmacy, 478, Old London Road, Ore, Hastings, Sussex, TN35 5BL. *Tel:* 01424 423314. May 2000

Laycock Chemists

Opening hours: Mondays to Saturdays 9am to5.30pm; closed Sundays.

Address: Laycock Chemists, 494 & 496 Old London Road, Ore, Hastings, Sussex, TN35 5BL. *Tel/Fax*: 01424 436778. Jul 2000

Robertsbridge

Robertsbridge Pharmacy

Opening hours: Mondays, Wednesdays & Thursdays 9am to 5.30pm; Tuesdays & Fridays 9am to 6.30pm; Saturdays 9am to 1pm; closed Sundays.

Address: Robertsbridge Pharmacy, 17-19, High Street, Robertsbridge, Sussex, TN32 5AE. *Tel*: 01580 880267. *Fax:* 01580 881161. Jul 2000

Rotherfield

St Denys Pharmacy

Pharmacist: Mr Charles Williams, MR PharmS, B Pharm. Opening times:

Mon . . . . 9am to 1pm, 2pm to 6.30pm.
Tues . . . . 9am to 1pm, 2pm to 6.30pm.
Wed . . . . 9am to 1pm, closed in pm.
Thur . . . . 9am to 1pm, 2pm to 6.30pm.
Fri . . . . 9am to 1pm, 2pm to 6pm.
Sat . . . . 9am to 1pm.

Address: St Denys Pharmacy, 24, High Street, Rotherfield, Sussex, TN6 3LJ. *Tel*: 01892 852352. Jul 2000

Rye

Boots The Chemists

Address: Boots The Chemists, 18-20, High Street, Rye, Sussex, TN31 7JF. *Tel*: 01797 222308. May 2000

Moss Chemists

Shop opening times are Mondays to Fridays from 9.00am to 5.30pm, with alternate weeks 6.30pm closing (see press for details). Open on Saturdays from 9.00am to 5.30pm and on Sundays from 11.00am to 1.00pm.

Address: Moss Chemists, 17, High Street, Rye, Sussex, TN31 7JF. *Tel/Fax*: 01797 222241. Jul 2000

Tenterden

Boots The Chemists

Opening hours: Mondays to Saturdays 9am to 5.30pm; closed Sundays.

Address: Boots The Chemists, 1, Eastwell High Street, Tenterden, Sussex, TN30 6AH. *Tel:* 01580 763239. Jul 2000

N C C Chemists

Opening hours: Mondays to Fridays 9am to 5.30pm; Saturdays 9am to 5pm; closed Sundays.

Address: NCC Chemists Ltd, 35, High Street, Tenterden, Kent, TN30 6BJ. *Tel*: 01580 763313. Jul 2000

Wadhurst

Martel, P J & R

Address: P J & R Martel Ltd, The Pharmacy, High Street, Wadhurst, TN5 6AP. *Tel*: 01892 782058. 5154

Further Information

Getting The Most From Your Pharmacist

Factsheet published by Mind, 1996, price £0.50 available from Mind, 020 8221 9666.

Health Information Service

The HIS is a free and confidential 24-hour service. You can speak to staff during office hours, and you can listen to any of hundreds of tapes at any time, e.g: *Pharmacists* (Tape 253); *NHS benefits for prescriptions/dentists* (Tape 389).

Address: The College of Health, St Margaret's House, 21, Old Ford Road, London, E2 9PL. *Freephone*: 0800 66 55 44. [5367]

Websites

Pharmacy2u

An internet pharmacy, launched Nov. 99, which sells private prescriptions such as anti-obesity drugs, the impotence remedy Viagra as well as over-the-counter products. Would-be purchasers must supply prescriptions from their own doctors for some preparations.

Managing director is Daniel Lee. Users of the service must first e-mail the name and quantity of the prescribed drug. If they are satisfied with an e-mailed price quote, they post their prescription to the pharmacy.

Customers who want to buy non-prescription medicines must answer a questionnaire. This is examined by a pharmacist, who decides if the sale should go ahead.

Clients who want advice on a drug or about their symptoms can call a freephone number and talk to one of the online pharmacists. The service costs £2.50 but is free for orders over £40. *Website:* www.phamacy2u.co.uk. Freephone: 0800 100 2531. [5197, 5204]

Allcures

An internet pharmacy. *Website:* www.allcures.com

Complaining

Most mental health professionals will listen to your point of view and try to provide a good service. But things can go wrong ... which is when you may need to check out the advice in this chapter.

Most mental health professionals will listen to your point of view and try to provide a good service. But things can go wrong, or you may disagree with decisions they make.

If this happens, first try talking to the person concerned, or to the senior person on duty at the time. If you don't get anywhere, you should consider making a complaint.

It may be helpful to talk it over with somebody from the Advocacy Service, Hastings Mind, or the Community Health Council who can all help you in making a complaint. [5224]

Doctors & other professionals

The General Medical Council (GMC) licenses all doctors to practise medicine in the UK. Their purpose is summed up in the phrase 'Protecting patients, guiding doctors.' The law gives them four main functions: keeping up-to-date registers of qualified doctors; fostering good medical practice; promoting high standards of medical education; dealing firmly and fairly with doctors whose fitness to practise is in doubt.

If you have a complaint about your doctor or a member of the practice staff, try speaking to the individual concerned or to the practice manager first.

If you think your doctor (or another health professional) has behaved unethically, unprofessionally or incompetently, complain directly to their professional body.

For doctors this is the General Medical Council, for address, see below.

For nurses this is the UK Central Council

5224 Jun 1999; 6005 Jul 2000

Local Councillors

If your complaint is about the lack of a service, your local councillor is the best person to contact.

Members of Parliament

Hastings & Rye

Michael Foster, DL, MP. *Address:* Ellen Draper Centre, 84, Bohemia Road, St Leonards, Sussex, TN37 6RN. *Tel:* 01424 460070. *Fax:* 01424 460072. [Jul 2000]

Bexhill & Battle

Charles Wardle, MP. *Address:* The House of Commons, London, SW1A 0AA.

NHS

Complaints about NHS services should be directed to the local Community Health Council, (please see the 'Community Health Councils', page 303. Alternatively, you can contact the Consumer Relations Officer at the Conquest Hospital, see below, page 146.

Ombudsman

If you have exhausted the complaints procedures open to you and are still dissatisfied, you can complain to the relevant ombudsman. For complaints about health services contact the Health Services Ombudsman. For complaints about council services contact the Local Government Ombudsman. 5224

Social Services

If you have a complaint about any aspect of Social Services, the following procedure is recommended.

Step 1. Talk to the staff concerned and try to get the problem sorted out. If you are not satisfield, telephone or write to the manager concerned, telling them what the problem is and what you have done so far. You will get a response within two weeks.

Step 2. If the problem is not resolved, write to or telephone the customer liaison officer, who is there to help you through the complaints process and will arrange for your complaint to be investigated.

Step 3. If you are still not satisfied, write again to the customer liaison officer and ask for a review panel meeting, at which two councillors and an independent person will consider your complaint and how it has been dealt with. The panel will make recommendations to the Director of Community Services, who has a legal duty to reply. 5224

Voluntary & private organisations

If possible, discuss your concerns with the person involved to try and sort the problem out straight away. Most reputable organisations will have a complaints procedure in place: usually putting your complaint in writing.

If you cannot get a satisfactory outcome locally and the organisation concerned is a member of a larger organisation or umbrella body, you can try complaining to the head office. If you are unhappy with a particular individual, such as a counsellor, it may be that they are a member of a professional body with a code of practice (such as the British Association for Counselling); if so you can make a complaint to the professional body. 5224

Local Organisations

East Sussex County Council

Address: ESCC, Pelham House, St Andrew's Lane, Lewes, BN7 1UN. *Tel:* 01273 481000. Jul 2000

Hastings & Rother NHS Trust

If you are not satisfied with any of the services you receive in hospital, as an outpatient, or in the community, firstly discuss your concerns with staff at the clinic, department or ward where you are being seen or treated. They should try to sort the problem out. If you are not satisfied, ask to speak to the manager of the department. If the matter is not resolved, or if you prefer to put your concerns in writing, write to the manager or the chief executive. 5224

The Consumer Relations Department deals with enquiries and complaints for all services provided by the NHS Trust. Contact: Frances Bates, Consumer Relations Manager. Hours: Mondays to Fridays 8.30am to 5.00pm.

Address: Consumer Relations Department, Hastings & Rother NHS Trust, Conquest Hospital, The Ridge, St Leonards-on-Sea, East Sussex, TN37 7RD. *Tel:* 01424 758092/758093. Jul 2000

Rother District Council.

Address: Rother District Council, Town Hall, Bexhill, Sussex, TN39 3JX. *Tel:* 01424 787878. *Fax:* 01424 787879. *Rother helpline:* 0800 393964. *Emergency:* 01424 787868. Jul 2000

National Organisations

General Medical Council

Address: General Medical Council, 178, Great Portland Street, London, W1N 6JE. *Tel:* 020 7580 7642. *Fax:* 020 7915 3641. *E-mail:* gmc@gmc-uk.org *Website:* www.gmc-uk.org

Health Services Ombudsman

Address: Health Services Ombudsman, Millbank Tower, Millbank, London, SW1P 4QP. *Tel:* 020 7217 3000. Jul 2000

Local Government Ombudsman

The local government Ombudsman is an independent person who investigates complaints against local authorities and certain other bodies. Covering all of England, he investigates complaints about most council matters, including housing, social services and council tax.

The council must have a chance to deal with the complaint first but, if you are not satisfied with the action taken by the council, you can send a written complaint to the Ombudsman. You may get someone to complain for you as long as they have your permission to represent you.

Contact name: Mr Jerry White, Local Government Ombudsman. *Address:* The Oaks, No. 2 Westwood Way, Westwood Business Park, Coventry, CV4 8JB. *Tel:* 024 7669 5999. *Adviceline:* 0845 602 1983. *Fax: 024 7669 5902. E-mail:* via website. *Website:* www.open.gov.uk/lgo May 2000

A leaflet called *'Complaint about the council? How to complain to the local government Ombudsman'* is available from council offices, citizens' advice bureaux or direct from the Ombudsman's office.

UK Central Council

Address: UK Central Council for Nursing, Midwifery, and Health Visiting, 23, Portland Place, London, W1N 3AF. *Tel:* 020 7637 7181. 5224 Jun 1999; 6005 Jul 2000

Further Information

A remedy for medical complaints

A practitioner's guide to complaints procedures, written by Rosamund Rhodes-Kemp. 'A practical, user- friendly guide to the new procedures involved when making a formal complaint against the NHS and other bodies offering medical treatment, from alternative therapists to private health-care organisations'.

Published by Sweet & Maxwell, 1999, ISBN 0-421-60000-4. 238 pages. Price £39.00. Available from Mind Mail Order Service. *Tel:* 020 8221 9666. 5088

Health Information Service

The HIS is a free and confidential 24-hour service. You can speak to staff during office hours, and you can listen to any of hundreds of tapes at any time, e.g: *Complaints about primary care services (GPs, dentists, opticians & pharmacists)* (Tape 285); *Complaints about hospitals & community health services* (Tape 286). *Address:* The College of Health, St Margaret's House, 21, Old Ford Road, London, E2 9PL. *Freephone:* 0800 66 55 44. 5367

See also these chapters ...

Advocacy, page 154.
Community Health Councils, page 303.
Media Issues, 226.
Your Rights, 269.

Counselling & Therapy

One of the main aims of counselling is to guide us from feeling victims of circumstances to feeling we have some control over our lives. [Hetty Einzig]

Counselling & therapy

Some people use the terms 'counselling' and 'psychotherapy' interchangeably; others, from well-established tradition, distinguish between them. There is much overlap between the two and fortunately the distinction is not a matter which need greatly concern anyone seeking help.

Counselling is a contractual arrangement when a counsellor meets a client in privacy and confidence to explore a difficulty, distress they may be experiencin; perhaps their dissatisfaction with life, or loss of a sense of direction or purpose. To quote from Hetty Einzig (see below) 'one of the main aims of counselling is to guide us from feeling victims of circumstances to feeling we have some control over our lives.'

Counselling will help you make decisions but a counsellor will not tell you what to do.' [5051]

What is counselling?

The overall aim of counselling is to provide an opportunity for the client to work towards living in a way he or she experiences as more satisfying and resourceful. The term 'counselling' includes work with individuals, pairs or groups of people often referred to as 'clients'. The objectives of particular counselling relationships will vary according to the client's needs.

Counselling may be concerned with developmental issues, addressing and resolving specific problems, coping with loss or bereavement, making decisions, coping with crisis, developing personal insight and knowledge, working through feelings of inner conflict or improving relationships with others.

The counsellor's role is to facilitate the client's work in ways which respect the client's values, personal resources and capacity for choice within his or her cultural context.

Counselling involves a deliberately undertaken contract with clearly agreed boundaries and commitment to privacy and confidentiality. It requires explicit and informed agreement. [5076]

Choosing a counsellor

The BAC publishes a *Directory* which lists reputable practitioners. Please contact the BAC for a free copy of the local section of the directory. There are, unfortunately, some technical words used in the descriptions of each counsellor. The BAC gives the following explanations of some of these terms:

Supervision

A counsellor 'in supervision' means one who meets regularly with a colleague to talk over the work, for support and discussion of the problems in complete confidentiality. All BAC members and most counsellors are in supervision. Psychotherapists and psychologists do not always see a need for supervision once they have reached registered status.

Personal therapy
Counsellors and psychotherapists place great importance on their own 'personal therapy', as it helps them experience the role of the client, increasing their understanding of themselves and others.

Theoretical approach
In general, the 'theoretical approach' is less important than the quality of the counsellor but for some problems this is a consideration and will be reflected in the information provided about each counsellor. [5051]

The different theoretical approaches are described on pages 176. [5849]

First contact
Your first contact with your chosen counsellor may be by telephone. Often you will get an answerphone as these instruments are frequently used to avoid interruption during counsellor sessions. Do not be put off by this - the counsellor will telephone you if you leave your name and number. Counsellors are very flexible and appointments can usually be made to suit you. [5051]

Confidentiality
All that takes place between counsellor and client is treated with respect and discretion and agreement is usually made during the first session about confidentiality. If circumstances change, the client's consent will be sought for an alteration to this agreement. [5051]

Questions to ask
When choosing a counsellor some questions you can ask or check are:

qualifications (diploma in counselling or psychotherapy is the usual minimum qualification);

membership of a professional organisation, e.g. British Association for Counselling;

accreditation or registration with an organisation;

code of ethics worked to;

experience - length and breadth;

type of counselling offered e.g. person centred, psychodynamic;

ongoing supervision: whether the counsellor or therapist is in ongoing supervision. [Jun 2000]

How many sessions?
This depends on you, the counsellor and the problem. While deep rooted problems will need maybe a weekly session for several months, short term counselling for a specific problem may take only a few weekly sessions. A 'session' is usually fifty minutes. A review of progress is made usually after not more than six sessions. [5051]

How much does it cost?
Most counsellors and pyschotherapists believe that some payment, however small, reflects the client's committment to the process. It is all too easy to miss sessions if the going gets tough and frequently clients find the counselling process quite painful before the benefits are felt. Charges may be open to negotiation if there is a genuine problem about paying. Agreement about payment should be made during the first session. [5051]

The right counsellor for you
If you are not sure about the first counsellor you see, it is better to arrange to see another one. Having confidence in your counsellor is very important and will enable you to get the best out of the work you do together. [5051]

Trust yourself
The final judge of whether a counsellor is right for you can only be yourself and you must trust your own instincts. Talk to a counsellor and don't be afraid to ask questions or request further information. Then ask yourself if you would feel comfortable telling this person intimate details of your life. Do you feel safe with them, do you like their manner towards you and could you be completely open with them? [5051]

Code of Ethics

The following is a summary of the British Association for Counselling's Code of Ethics, published April 1998:

Values

Counsellors' basic values are integrity, impartiality and respect.

Responsibility

All reasonable steps should be taken to ensure the client's safety during counselling sessions. Counselling is a non-exploitative activity. Counsellors must take the same degree of care to work ethically whatever the setting or the financial basis of the counselling contract.

Anti-discriminatory practice

Counsellors must consider and address their own prejudices and stereotyping and ensure that an anti-discriminatory approach is integral to their counselling practice.

Confidentiality

Counsellors offer the highest possible levels of confidentiality in order to respect the client's privacy and create the trust necessary for counselling.

Contracts

The terms and conditions on which counselling is offered shall be made clear to clients before counselling begins. Subsequent revision of these terms should be agreed in advance of any changes.

Boundaries

Counsellors must establish and maintain appropriate boundaries around the counselling relationship. Counsellors must take into account the effects of any overlapping or pre-existing relationships.

Competence

Counsellors shall take all reasonable steps to monitor and develop their own competence and to work within the limits of that competence. Counsellors must have appropriate, regular and ongoing counselling supervision. 5076

Code of Practice

The following is a summary of the British Association for Counselling's *Code of Practice*, published April 1998:

Introduction

This code applies the values and ethical principles outlined above to more specific situations which may arise in the practice of counselling. The sections and clauses are arranged in the order of the ethics section and under the same headings. No clause or section should be read in isolation from the rest of the Code.

Issues of responsibility

The counsellor-client relationship is the foremost ethical concern. However, counselling does not exist in social isolation. Counsellors may need to consider other sources of ethical responsibility. The headings in this section are intended to draw attention to some of these. *Counsellors take responsibility for clinical/therapeutic decisions in their work with clients. Responsibility to the client.*

Client safety

Counsellors must take all reasonable steps to ensure that the client suffers neither physical nor psychological harm during counselling sessions. Counsellors must not exploit their clients financially, sexually, emotionally, or in any other way. Suggesting or engaging in sexual activity with a client is unethical. Counsellors must provide privacy for counselling sessions.

The sessions should not be overheard, recorded or observed by anyone other than the counsellor without informed consent from the client. Normally any recording would be discussed as part of the contract. Care must be taken that sessions are not interrupted.

Client self-determination

In counselling, the balance of power is unequal and counsellors must take care not to abuse their power. Counsellors do not

Q & A

Q. How many counsellors does it take to change a light bulb?
A. Only one, but the light bulb must want to change.

normally act on behalf of their clients. If they do, it will be only at the express request of the client, or else in exceptional circumstances. Counsellors do not normally give advice.

Counsellors have a responsibility to establish with clients, at the outset of counselling, the existence of any other therapeutic or helping relationships in which the client is involved and to consider whether counselling is appropriate. Counsellors should gain the client's permission before conferring in any way with other professional workers.

Breaks and endings

Counsellors work with clients to reach a recognised ending when clients have received the help they sought or when it is apparent that counselling is no longer helping or when clients wish to end. External circumstances may lead to endings for other reasons which are not therapeutic. Counsellors must make arrangements for care to be taken of the immediate needs of clients in the event of any sudden and unforeseen endings by the counsellor or breaks to the counselling relationship. Counsellors should take care to prepare their clients appropriately for any planned breaks from counselling. They should take any necessary steps to ensure the well-being of their clients during such breaks. 5076

Counselling Terms

In this section an attempt is made to explain some of the technical words found throughout counselling and therapy. With each explanation there follows a list of the practitioners who have indicated that they use the methods described.

Analytical therapy

This therapy is designed to break down the problem into its root cause origin. Put forward by Carl Jung originally, and designed to reduce the problem down to its fundamental causes.

Counsellors: Carol Geer (Wadhurst); Genevieve Picquart (Hove); Lawrence Suss (Brighton).

Art therapy

Art therapy is the use of art materials in a therapeutic setting, accompanied by a qualified therapist, in order to achieve self expression without necessarily using words. 5217

What is an art therapist?

An art therapist is a qualified artist who has taken further training in psychiatry, psychology and psychotherapy in order to gain a better understanding of human behaviour and mental processes.

Art processes

Qualified art therapists have an understanding of art processes, are proficient in the area of non-verbal communication and are able to provide a trusting and facilitating environment in which patients or clients feel safe to express strong, difficult or embarrassing emotions.

Art therapists' professional body is BAAT (see below).

Areas

Art therapists are increasingly being employed in a great diversity of areas and settings including: stroke rehabilitation units, psychiatry, learning difficulties, autistic adults and children, palliative care, special and mainstream education, social services, secure units and prisons.

Assessment

Usually an assessment is made over two or three sessions to see if art therapy is the most suitable type of treatment for the individual. Then an agreement is reached as to the duration of the treatment and its main goals.

Materials
A range of art materials is made available and the artwork produced helps to access deeply felt emotions, which are often beyond the reach of words. For more information please contact BAAT.

BAAT
Address: BAAT, Mary Ward House, 5, Tavistock Place, London, WC1H 9SN. *Tel:* 0207 383 3774. *Fax:* 0207 387 5513. *E-mail:* baat@gateway.net *Website:* www.baat.co.uk [5217]

Art therapists
Margaret Taylor (Hastings); Jill Halpin (Rye Harbour). Hazel Redsull, (Northiam). See also Sandy Adey, (Hastings), who has 'for some time run groups focusing on the therapeutic use of art'.

See also ...
'Art' (under 'Alternative Therapies') and 'Person-centred art therapy' (in this section).

Behavioural therapy
This therapy is based on the assumption that any inappropriate behaviour can be objectively treated independently of the rest of the client's behaviour. *Counsellors:* Prue Doherty (Bexhill); Wendy Lidster (Hove); Madeleine Richardson (Brighton).

Bioenergetics
A form of psychotherapy derived from the theories of Wilhelm Reich. It focuses on the functioning of the person as an organism and the relationship of its functions to emotional stability and well-being. *Counsellors:* Genevieve Picquart (Hove).

Brief therapy.
See under 'Solution-focused therapy'.

Client-centred therapy
See under 'Person-centred therapy'.

Cognitive therapy
What is cognitive therapy?
Cognitive therapy is a form of problem solving. It is based on the principle that the ways that people think about their experiences may produce emotional problems. For instance, if a person undervalues themselves and always sees the bad side of things, they are more likely to become depressed. If a person assumes that they cannot cope with circumstances, or that people are very critical of them, they are likely to become anxious.

Cognitive therapy helps people to identify and change unhelpful ways of thinking and to learn more effective ways of solving problems.

Who can it help?
Research has shown that cognitive therapy helps depression, anxiety and eating disorders. Generally, it is not suitable for severe psychiatric disorders such as schizophrenia.

Cognitive therapy is most suited to people who want to learn methods for coping with and reducing symptoms. It focuses on 'here and now' experiences. Developing insight, or resolving childhood problems are not the main goal of therapy.

What is involved?
Most courses of cognitive therapy last from 8 to 20 sessions, each lasting 50 minutes. Clients take an active part and carry out homework between sessions.

The early stages involve firstly identifying problems and then learning methods for coping with them. Clients record their negative thoughts in relation to stressful situations. Through discussion and action they test whether or not these ways of thinking are accurate, and learn to use more realistic and helpful ones. The later stages of therapy deal with the prevention of future problems. Unhelpful 'rules for living', which may create emotional problems, are discovered (e.g. I can only be happy if I'm successful at everything I do).

These are challenged and other, more flexible ways of thinking and acting are developed.

How can I get therapy?
Various mental health professionals practise cognitive therapy. The therapist could be a clinical psychologist, psychiatrist or nurse therapist. Your general practitioner should be able to refer you to a suitable therapist in your area.

The local NHS provides Cognitive Therapy at the Department of Clinical Psychology.

Address: Department of Clinical Psychology, Braybrooke House, 9, Holmesdale Gardens, Hastings, East Sussex, TN34 1LY. *Tel*: 01424 435066. 5227

Publications & information
'Cognitive Behaviour Therapy' by George Stewart. Published by MIND Information Unit, September 1999. Available from Mind Mail Order Service. *Tel*: 020 8221 9666.
'Cognitive Therapy & the Emotional Disorders' by Aaron T Beck. Published by Penguin, 1989.

Egan
The counsellor helps the client explore themselves and their issues, helps them come to a deeper understanding and then helps them plan how to use their strengths to live more resourcefully. Jun 2000

Family therapy
The counsellor works with the family as a unit. Jun 2000
Nigel Short (Hastings).

Eclectic
An approach not following any one procedure, but selects and uses whatever is considered best in all systems. No one theoretical approach is regarded as universally applicable in an attempt to reconcile any differences between competing theoretical positions in the search for harmony. The therapist will use whatever therapeutic procedures seem most applicable to the case. It is a general and informal approach.

Counsellors: Joy Cobban (Eastbourne); Prue Doherty (Bexhill); Jen Popkin (St Leonards); John Stedman (Hove).

Existential
This form of therapy is highly subjective and focuses on the immediate situation. It differs from most other therapies in an avoidance of intellectual explanation or interpretation. The focus is on the immediate reality shared by client and therapist.

Practitioners: Philippa Cannan (Lewes); Sally McLaughlin (Hastings); Peter Stehle (Winchelsea).

Gestalt therapy
A form of psychotherapy associated with Fritz Perls. It is based on the Gestalt concepts of unity and wholeness in an attempt to explain how the brain sees the world. Treatment is conducted individually and in groups and focuses on the broadening of a person's awareness of self by using past experiences, memories, emotional states and bodily sensations contributing to the person forming a meaningful whole viewpoint rather than a bit of their reality.

Counsellors: Sandy Adey (Hastings); Christine Coxhead (Bexhill); Joy Cobban (Eastbourne); Jenny Deadman (Hove); Jilly Hall (Hastings); Mary Jenkins (Hastings); Monika Jephcott (Uckfield); Pauline Mackay-Danton (Hastings); Sally McLaughlin (Hastings).

Humanistic
Based on the theories of Abraham Maslow, Humanistic therapy is concerned with higher human motives of self-development, knowledge and understanding as well as the basic instincts for the necessities of life. It

looks at how these needs are causative at different levels of behaviour towards satisfying these needs. Other theorists associated with this category are Carl Rogers, Alfred Adler, Rollo May and Kelly.

Counsellors: Lorna Couldrick (Bexhill); Sue Cottrell (Hove); Francesca Inskipp (St Leonards); Mary Jenkins (Hastings); Wendy Lidster (Hove); Sally McLaughlin (Hastings); Madeleine Richardson (Brighton).

Hypnotherapy

A general term for any psychotherapy that makes use of hypnosis. Hypnotherapy is generally classified as a directive therapy since hypnosis tends to produce a passivity during which the client accepts directions from others. *Practitioners:* Heathfield Centre (Heathfield); Brenda Riley (St Leonards); Mel Stockdale (Battle). [5093]

Integrative therapy

The counsellor integrates two or more theories to suit individual clients. [5849 Jun 2000]

Counsellors: Sandy Adey (Hastings); Philipa Cannan (Lewes); Susan Chiswell Jones (Brighton); Stephen Clifford (Bexhill); Sue Cook (Battle); Christine Coxhead (Bexhill); Sue Cottrell (Hove); Mary Jenkins (Hastings); Monika Jephcott (Uckfield); Wendy Lidster (Hove); Pauline Mackay-Danton (Hastings); Edna Murdoch (Hove); Jen Popkin (St Leonards); Madeleine Richardson (Brighton); Gillian Rock (Brighton); Val Simanowitz (Lewes).

Music therapy

Practitioners: Beryl Hope (St Leonards).

Object relations

This therapy covers the emotional bonds between oneself and another which typically expresses capacity to love and care for another as against interest and love for the self. It is an ego-psychology which attempts to explain and understand how people relate to the outside world and others in it. *Counsellors:* Michael Bulman (Lewes); Anthony Anderson (Bexhill).

Person-centred art therapy

A form of art therapy developed by Lisa Silverstone, using the ideas of person centred counselling as originated by Carl Rogers. There are practitioners in this area who hold a Certificate in Person Centred Art Therapy. Practitioners of Person-centred art therapy can be found at Elphinstone Family Centre; Tall Trees, Bexhill; NSPCC, and the Family Support Practitioner Team. [5371]

Person-centred therapy

Also called 'client-centred' or 'Rogerian therapy'. A form of psychotherapy developed by Carl Rogers. It is non-directive and reflective. It does not interpret or advise except to encourage or clarify points. It is based in an encouraging, non-judgemental environment and aims to self-empower the clients into arriving at the best solution for themselves.

Counsellors: Susan Chiswell Jones (Brighton); Christine Coxhead (Bexhill); Joy Cobban (Eastbourne); Val Cunningham (KCPU Tunbridge Wells); Prue Doherty (Bexhill); Francesca Inskipp (St Leonards); Lynn Jackson (Brighton); Mary Jenkins (Hastings); Pauline Mackay-Danton (Hastings); Graham Molyneux (Brighton); Genevieve Picquart (Hove); Val Simanowitz (Lewes).

Psychodynamic therapy

This therapy covers all types of motivational counselling. It covers all those that have motivation and drive central in their concepts.

Counsellors: Michael Bulman (Lewes); Susan Chiswell Jones (Brighton); Lorna Couldrick (Bexhill); Jenny Deadman (Hove); Rosemary Dixon-Nuttall (Crowborough); Prue Doherty (Bexhill);

Carol Geer (Wadhurst); Monika Jephcott (Uckfield); Wendy Lidster (Hove); Genevieve Picquart (Hove); Roger Powe (Brighton); Madeleine Richardson (Brighton); John Rignell (Brighton); Gillian Rock (Brighton); John Stedman (Hove); Lawrence Suss (Brighton); Melanie Withers (Brighton).

Psychoanalysis
This therapy is usually based on Freud's theories of the mind. It could also be based on Adler's or Jung's theories. It explores the underlying motivations of behaviour in an attempt to trace it back to it origins usually in childhood. It relies heavily upon interpretation, unconscious motivation and a search for deep causes often conducted through associational interpretation. It is long term and usually involves several sessions weekly. 5849 Jun 2000

Counsellors: Anthony Anderson (Bexhill); Rosemary Dixon-Nuttall (Crowborough).

Psychodrama psychotherapy
Practitioner: Hugh Maxwell (Hastings).

Psychotherapy
This is a general term that covers any technique used on any mental, emotional or behavioural disorder. The term is neutral as regards the theoretical basis adhered to.

Counsellors: Gail Alexander (Brighton); June Broadhurst (Brighton); Daryl Cohen (Hove); Jessica Fox (Hove); Eogain Gallagher (Brighton); Alegra Garner (Hove); Betty Gilbert (Brighton); Jilly Hall (Hastings); Jill Halpin (Rye Harbour); Francoise Hutton (Lewes); Leslie Ironside (Brighton); Catherine Kaplinsky (Lewes & Ticehurst); Jennifer Leeburn (Lewes); Barbara Lloyd (Brighton); Peter Masani (Lewes); Lindsay Miller (Hove); Ben Mooncie (Hastings); Richard Morgan-Jones (Eastbourne); Jean Mulvey (Lewes); Frances Neilson (Brighton); Brenda Riley (St Leonards); Nina Russell (Hove); John Stedman (Hove); Mel Stockdale (Battle); Clare Tredgold (Brighton); Anne Tyndale (Brighton); George Ward (Brighton); Robert Withers (Brighton).

Psychosynthesis
The counsellor works to help the client synthesize mind, body, emotions and soul. Jun 2000 *Counsellor:* Francesca Inskipp (St Leonards).

Rogerian therapy
See under 'Person-centred therapy'.

Solution-focused therapy
Also known as 'Brief therapy'. The counsellor works to help the client find their strengths and focus on solutions in five or six sessions or less.
Jun 2000

Systemic psychotherapy
Practitioners: Elli Buffery (Westfield); Simon Howell (St Leonards).

Systemic therapy
Counsellors: Wendy Lidster (Hove); Madeleine Richardson (Brighton).

Transactional analysis
A form of therapy originally developed by Eric Berne, usually practised in an individual or group setting in which the goal is to achieve a mature, adaptive and realistic attitude towards life over a mal-adaptive child's behaviour.

Counsellors: Philipa Cannan (Lewes); Val Cunningham (KCPU Tunbridge Wells); Susan Chiswell Jones (Brighton); Christine Coxhead (Bexhill); Mary Jenkins (Hastings); Monika Jephcott (Uckfield); Ben Mooncie (St Leonards); Peter Saunders (Hastings).

Free Counselling
The following organisations provide free counselling and therapy. Some can be approached directly, for others you must go through your GP.

H&RCS

Hastings & Rother Counselling Service. A charity which has been established for seven years. People from all walks of life are seen and one of the central aims is to provide a general counselling service for those in receipt of benefit or on low income. Clients can refer themselves and long term and short term counselling is offered on a weekly basis. Clients can donate whatever they can afford. *Contact:* Mrs Rose Webster.

Address: Hastings & Rother Counselling Service, 73, London Road, St Leonards-on-Sea, East Sussex, TN37 6AR. *Tel:* 01424 428300. 5867 Jun 2000

Dept of Clinical Psychology

For further information please see 'Psychology' chapter, page 343.

Face to Face

For information please see the 'Counsellors & Therapists' chapter, page 193.

H&RCS

Hastings & Rother Counselling Service. See the 'Counsellors & Therapists' chapter, page 194.

Heathfield Centre

For further information please see the 'Counsellors & Therapists' chapter, p 194

Pinehurst Centre

Please see 'Counsellors & Therapists' chapter, page 199.

Relate (South East Sussex)

Please see under the 'Family Problems' chapter, page 69.

Counselling Specialities

The following categories are those which the counsellors and therapists have themselves used to describe their specialities.

Abuse

Philipa Cannan (Lewes); Susan Chiswell Jones (Brighton); Joy Cobban (Eastbourne); Sue Cook (Battle); Sue Cottrell (Hove); Counselling Centre (St Leonards); Jenny Deadman (Hove); Lynn Jackson (Brighton); Genevieve Picquart (Hove); Jen Popkin (St Leonards); Madeleine Richardson (Brighton); Gillian Rock (Brighton).

Addictions

Susan Chiswell Jones (Brighton); Joy Cobban (Eastbourne); Monika Jephcott (Uckfield); Jen Popkin (St Leonards); Frankie Sidhu (Brighton).

All types of clients

Anthony Anderson (Bexhill); Sue Cook (Battle); Val Cunningham (KCPU Tunbridge Wells); Jenny Deadman (Hove); Jilly Hall (Hastings); Francesca Inskipp (St Leonards); Pauline Mackay-Danton (Hastings); Paul Morgan (Brighton); Roger Powe (Brighton); Madeleine Richardson (Brighton); Peter Saunders (Hastings); Val Simanowitz (Lewes); Mel Stockdale (Battle); Kay Thompson (Hastings).

Anxiety and fears

Michael Bulman (Lewes); Val Cunningham (KCPU Tunbridge Wells); Monika Jephcott (Uckfield); Kent Counselling and Psychotherapy Unit; Wendy Lidster (Hove); Sally Mclaughlin (Hastings); Graham Molyneux (Brighton); Ben Mooncie (Hastings); Madeleine Richardson (Brighton); Frankie Sidhu (Brighton); Val Simanowitz (Lewes); Melanie Withers (Brighton).

Bereavement

Susan Chiswell Jones (Brighton); Joy Cobban (Eastbourne); Sue Cottrell (Hove); Lorna Couldrick (Bexhill); Val Cunningham (KCPU Tunbridge Wells); Rosemary Dixon-Nuttall (Crowborough); Prue Doherty (Bexhill); Lynn Jackson

(Brighton); Graham Molyneux (Brighton); Edna Murdoch (Hove); Genevieve Picquart (Hove); Roger Powe (Brighton); Gillian Rock (Brighton); Frankie Sidhu (Brighton); John Stedman (Hove); Melanie Withers (Brighton).

Children and adolescents
Lesley Ironside (Brighton); Ben Mooncie (Hastings).

Co-counselling
Monika Jephcott (Uckfield).

Cognitive analytic therapy
Cognitive analytic therapy (CAT), was devised by Anthony Ryle in his book 'Cognitive Analytic Therapy: active participation in change'; published 1991 by Wiley. Mar 2000

Creativity problems
Michael Bulman (Lewes); Jill Halpin (Rye Harbour); Lynn Jackson (Brighton); Wendy Lidster (Hove); Pauline Mackay-Danton (Hastings); Frankie Sidhu (Brighton).

Crisis management
Jill Halpin (Rye Harbour).

Critical incident de-briefing
Jen Popkin (St Leonards).

Depression
Steve Clifford (Bexhill); Val Cunningham (KCPU Tunbridge Wells); Prue Doherty (Bexhill); Pauline Mackay-Danton (Hastings); Sally Mclaughlin (Hastings); Ben Mooncie (Hastings); Genevieve Picquart (Hove); Gillian Rock (Brighton); Val Simanowitz (Lewes).

Eating disorders
Susan Chiswell Jones (Brighton); Jane Dale (Brighton/Hove); Prue Doherty (Bexhill); Monika Jephcott (Uckfield); Jen Popkin (St Leonards); Val Simanowitz (Lewes); Melanie Withers (Brighton).

Educational issues
Roger Powe (Brighton).

Elderly problems
Mary Jenkins (Hastings).

Family problems
Dr Marie Botha (Tunbridge Wells); Joy Cobban (Eastbourne); Sue Cook (Battle); Michael Montier (Tunbridge Wells); Paul Morgan (Brighton); Deirdre Schueppert (Tunbridge Wells).

French speaking
Genevieve Picquart (Hove); Melanie Withers (Brighton).

German speaking
Monika Jephcott (Uckfield).

Health related issues
Lorna Couldrick (Bexhill); Rosemary Dixon-Nuttall (Crowborough).

HIV/Aids
Philipa Cannan (Lewes).

Identity problems
Michael Bulman (Lewes); Sue Cottrell (Hove); Jenny Deadman (Hove); Monika Jephcott (Uckfield); Madeleine Richardson (Brighton).

Inter-cultural issues
Val Simanowitz (Lewes).

Italian speaking
Michael Bulman (Lewes).

Learning disablilites
Joy Cobban (Eastbourne); Lorna Couldrick (Bexhill); Prue Doherty (Bexhill); Lynn Jackson (Brighton); Jen Popkin (St Leonards).

Men
John Rignell (Brighton).

Minority groups
This includes religious groups. Sally

Mclaughlin (Hastings); John Rignell (Brighton); John Stedman (Hove).

Obsessional disorders
Graham Molyneux (Brighton).

Oppressed Groups
Val Simanowitz (Lewes).

Organisations
Michael Bulman (Lewes); Prue Doherty (Bexhill); Jen Popkin (St Leonards); Madeleine Richardson (Brighton).

Personal growth
Joy Cobban (Eastbourne); Sue Cook (Battle); Lorna Couldrick (Bexhill); Christine Coxhead (Bexhill); Jenny Deadman (Hove); Carol Geer (Wadhurst); Jill Halpin (Rye Harbour); Mary Jenkins (Hastings); Wendy Lidster (Hove); Pauline Mackay-Danton (Hastings); Graham Molyneux (Brighton); Val Simanowitz (Lewes); Lawrence Suss (Brighton).

Phobias
Michael Bulman (Lewes); Lynn Jackson (Brighton); Monika Jephcott (Uckfield); Wendy Lidster (Hove); Sally McLaughlin (Hastings); Graham Molyneux (Brighton); Ben Mooncie (Hastings); Madeleine Richardson (Brighton); Frankie Sidhu (Brighton); Val Simanowitz (Lewes); Melanie Withers (Brighton).

Refugees
Val Simanowitz (Lewes).

Relationship problems
Dr Marie Botha (Tunbridge Wells); Michael Bulman (Lewes); Philipa Cannan (Lewes); Susan Chiswell Jones (Brighton); Joy Cobban (Eastbourne); Sue Cook (Battle); Sue Cottrell (Hove); Christine Coxhead (Bexhill); Jenny Deadman (Hove); Prue Doherty (Bexhill); Carol Geer (Wadhurst); Lynn Jackson (Brighton); Mary Jenkins (Hastings); Monika Jephcott (Uckfield); Wendy Lidster (Hove); Pauline Mackay-Danton (Hastings); Sally Mclaughlin (Hastings); Graham Molyneux (Brighton); Michael Montier (Tunbridge Wells); Edna Murdoch (Hove); Genevieve Picquart (Hove); Jen Popkin (St Leonards); Roger Powe (Brighton); Madeleine Richardson (Brighton); Gillian Rock (Brighton); Deirdre Schueppert (Tunbridge Wells); Frankie Sidhu (Brighton); John Stedman (Hove); Lawrence Suss (Brighton); Melanie Withers (Brighton).

Sex-related problems
Includes fertility problems. *Counsellors:* Michael Bulman (Lewes); Joy Cobban (Eastbourne); Sue Cottrell (Hove); Lorna Couldrick (Bexhill); Christine Coxhead (Bexhill); Wendy Lidster (Hove); Genevieve Picquart (Hove); Roger Powe (Brighton); Madeleine Richardson (Brighton); Frankie Sidhu (Brighton); John Stedman (Hove); Kay Thompson (Hastings).

Sexual minorities
Michael Bulman (Lewes); Philipa Cannan (Lewes); Christine Coxhead (Bexhill); Pauline Mackay-Danton (Hastings); Sally Mclaughlin (Hastings); Edna Murdoch (Hove); Genevieve Picquart (Hove); Frankie Sidhu (Brighton).

Spanish speaking
Genevieve Picquart (Hove).

Stress
Susan Chiswell Jones (Brighton); Joy Cobban (Eastbourne); Sue Cook (Battle); Val Cunningham (KCPU Tunbridge Wells); Prue Doherty (Bexhill); Carol Geer (Wadhurst); Mary Jenkins (Hastings); Wendy Lidster (Hove); Ben Mooncie (Hastings); Roger Powe (Brighton); Madeleine Richardson (Brighton); Gillian Rock (Brighton); Melanie Withers (Brighton).

Suicidal tendencies
Joy Cobban (Eastbourne);

Trauma
Philipa Cannan (Lewes); Susan Chiswell Jones (Brighton); Joy Cobban (Eastbourne); Sue Cook (Battle); Val Cunningham - KCPU (Tunbridge Wells); Jenny Deadman (Hove); Kent Counselling and Psychotherapy Unit Madeleine Richardson (Brighton); Lawrence Suss (Brighton).

Victims of crime
This includes victims of violence. *Counsellors:* Philipa Cannan (Lewes); Susan Chiswell Jones (Brighton); Jen Popkin (St Leonards); Gillian Rock (Brighton).

Visually impaired
Gillian Rock (Brighton).

Wheelchair access
Marie Botha (Sevenoaks); Mrs June Broadhurst (Brighton); Steve Clifford (Bexhill); Dr Francoise Hutton (Hove); Catherine Kaplinsky (Ticehurst); Richard Morgan-Jones (Eastbourne); Jen Popkin (St Leonards); Hazel Redsull (Northiam).

Women
Joy Cobban (Eastbourne); Lynn Jackson (Brighton); Mary Jenkins (Hastings); Val Simanowitz (Lewes).

Work related issues
Susan Chiswell Jones (Brighton); Joy Cobban (Eastbourne); Wendy Lidster (Hove); Roger Powe (Brighton).

National Organisations

Albany Trust
A professional therapy service for individuals and couples needing emotional and psychological help. The Albany Trust is a charitable foundation established in 1958 to promote psychosexual health and emotional well-being through counselling, education and research. Contact: Carol Zimmeren, Referrals Co-ordinator.

Address: Albany Trust, The Art of Yoga & Health, 280, Balham High Road, London, SW17 7AL. *Tel*: 020 8767 1827. 6057 Oct 99; Jun 2000

APAC
Association of Psychotherapists and Counsellors. APAC operates throughout the UK with headquarters in London. APAC at Fern Hill Centre is one of the country's leading training institutions in play therapy. All their courses are accredited by Play Therapy International. They run day weekend certificate and diploma courses for anybody who works with children and wants to increase their skills in play therapy. APAC has a database containing several hundred fully accredited psychotherapists, chartered psychologists, psychiatrists and counsellors together with their specialist areas of experience.

About 70 of these are in this area. Among the problems which can be addressed are: addiction, anxiety, bullying, bereavement, children's mental health, depression, eating disorders, employment opportunities, family problems, manic depression, phobias, post natal illness, sexual issues, stress.

All therapists are accredited counsellors of the British Association for Counselling or registered therapists with the UK Council for Psychotherapy."

Address: (Sussex): Fern Hill Centre, Fern Hill, Fairwarp, Uckfield, Sussex, TN22 3BU. *Tel*: 01825 712312. *Fax*: 01825 713679. *E-mail*: mokijep@aol.com *Website*: www.counsellingnet.co.uk

Address (London): Association of Psychotherapists and Counsellors, 10, Harley Street, London, W1N 1AA. *Tel*: 020 7467 8435. Jul 2000

British Assn for Counselling

The British Association for Counselling (BAC), is the main body in the UK representing counselling at national and international levels. The Association aims to promote counselling and to raise the standards of training and practice. Registered charity 298361.

BAC Directory

The BAC publishes *The U.K. Counselling and Psychotherapy Resources Directory*. Entry to this publication is restricted to practitioners on the UK Register of Counsellors, the BCP and UKCP Registers of Psychotherapists, the British Psychological Society (BPS) Register of Psychologists, COSCA accredited members and practicing BAC members who are properly supervised. This means that all practitioners listed are covered by a Code of Ethics and Practice and a Compaints procedure. This will give you confidence in selecting a suitable therapist. To obtain a copy of the Directory, please contact BAC. 5051 May 2000

Address: 1, Regent Place, Rugby, Warwickshire, CV21 2PJ. *Tel*: 01788 550899. *Fax*: 01788 562189. *Minicom*: 0178 8 57 2838.

E-mail: bac@bac.co.uk *Website*: www.counselling.co.uk 5051 May 2000

British Assn of Psychotherapists

The British Association of Psychotherapists (BAP) is a long standing professional organisation of psychotherapists with members nationwide, affiliated to the British Confederation of Psychotherapists Register. It offers training, courses and workshops in adult and child psychotherapy. The clinical service offers assessment and referral for children and adults requiring psychotherapy. *Chief executive:* Elise Ormerod. Registered Charity No. 281720.

Address: British Association of Psychotherapists, 37, Mapesbury Road, London, NW2 4HJ. *Tel*: 020 8452 9823. *Fax:* 020 8452 5182. *E-mail:* mail@bap-psychotherapy.org *Website:* www.bap-psychotherapy.org May 2000

British Confederation

The British Confederation of Psychotherapists publishes a list of 1,300 practitioners, i.e. psychoanalysts, analytical psychologists, psychoanalytic psychotherapists, child psychotherapists, with addresses and telephone numbers; please telephone for a free copy. Senior Administrator: Susan H Lucks. 6078 Jul 2000

Address: The British Confederation of Psychotherapists, 37, Mapesbury Road, London, NW2 4HJ. *Tel:* 020 8830 5173. *Fax:* 020 8452 3684. *E-mail:* mail@bcp.org.uk *Website:* www.bcp.org.uk 6001 Jul 2000

British Psychological Society

Address: British Psychological Society, St Andrews House, 48, Princess Road East, Leicester, LE1 7DR. *Tel*: 0116 254 9568. May 2000

Counsel and Care

Covering all areas of the UK. Chief Executive: Martin Green; Deputy Chief Executive: Les Bright.

Address: Counsel and Care, Twyman House, 16, Bonny Street, London, NW1 9PG. *Tel*: 020 7485 1550. *Helpline*: 0845 300 7585 (10.30am to 4pm); *Fund Raising/Membership:* 020 7485 4513. *Fax:* 020 7267 6877. *E-mail:*advice@counselandcare.demon.co.uk. Registered Charity No. 203429 May 2000

Psychiatry Research Trust

Registered charity number 284286.
Address: Psychiatry Research Trust, De Crespigny Park, London, SE5 8AF. *Tel:* 020 7703 6217. May 2000

PACE

Project for Advice, Counselling and Education. *Address*: PACE, 34, Hartham Road, London, N7 9JL. *Tel:* 020 7700 1323. Jul 2000

Royal College of Psychiatrists

Address: Royal College of Psychiatrists, 17, Belgrave Square, London, SW1X 8PG. *Tel*: 020 7235 2351. *Fax:* 020 7245 1231. *Direct Fax:* 020 7235 1935.
Registered Charity No. 228636. May 2000

UK Council for Psychotherapy

Registered Charity No. 1058545.
Address: UKCP, 167-169, Great Portland Street, London, W1N 5FB. *Tel:* 020 7436 3012. *Fax:* 020 7436 3013. *E-mail:* ukcp@psychotherapy.org.uk *Website:* www.psychotherapy.org.uk 5449

UK Register of Counsellors

Address: UK Register of Counsellors, PO Box 1050, Rugby, CV21 2HZ. *Tel:* 01788 568739. May 2000

Women's Therapy Centre

Address: Women's Therapy Centre, 10, Manor Gardens, London, N7 6JS. *Tel*: 020 7263 6200. May 2000

Westminster Pastoral Foundation

WPF Counselling and Psychotherapy provides individual counselling and group psychotherapy on a sliding scale of fees. It is a self referral service. WPF Counselling also trains counsellors and psychotherapists. It has a network of some forty-five affiliated and associated counselling centres in the UK. *Contact:* Simon Pike, clinical manager.

Address: Westminster Pastoral Foundation Counselling, 23, Kensington Square, London, W8 5HN. *Tel*: 020 7361 4800. 5051, 5986 May 2000

Further Information

Counselling & Psychotherapy - Is It For Me?
By Hetty Einzig, obtainable from the British Association for Counselling, address above 5051

Counselling Factsheet
By Katherine Darton. Published by Mind Information Unit, Sept. 1999. £0.35. Available from Mind Mail Order Service. *Tel*: 020 8221 9666.

Feeling Good, the New Mood Therapy
By David D Burns. Published by Penquin Books. Price £5.95. A book on cognitive therapy.

Getting the Best From Your Counsellor or Psychotherapist
Published by Mind. Price £1.29, including postage and packing. Available from Mind Mail Order Service. *Tel*: 020 8221 9666.

Health Information Service
The HIS is a free and confidential 24-hour service. You can speak to staff during office hours, and you can listen to any of hundreds of tapes at any time, e.g: *Counselling for marriages & relationships* (Tape 269); *Talking treatments* (Tape 454).

Address: The College of Health, St Margaret's House, 21, Old Ford Road, London, E2 9PL. *Freephone*: 0800 66 55 44.

Mind Over Mood
*M*ind Over Mood - Change how you feel by changing the way you think. By Dennis Greenberger & Christine A Padesky. A step-by-step guide to managing your moods by using the tools of cognitive therapy. This

manual offers practical steps to feeling better and making the changes you want in your life.

Published by The Guilford Press, 1999. ISBN: 0-89862-128-3. 243 pages. Price £15.99. Available from Mind Mail Order Service. *Tel*: 020 8221 9666. [5221]

Psychological Methods of Treatment

By Dr Brenda Lintner. 8-page booklet published by Sane, 1993.

Psychotherapy

An introductory text on psychotherapy is Anthony Storr's 'Introduction to Psychotherapy'.

Psychotherapy Factsheet

By George Stewart. Published by Mind Information Unit, April 1998. £0.35p. Available from Mind Mail Order Service. *Tel*: 020 8221 9666.

Abbreviations.

ACTP. Advanced Certificate in Applied Transpersonal Psychotherapy.
AFT. Assoc. for Family Therapy & Systemic Practice in the UK.
AssMORAH. Associate Member of Advanced Hypnotherapists.
BA (Psychol).
BAABP. Cert. Analytical Body Psychotherapy. ??
BAAT. Brit. Assoc. Art Therapy.
BABCP. Brit. Assoc. for Behavioural and Cognitive Psychotherapies.
BAC AccC.
BAC. British Association for Counselling.
BACAccT. British Association for Counselling Accredited Trainer.
BICA. British Infertility Counselling Association.
BPA. British Psychodrama Assoc.
C. Psychol. Chartered Psychologist.
Cert. Family Systems (St George's).
CQSW. Certificate of Qualification in Social Work.
CTA. Certified Transactional Analyst.
CTP. Centre for Transpersonal Psychology.
CUKCP.
DHP. Diploma in Hypnotherapy & Psychotherapy.
Dip Couple Therapy (Maudsley).
Dip. CG.
Dip. Cognitive Therapy/Hypnotherapy (BHR) Practitioner NLP 1994.
Dip. Couns. (CSCT).
Dip. Memb. IPC (WPF).
Dip. Soc. Admin.
Dip. THP N-Shap.
Dip. TMHA.
DipSW. Diploma in Social Work.
DST. Diploma in Systemic Therapy.
FMA Acc.
FMA. Family Mediation ?
FPC. Foundation for Psychotherapy & Counselling
FRSM.
IFT. Institute of Family Therapy.
IPC (FPC).
IPC/WPFI 1983.
IPLC. Diploma in Supervising Person-Centred Practice.
KCPU. Kent Counselling & Psychotherapy Union.
M.Cl.Sc. Master of Clinical Science in Psychotherapy.
MA Couns. Psychol.
MACP. Member of the Association of Child Psychotherapists.
MAssNLP. Associate Member of NLP.
MBIM.
MBSECH. Member of Brit. Soc. for Experimental & Clinical Hypnosis.
MCRAH.
Memb. EATA.
Memb. GAS (Lon.) BAPPS.
MLitt.
MNCP. Member of the National Council for Psychotherapy.
MNRHP. Member of the National Register of Hypnotherapists & Psychotherapists.
MORAH.
NAP. National Association of Psychotherapists.
NHS. National Health Service.
NLP. Neurolinguistic Programming.
NMGC.
PCGE. Post Graduate Certificate, Education.
PGCCP.Post Graduate Certificate in Counselling & Psychotherapy.
PGDip Couns.
PgDPP. Postgraduate Diploma, Psychodynamic Psychoanalytic Psychotherapy.
PhD. Counselling Psychotherapy.
Prof. Memb. IPC.
PTSTA. Provisional Teaching & Supervising TA.
RATh. Registered Art Therapist.
RCSCP. Regents College School of Psychotherapy & Counselling.
RMN. Registered Mental Nurse.
RNMH. Registered Nurse for the Mentally Handicapped.
SRAT. State Registered Arts Therapist.
TA. Transactional Analyst.
TSP. Tavistock Society of Psychotherapists.
TSTA.
UKCP. UK Council for Psychotherapy.
UKRC.UK Reg. Ind. C.

Acknowledgements

Our grateful thanks to Margaret Taylor, art therapist, for editorial assistance with the art therapy section, and to Mary Cairns, psychotherapist, and Francesca Inskipp, counsellor & counselling supervisor, for general assistance with this chapter.

Counsellors & Therapists

The people and organisations listed in this section are practising counsellors and therapists working in this area. Some are included who work outside Hastings & Rother, as it may be that you cannot find a suitable counsellor locally. If you want to quickly find the names of counsellors practising in your town, please see the table, 'Counsellors by location', at the end of this section.

It must be stressed that Mind does not recommend or endorse any of the practitioners listed here. Please see 'Choosing a Counsellor' (page 173) and 'Questions to ask' (page 174).

Adey, Sandy

Sandy is an integrative counsellor and trainer. She offers counselling for individuals, couples, families, and groups. She is also a trainer of counselling skills, and has a particular interest in the therapeutic value of art therapy. She is a supervisor and mediator (especially conflict resolution in organisations). She is also running an on-going therapy group. Clients may contact Sandy Adey direct or through their GP. Hours are 9am to 6.30pm, and some evenings. She also practices in Eastbourne. Fees will be discussed directly with the client.

Qualifications: PGDip Couns; MA Couns. Psychology. *Address*: Sandy Adey, 16, Priory Road, Hastings, Sussex, TN34 3JH. *Tel*: 01424 712968. Aug 2000

Anderson, Anthony

Anthony is a psychoanalytical therapist and his theoretical basis is object relations. His clients are generally referred. They include people with emotional difficulties, anxiety and stress of all kinds. Fees are £15 - £25 per session negotiable at the initial meeting.

Qualifications: UKCP; M.Cl.Sc.Clinical; PgDPP. *Address*: Anthony J Anderson, Bexhill, Sussex, TN40 2HP. *Tel*: 01424 734027. Jul 2000

Beech Group

This is a group of highly qualified and experienced counsellors. They include counselling psychotherapy for individuals, couples, teenagers, children and families. The group offers supervision for trainee counsellors, experienced counsellors, groups and health and social care workers. Training is also given in counselling skills, dealing with eating disorders, working with sexual problems, communicating with teenagers and coping with anger.

Mediation is available for families in conflict, separating couples and resolving conflict in the workplace. Corporate services are available for employee support, interpersonal skills, initiating change and facilitating teamwork. Low cost counselling is available for those on low income, those who are unemployed and also for students. Madeleine Richardson, Principal & Psychotherapist (see separate entry for full details).

Address: Jane Rimmington, The Beech Group of Counsellors, 221, Preston Road, Brighton, Sussex, BN1 6SA. *Tel/Fax*: 01273 504385. *E-mail:* beechgroup@onet.co.uk May 2000

Botha, Dr Marie E

Qualifications: These include MB Ch.B, Bachelor of Medicine, Bachelor of Surgery; Dip FPC, Foundation for Psychotherapy and Counselling; UKCP Registered. She offers psychodynamic counselling and group analytic psychotherapy. Her fees are £15 - £30, negotiated, for individual sessions. £15 (per person) for group sessions. There is wheelchair access.

Address: Dr Marie Botha, 70, Bradbourne Road, Sevenoaks, Kent, TN13 3QA. *Tel*: 01732 455903. (See also entry for Tunbridge Wells Counselling Centre). Aug 2000

Broadhurst, June Elizabeth

Analytic Psychotherapist, British Association of Psychotherapists (Jungian).

June is an analytical psychotherapist working with adults on an individual basis, usually once or twice a week, or sometimes more, wanting help with relationships or personal problems. June bases therapy on the relationship with the therapist to explore feelings and difficulties, linking conscious and unconscious thoughts and feelings, and past and present experiences.

Address: Mrs June Broadhurst, The British Association of Psychotherapists, 90, Coventry Street, Brighton, BN1 5PQ, East Sussex. *Tel:* 01273 562321. (There is wheelchair access). 5798 May 2000

Buffery, Elli Patricia

Systematic psychotherapist. Address: The Old Stables, Cottage Lane, Westfield, Sussex, TN35 4QG. 5409

Bulman, Michael

Michael is a general counsellor and also provides long-term counselling. He deals with anxiety, phobias, identity, relationship and sexuality problems. He works with individuals and can speak Italian. His clientele includes students and trainees, creative people and sexual minorities. He is in personal therapy and ongoing supervision himself. His theoretical approach is psychodynamic and object relations. Michael's fees are £20 - £30 per session, but reduced in cases of hardship.

Qualifications: these include BAC AccC; Advanced Diploma in Psychodynamic Counselling (WPF 1997); Prof Memb IPC. Code of Ethics: BAC.

Address: Michael Bulman, Trevor House, The Street, Glynde, Sussex, BN8 6SX. *Tel*: 01273 858695. *E-mail:* michael_bulman@hotmail.com May 2000

Cannan, Philipa

Philipa is a general counsellor, psychotherapist and counselling supervisor. She deals with abuse, HIV and AIDS, trauma, relationship problems and stress. She provides short-term and long-term counselling. She works with individuals, couples, groups and organisations. Her clientele includes sexual minorities, victims of crime and violence, students and trainees, indeed anyone who needs counselling. She is in personal therapy and ongoing supervision herself. Her theoretical approach is integrative, transactional analysis, and existential. Philipa's fees are £35 per session but are negotiable.

Qualifications: these include BAC AccC; BA (Hons); Dip Soc Admin; PG Dip Couns; Advanced TA Clinical Training (2yrs); Family Mediation (FMA). Code of Ethics: BAC. Registration: UKRC Reg. Ind. Counsellor.

Address: Philipa Cannan, The Hollows, Wellgreen Lane, Kingston, Lewes, Sussex, BN7 3NR. *Tel*: 01273 476063. May 2000

Chiswell Jones, Susan

Susan is a general counsellor and counselling supervisor. She deals with relationship problems, bereavement, abuse, trauma, addictions, eating disorders, work related issues and stress. She works with individuals, couples and groups. Her clientele includes helping and caring professionals, victims of crime or violence, students and trainees. She has ongoing personal therapy and supervision. Susan's theoretical approach is integrative, person-centred, transpersonal and informed by psychodynamic insights. Fee is £28, negotiable.

Qualifications: these include BAC AccC; BA (Hons); PGCE; Dip Couns (Brighton Univ 1995); Gestalt Training; MA Couns Psychol (Brighton & Sussex Univ) 1994, Cascade Supervision Training 1995/6. Code of Ethics: BAC. Registration: UKRC Reg Ind Counsellor.

Address: Susan Chiswell Jones, 205, Osborne Rd, Brighton, BN1 6LT. *Tel*: 01273 541985. May 2000

Clifford, Steve

Steve is a general counsellor and therapist. His theoretical approach is integrative. Fees are from £30 per session. The premises have wheelchair access. Stephen has also set up a new internet site called "Fightdepression" which goes live in Autumn 2000. It is a site dedicated to bringing you the latest treatment and therapy options available in the UK. [Please see the chapter 'Depression' for details]. *Qualifications*: these include Dip Couns PGCCP (Surrey Univ); ACTP; RMN; RNMH.

Address: Steve Clifford, TLC Primary Healthcare, Summer House, 56A, Cranston Ave, Bexhill, Sussex, TN39 3NN. *Tel*: 01424 220189. Jul 2000

Cobban, Joy

Joy is a general counsellor. She deals with relationship problems, abuse, bereavement, traumas, addictions, sex and work related issues such as stress, and also counsels in personal growth. She works with individuals, couples, families and groups. Her clientele includes carers, people who have attempted suicide, helping and caring professionals, people with disabilities and women in particular. Joy has experience of crisis and traumatic incident debriefing. She is in personal therapy and ongoing supervision herself. Her theoretical approach is Rogerian, Gestalt, Egan and Eclectic. Joy's fees are £15 - £25 per *session.*

Qualifications: these include Dip Couns; Al Accred (VACTS). Code of Ethics: BAC.

Address: Joy Cobban, Chandlers, 85, Pashley Road, Eastbourne, Sussex, BN20 8EA. *Tel*: 01323 638440. May 2000

Cohen, Dr Daryl

Qualifications: Medically qualified practitioner; MRC Psych; Psychoanalyst (British Psycho-Analytical Society).

Psychoanalytic Psychotherapist (Assoc. for Psychoanalytic Psychotherapy in the NHS).

Address: Dr Daryl Cohen, 18, Wolstonbury Road, Hove, East Sussex, BN3 6EJ. *Tel:* 01273 734020 / 01273 464523.

Consultant Psychotherapist, South downs Health NHS Trust.

Address: Dr Daryl Cohen, District Psychotherapy Service, Hove Polyclinic, Nevill Avenue, Hove, East Sussex, BN3 7HY. *Tel:* 01273 242017. 5798

Cook, Sue

Sue is a general counsellor, psychotherapist and counselling supervisor. She deals with abuse, personal growth, relationship problems, trauma and stress. She works with individuals, couples, families, and groups. She counsels on both a short-term and long-term basis. She has hard personal therapy and is in ongoing supervision. Her clients are everyone and her theoretical approach is integrative. Sue's fees are £35 per session.

Qualifications: these include BAC Senior Practitioner; NMGC; CRUSE; Training in Grief Therapy; Assertiveness; Youth Counselling; Gestalt; Memb British Assoc for Performing Arts Medicine. Code of Ethics: BAC. Registration: UKRC Reg Ind Counsellor.

Address: Sue Cook, Woods Place, Mill Lane, Whatlington, Battle, Sussex, TN33 0ND. *Tel*: 01424 775337. *Fax:* 01424 775063. *E-mail:* woodsplace@kirion.net May 2000

Cottrell, Sue

Sue is a general counsellor, psychotherapist and counselling supervisor. She deals with relationship problems, abuse, bereavement, identity and sexuality problems. She counsels short-term and long-term. She takes individuals, couples and groups and has ongoing supervision. Her theoretical approach is integrative and humanistic. Sue's fees are £30 (individuals) - £45 (couples) per session.

Qualifications: These include UKCP; MSc Integrative Psychotherapy (1999); BAC

AccC; BA Social Science 1989; Dip & Adv Dip Gestalt; Contribution Training & Feminist Psychotherapy (Pellin 1986/7); Integrative Psychotherapy (Metanoia 1998).Code of Ethics: BAC. Registration: UKRC Reg Ind Counsellor.

Address: Sue Cottrell, 50, Waldegrave Road, Brighton, BN1 6GE. *Tel:* 01273 507776. *E-mail:* suecottrell@hotmail.com Jun 2000

Couldrick, Lorna

Lorna is a general counsellor and counselling supervisor. She offers short-term focused counselling to help in times of crisis (e.g. post trauma, bereavement, ill health, relationships, sexual issues) or long-term for personal development. She works with individuals. Her clients include people on Employee Assistance Programmes, the unemployed, those with illness or disability, student counsellors, those in the caring professions etc. Her approach is humanistic and psychodynamic. Lorna's fees are £15 - £30 per session, but are negotiable for the low-waged.

Qualifications: these include BAC AccC; Dip Couns; Forensic Psychotherapy Training; Supervision Training & Experience; State Registered Occupational Therapist. Code of Ethics: BAC. Registration: UKRC Reg Ins Counsellor.

Address: Lorna Couldrick, 66, Martyns Way, Bexhill, Sussex, TN40 2SH. *Tel*: 01424 215205. May 2000

Counselling Centre

A service provided by NSPCC East Sussex. This is a very significant well established local resource in partnership with local PCGs and provides counselling services for adults who were abused as children, and abused children and their families. Informed enquiries are welcomed. Contact: Ron Fellows. Hours: Mondays to Fridays 9.00am to 5.00pm.

Address: Counselling Centre, 2, Sedlescombe Road South, St Leonards-on-Sea, Sussex, TN38 0TA. *Tel*: 01424 728500. May 2000

Counselling Partnership

See under 'Rae, Frances'

Cox, Christine

Christine describes her work as "person centred counselling, cognitive and behavioural therapy, hypnotherapy for stress, anxiety and emotional problems." Fees: 90 minute session - £30; 60 minute session - £25. *Qualifications*: BA Honours; MNRHP; DHP; Certificate in Stress Management from the Centre for Stress Management.

Address: Christine Cox, 28, Fern Road, St Leonards, Sussex, TN38 0UH. *Tel:* 01424 424797. May 2000

Coxhead, Christine

Christine is a general counselling and counselling supervisor. She deals with relationship and sexuality problems, and with personal growth. She counsels for both short-term and long-term periods. She works with individuals, couples and groups. Her own therapy and supervision is ongoing. Clients include students, sexual minorities and young people. Christine's theoretical approach is integrative. Her fees are £30 for individuals, £35 for couples and £15 for groups. *Qualifications:* these include Dip Integrative Couns (Wealden College); Dip Supervision (Wealden College). Code of Ethics: BAC.

Address: Christine Coxhead, 36, Withyham Road, Cooden, Bexhill, Sussex, TN39 3BA. *Tel*: 01424 843604. *E-mail:* golfer@bluecarrotts.com May 2000

Crellin, Clare

Adult psychotherapy, counselling. Clare offers a service in psychoanalytical psychotherapy, cognitive therapy, assessments and neuropsychological assessments for adults and those over 65 years of age. She is a specialist in PTSD therapy. Clare's fees at present are £40 per clinical hour.

Qualifications: BA Hons. Psychology; Masters in Clinical Psychology, M.Clin. Psychology; Accredited Psychotherapist NAP i.e. psychologists with additional psychotherapy training; Psychoanalyst UKCP; AFBPsS, NAP. *Tel:* 01825 712139. Aug 2000

Cunningham, Valerie

Valerie and her associates provide a service in counselling, psychotherapy, supervision and training in transactional analysis. Their work includes most areas and especially bereavement, anxiety, depression, relationship issues and post traumatic stress. *Qualifications*: Dip. A.T., RATh; CTA; PTSTA; BACAccT. Fees are negotiated from £35 per session. Training course fees on application.

Address: Valerie Cunningham, Senior Tutor KCPU, Kent Counselling and Psychotherapy Union (KCPU), 19, Birling Road, Tunbridge Wells, Kent, TN2 5LX. *Tel*: 01892 529903. *E-mail*: val@kcpu.org.uk *Website:* www.kcpu.uk (Please see separate entry for KCPU in this chapter). Aug 2000

Deadman, Jenny

Jenny is a BAC accredited counsellor and a WPF trained supervisor and she has a psychology degree. She works with individual clients who are having emotional difficulties and are working through relationship problems, bereavement, anxiety problems and depression, or may need counselling as part of a training course. She works in a psychodynamic and a gestalt approach. Her fees are £25 per session with some reductions available.

Qualifications: these include BA Hons Psychology; Dip Couns; Rochester Foundation training in Gestalt Therapy; PG training in Psychodynamic Couns. Code of Ethics: BAC.

Address: Jenny Deadman, 22, Cromwell Rd, Hove, Sussex, BN3 3EB. *Tel*: 01273 777760. May 2000

Dixon-Nuttall, Rosemary

Rosemary is a general psychotherapist, counsellor and counsellor supervisor. She deals with stress, bereavement, eating disorders, personal growth and health related issues. She works long and short term or focused, with individuals and groups. She also does consultation work for carers/staff. She has had personal therapy and has ongoing supervision regularly. Her theoretical approach is psychoanalytical and psychodynamic. Fees are £30 per session, negotiable.

Qualifications: these include senior registered practitioner BAC; Dip Memb FPC (WPF) 1984; group psychotherapist 1986; Prof. Memb AGIP 1998; Dip Couns Supervision (WPF 1994); Memb GAS (Lon), BAPPS. Code of Ethics: BAC, AGIP, FPC. Registration: UKCPP; Reg group & individual psychotherapist; UKRC Reg individual & organisational counsellor.

Address: Rosemary Dixon-Nuttall, 30, Brooklands Avenue, Crowborough, East Sussex, TN6 3BP. *Tel*: 01892 663192. Jun 2000

Doherty, Prue

Prue works for various organisations and has a private practice providing therapy, short or long-term, for adults aged 16+. Various approaches are used to suit the individual at the time. Prue is a general counsellor and counselling supervisor. She deals with bereavement, depression, eating disorders, relationship and stress counselling. She works with all types of individuals, couples, groups and organisations, and offers supervision and training also.

Writing is sometimes introduced into the therapy as a technique. She is in ongoing therapy and supervision herself. Her clients include students, people with learning disabilities, helping and caring professionals and young people. Her theoretical approach is eclectic, person-centred, cognitive, behavioural and psychodynamic. Prue's fees are £25-35 per session. Clients need to get to Prue's address in Bexhill, except for exceptional circumstances.

Qualifications: these include BAC AccC; Dip Couns (London 1990); Memb Inst of Linguists. Post Grad. Dip. Creative Writing & Personal Development (1999). Code of Ethics: BAC. Registration: UKRC Reg Ind Counsellor.

Address: Prue Doherty, 150, Cooden Drive, Bexhill, Sussex, TN39 3AW. *Tel*: 01424 214605. May 2000

Face to Face

Free confidential counselling service for 16-25 year olds. *Address*: Face to Face, 5, Queens Road, Hastings, TN34 1QP, Sussex. *Tel*: 01424 466366. Self-referral by telephone or letter. Jul 2000

Fox, Jessica

Psychoanalytic Psychotherapist (London Centre for Psychotherapy). *Address:* Mrs Jessica Fox, Flat 2, 15, Adelaide Crescent, Hove, East Sussex, BN3 2JF. *Tel:* 01273 732177. 5798 Jun 2000

Gallagher, Eogain R

Qualifications: Psychoanalytic Psychotherapist, London Centre for Psychotherapy.

Address: Mr Eogain R. Gallagher, Flat 5, 17, Melville Road, Brighton, BN3 1TH, East Sussex. *Tel:* 01273 279805. 5798

Garner, Alegra

Analyst (Jungian), Society of Analytical Psychology; BAAP. Provides supervision for people in training. 5798, 6010 Jul 2000

Address: Mrs Alegra Garner, 37, Carlisle Road, Hove, East Sussex, BN3 4FP. *Tel:* 01273 249190. *Fax:* 01273 249191.

Gatehouse Therapy Centre

See under Hazel Redsull in this chapter. Jun 2000

Geer, Carol

Carol is a general counsellor and counselling supervisor. She deals with personal growth, relationship and stress issues. She offers both short-term and long-term counselling. She works with individuals and couples and her own personal therapy and supervision is ongoing. Her clientele are helping and caring professionals, carers, students and includes women. Her theoretical approach is psychodynamic and analytical. Carol's fees are £18 - £30 per session.

Qualifications: include BAC. AccC; Dip Memb IPC; Adv Dip Psychodynamic Couns (WPF 1991) PG Marital Interaction (WPF 1993); Cert Person-centred Art Therapy (1988); Dip Supervision 1997. Code of Ethics: BAC. Registration: UKRC Reg Ind Counsellor.

Address: Carol Geer, Elderwood, Wallcrouch, Wadhurst, Sussex, TN5 7JJ. *Tel*: 01580 200730. *E-mail:* carol@geer.fsnet.co.uk May 2000

Gilbert, Betty

Analytical Psychologist (Jungian), The British Assoc. of Psychotherapists.

Address: Mrs Betty Gilbert, 24, Braybon Avenue, Brighton, BN1 8HG, East Sussex. *Tel:* 01273 502767. 5798

Hall, Jilly.

A private practice offering counselling and psychotherapy for individuals, couples and groups. She offers training in counselling skills for statutory and voluntary agencies. Jilly offers individual or group supervision. An assessment session is offered initially. Hours: Monday to Friday mornings, afternoons and evenings. Her theoretical basis is Gestalt. Jilly's fees are £28 per session.

Qualifications: BAC Accred. Trainer; Dip. Couns; Dip. Psychotherapy (UKCP).

Address: Jilly Hall, 22, Collier Road, Hastings, Sussex, TN34 3JR. *Tel*: 01424 431154. May 2000

Halpin, Jill

Jill is an analytical psychotherapist and art psychotherapist. She provides developmental and crisis therapy on an intensive, long-term basis by preference. Her aim is to be available to people in order to facilitate growth and development in an open and non-judgemental way. Jill's fees are £30 per session but are negotiable to lower wage earners. *Qualifications:* Member of the Guild of Psychotherapists (London); training analyst for a number of people training at the University of Kent.

Address: Mrs J Halpin, Stonerunner Cottage, Rye Harbour, Sussex, TN31 7TT. *Tel*: 01797 224351. Jul 2000

Heathfield Centre

This centre provides hypnotherapy and psychotherapy. *Contact:* Ken Gilmore. *Address*: Heathfield Centre, Culverden, Hailsham Road, Heathfield, Sussex, TN21 8ET. *Tel*: 01435 862380. *Note:* Details not verified at August 2000.

Hope, Beryl

Music therapist and counsellor. Beryl specialises in working with adults who were abused as children, but helps people who have all kinds of problems.

Beryl's work is basically Person Centred, but she also uses Gestalt, Brief Therapy and Cognitive Therapy according to each individual person's needs. Sometimes a person may benefit from Music or Art Therapy, both of which she incorporates into her work. Counselling may be on a short-term or long-term basis for individual adult clients. Sessions last one hour and Beryl uses a sliding scale of fees.

As a member of the British Association for Counselling, Beryl is committed to its Code of Ethics. She is also a member of Sussex Counselling, and the British Society for Music Therapy.

Address: Burnt Oak Cottage, Grove Lane, Iden, Rye, East Sussex, TN31 7QA. *Tel:* 01797 280481. *E-mail:* bbhope@msn.com May 2000

Howell, Simon

Simon is a Systemic psychotherapist.

Address: NSPCC, 2, Sedlescombe Road South, St Leonards, Sussex, TN38 0TA. *Tel:* 01424 428833. 5409

H&RCS

Hastings & Rother Counselling Service offers clients the opportunity to talk in confidence with a trained counsellor who is not personally involved and a chance to explore their situation from all angles. Help is offered whilst working on their own best course of action and support given while any change is being made. It is voluntary, non-fee charging service, reliant on donations from clients and others.

H&RCS has the support of psychiatrists, psychologists and senior counsellors. It conforms to the Code of Ethics & Practice of the British Association for Counselling. It also holds an annual programme of whole-day workshops. H&RCS offers confidential counselling to people at times of stress, change, disaster or bereavement, at any age or stage in their lives.

Counsellors and support staff donate their skills as unpaid volunteers. Clients donate whatever they can afford. Donations in cash or in kind are welcome.

Contact: Rose Webster. *Address*: Hastings & Rother Counselling Service, Ground Floor Flat, 73, London Road, St Leonards-on-Sea, East Sussex, TN37 6AR. *Tel*: 01424 428300. Jun 2000

Hutton, Dr Francoise

Qualifications: Medically qualified practitioner. MRC Psych. Analytical Psychologist (Jungian), The British Assoc. of Psychotherapists; Psychoanalytic Psychotherapist, Assoc. for Psychoanalytic Psychotherapy in the NHS. Consultant psychiatrist and psychotherapist.

Address; Dr Francoise Hutton, Ticehurst

Clinic, 14-18, New Church Road, Hove, East Sussex, BN3 4FH. (There is wheelchair access). *Tel:* 01273 747464. *TelFax:* 01273 473850. 5798 Jun 2000

Inskipp, Francesca

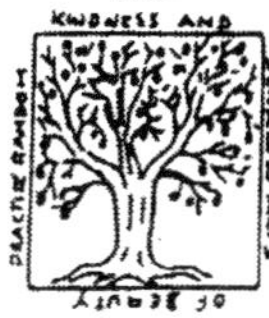

Francesca is a general counsellor and counselling supervisor. She works with both individuals and groups and her clientele are anyone who needs counselling. She is in personal therapy and ongoing supervision. Her theoretical approach is humanistic, person-centred and psychosynthetic. Francesca's fees are £25 negotiable per session and £30 for supervision.

Qualifications: include BAC Fellow; BAC Acc Supervision; Dip Couns (Keele 1971); Dip Psychosynthesis Couns & Therapy (PET 1990). Code of Ethics: BAC.

Address: Francesca Inskipp, 2, Market Terrace, St Leonards, Sussex, TN38 0DB. *Tel*: 01424 427948. May 2000

Ironside, Leslie

Child and adolescent psychotherapist. Qualifications: Tavistock Clinic training in child and adolescent psychotherapy leading to full membership of the Association of Child Psychotherapists. Fees: These are negotiated individually with the client.

Address: Leslie Ironside, 35, Clermont Terrace, Brighton, Sussex, BN1 6SJ. *Tel*: 01273 709660. May 2000

Jenkins, Mary

Mary is a general counsellor. She deals with people with relationship problems; stress and anxiety problems; identity and loss issues; also personal growth. She is in ongoing personal therapy and supervision. Clients include carers, the elderly, women, helping professionals; and young people. Her theoretical approach is humanistic, integrative (TA Gestalt and Person-Centred). Mary's fees are £25 with some concessions.

Qualifications: Dip Couns (Wealden Col); RGN. Mary abides by the BAC Code of Ethics.

Address: Mary Jenkins, 481, The Ridge, Hastings, East Sussex, TN34 2RT. *Tel*: 01424 754741. Jun 2000

Jephcott, Monika

Monika is a general counsellor, counselling supervisor, psychotherapist and psychotherapy supervisor. She deals with addictions, depression and anxiety, phobias, co-counselling, eating disorders, identity problems and relationship counselling. She works with individuals, couples, families and groups and speaks German as an alternative language. She is in ongoing personal therapy and supervision herself. Her theoretical approach is integrative, person centred, psychodynamic, TA, and gestalt. Monika's fees are £25-40 per session.

Qualifications: BA (Hons), Cert. Ed. Dip. Couns. BAC AccC. UKRC Reg. Code of Ethics: BAC & UKCP. *Registration:* UKRC Occupational Registered Counsellor. Registered Member of Counsellors in Primary Care.

Address: Monika Jephcott, Fern Hill Centre, Fern Hill, Fairwarp, Uckfield, TN22 3BU. *Tel*: 01825 712312. *Fax:* 01825 713679 *E-mail*: mokijep@aol.com Jul 2000

Kaplinsky, Catherine

Analyst (Jungian), Society of Analytical Psychology. Psychotherapist.

Barcombe address: Mrs Catherine Kaplinsky, Mill Brook, Barcombe Mills Road, Barcombe, Lewes, East Sussex, BN8 5BP. *Tel:* 01273 401167. *Fax:* 01273 400663.

Ticehurst address: Mrs Catherine Kaplinsky, Young Persons Unit, Ticehurst Hospital, Ticehurst, Wadhurst, East Sussex, TN5 7HU. (There is wheelchair access). *Tel:* 01580 200391. 5798

KCPU

Covering the counties of Kent, Sussex and Surrey, the Associates of the KCPU provide counselling, psychotherapy, supervision and training courses which include most areas of client difficulties. The underlying philosophy is for the respect, worth and dignity of individuals, and the fundamental belief that people have capacity to change.

The KCPU is optimistic and, when used by our Associates, demonstrates a profound respect for the person's autonomy. The aim is to apply these principles in a creative, flexible and responsible manner. Founder member: Valerie Cunningham; Secretary: Elizabeth Buckley.

Address: Kent Counselling & Psychotherapy Union, 19, Birling Road, Tunbridge Wells, Kent, TN2 5LX. *Tel:* 01892 529903. *E-mail:* val@kcpu.org.uk May 2000

Leeburn, Jennifer

Psychoanalytic Psychotherapist, The British Association of Psychotherapists.

Address: Mrs Jennifer Leeburn, 12, Priory Crescent, Lewes, East Sussex, BN7 1HP. *Tel:* 01273 476444. 5798

Lidster, Wendy

Wendy is a general counsellor, psychotherapist and counselling supervisor. She deals with relationship, sexuality and sex related issues, work related problems, and personal growth. She counsels anxiety, phobias, and stress. She works with individuals and couples. Her clientele includes creative people, helping and caring professionals, students and trainees. Wendy deals with both men and women. She has ongoing supervision for her work. Her theoretical approach is integrative, psychodynamic, behavioural, systemic and humanistic. Wendy's fees are £45 per session.

Qualifications: include BAC AccC; Dip Couns; BASMT Acc; FMA Acc; Relate Acc. Code of Ethics: BAC, BASMT. Registration: UKRC Reg Ind Counsellor, UKCP Reg Psychotherapist.

Address: Wendy Lidster, 19, Shirley Drive, Hove, Sussex, BN3 6NQ. *Tel:* 01273 330262. May 2000

Lloyd, Dr Barbara,

Psychoanalytic Psychotherapist, The British Association of Psychotherapists. *Qualifications:* B. Ph. D., FBPS.

Address: Dr Barbara B. Lloyd, 10, Withdean Road, Brighton, BN1 5BL, East Sussex. *Tel:* 01273 501252.

Reader in Social Psychology. *Address:* Dr Barbara Lloyd, University of Sussex, School of Social Sciences, Falmer, Brighton, BN1 9QN, East Sussex. *Tel:* 01273 678035. *Fax:* 01273 678466. 5798

Mackay-Danton, Pauline

Pauline is a general counsellor and counselling supervisor. She deals with depression, personal growth and relationship problems. She counsels on both a short-term and long-term basis. She works with individuals and groups and her clients include students or trainees, creative people, helping caring professionals, sexual minorities, and indeed anyone else. She is in ongoing personal therapy and supervision. Her theoretical approach is integrative, person-centred and gestalt. Pauline's fees are £25 per session. *Qualifications*: include BA; PG Dip Couns (Brighton); RSA Cert Couns Skills in Devel Learning; Primary Cert Supervision (SMC, Lon); Gestalt Psychotherapy Trainee (Gestalt Centre, Lon). Post-graduate Diploma in Gestalt Therapy. Code of Ethics: BAC.

Address: Pauline Mackay-Danton, 5, Godwin Rd, Hastings, Sussex, TN35 5JR. *Tel*: 01424 439300. May 2000

Masani, Peter

Analytical Psychologist (Jungian), The British Association of Psychotherapists.

Address: Mr Peter A. Masani, C. Psychol., 7, Clare Road, Lewes, East Sussex, BN7 1PN. Tel: 01273 474800. [5798]

McLaughlin, Sally

Sally offers short- and long-term individual counselling and family systems work which is usually done with groups and couples. Sally deals with depression, anxiety, relationship problems and with people who want to explore their lives and assess how they are living them. Her clients include women, men and sexual and other minorities. Sally is in ongoing therapy and supervision. Her fees are £10 - £30 and she offers some low cost places.

Qualifications: BA; MA Psychotherapy & Councselling; six years' training in Gestalt therapy and ongoing training in Gestalt and Family Systems. BAC Code of Ethics.

Address: Sally McLaughlin, Newenden, Croft Road, Hastings, Sussex, TN34 3HB. *Tel*: 01424 718026. *Fax:* 01424 426754. [May 2000]

Michaelson, Sue

Sue is a transpersonal psychotherapist.

Address: 34, St Mary's Terrace, Hastings, Sussex, TN34 3LR. *Tel:* 01424 429858. [5409]

Maxwell, Hugh

Hugh is a psychodrama psychotherapist.

Address: Westwood Day Hospital, Westwood House, 7, Holmesdale Gardens, Hastings, Sussex, TN34 1LY. [5409 May 2000]

Molyneux, Graham

Graham is a general counsellor and counselling supervisor. He deals with anxiety, phobias, obsessional disorders, bereavement, personal growth and relationship counselling. He works with individuals, couples, families and groups. He is in active therapy and supervision himself. His theoretical approach is person-centred and his fees are £28 per one hour session.

Qualifications: include BAC AccC; Dip in Person-Centred Couns (Metanoia 1996); IPCL; Memb BAPCA. Code of Ethics: BAC.

Address: Graham Molyneux, 3, Valley Drive, Withdean, Brighton, Sussex, BN1 5FA. *Tel*: 01273 566918 / 884614. *E-mail:* gmolyneux@avl.com [May 2000]

Montier, Michael

See under Tunbridge Wells Counselling Centre. [May 2000]

Mooncie, Ben

Ben practices in counselling and psychotherapy using transactional analysis. All his work is supervised and he attends ongoing clinical training. His clients include children, individuals, couples, people with learning disabilities and people in group therapy. He also takes sessions at the Pinehurst Centre in the evenings and at weekends. His fees are £25 per session.

Address: Ben Mooncie, The Professional Centre, 50, High Street, Old Town, Hastings, East Sussex, TN34 3EN. Also at The Pinehurst Centre, 3, Avondale Road, St Leonards, East Sussex, TN38 0SA. *Tel*: 01424 423687 (Pinehurst Centre); 01424 465050 (The Professional Centre).

Morgan-Jones, Richard

Psychoanalytic Psychotherapist, London Centre for Psycotherapy. Therapy supervision and team development.

Address: Richard Morgan-Jones, 25, Lewes Road, Eastbourne, East Sussex, BN21 2BY. *Tel:* 01323 647531. (There is wheelchair access). [5798 Jun 2000]

Mulvey, Jean

Psychoanalytical Psychotherapist and Analytical Psychologist (Jungian), Society of Analytical Psychology, International Association for Analytical Psychology, Confederation of Analytical Psychologists, Brighton Association of Analytic Psychotherapists.

Address: Mrs Jean Mulvey, Aldsworth, Lewes Road, Ringmer, East Sussex, BN8

5ER. *Tel/Fax:* 01273 812944.

Psychotherapist, Mid-Sussex NHS Trust. *Address:* Mrs Jean Mulvey, Department of Psychotherapy, Princess Royal Hospital, Haywards Heath, West Sussex, RH16 4EX. *Tel:* 01444 441881. 5798, 6004 Jul 2000

Munro, Frances

Frances is a stress counsellor. Her and her husband, Dr William Munro (see chapter 'Alternative Help - Autogenic Therapy), travel all over the country to offer their services on stress and other related health issues. *Qualifications:* B.Sc. Hons.

Address: Mrs Frances Munro, The Estana, Freezeland Lane, Bexhill, Sussex, TN39 5JD. *Tel:* 01424 219133. Aug 2000

Murdoch, Edna

Edna is a general counsellor, psychotherapist and counselling supervisor. Covering all of East Sussex, she offers stress management, psychotherapy, brief counselling and supervision for psychotherapists and counsellors. Edna deals with bereavement and relationship issues. She works with individuals such as students and trainees, helping and caring professionals, women, sexual minorities and young people. She is in ongoing personal therapy and supervision herself. Her theoretical approach is integrative. Edna's fees are £30 per session.

Qualifications: these include BAC AccC; Adv Dip Psychotherapy (Pellin); CTP. Code of Ethics: BAC.

Address: Edna Murdoch, 104, Tamworth Rd, Hove, East Sussex, BN3 5FH. *Tel/Fax*: 01273 735732. *E-mail:* e.murdoch@virgin.net May 2000

Muriel, Nick

Nick is a general counsellor and experienced group worker who has worked for many years with drug addiction, anger management, problems with relating to others, anxiety and stress. *Qualifications:* Cert. Ed, Post Graduate Diploma in Counselling.

Address: Nick Muriel, 39c, Carisbrooke Road, St Leonards-on-Sea, East Sussex, TN38 0JN. *Tel/Fax:* 01424 425923. *E-mail:* 106672.1130@compuserve.com 6008 Jul 2000

Neilson, Dr Frances

Analytical Psychologist (Jungian). *Address:* Dr Frances Neilson, 63, Beatty Avenue, Coldean, Brighton, BN1 9EP, East Sussex. *Tel:* 01273 260344. *Qualifications:* MRC Psych. Medically qualified practitioner.

Staff Grade Doctor (psychiatry). *Address:* Dr Frances Neilson, Mill View Hospital, Nevill Avenue, Hove, BN3 7HZ. *Tel:* 01273 696011. *Fax:* 01273 242046.

NHS psychotherapy. *Address:* Dr Frances Neilson, Hove Polyclinic, Nevill Avenue, Hove, BN3 7HY. *Tel:* 01273 696011. 5988

Oakley, Joy

Counsellor. Joy is a Member of the British Psychological Society. Qualifications: BA Hons. Psychology. Dip. Couns. (BAC recognised).

Address: Joy Oakley, 63, St Helen's Park Road, Hastings, Sussex, TN34 2JJ. *Tel:* 01424 420140. Jul 2000

O'Toole, Gerry

Member of the Beech Group; please see under 'Beech'.

Picquart, Genevieve

Genevieve is a general counsellor, psychotherapist. She deals with: anxiety; depression; panic attacks; relationship problems; bereavement; divorce; abuse (verbal, physical, sexual, ritual); eating disorders; sexual difficulties; phobias; and addictions. She works with individuals, couples and groups. She has been practising for 11 years and is in ongoing therapy and supervision herself. Her theoretical approach is psychodynamic, analytical body-psychotherapeutic, person centered. Genevieve's fees are £30 per hour session. She also speaks French and some Spanish.

Qualifications: include BAC AccC; Dip Couns (Crawley 1993); Cert Analytical Body Psychotherapy (BAABP 1991); Post Grad. Cert. of Advanced Studies in Psychosexual Counselling and Therapy (2000). Code of Ethics: BAC. Registration: UKRC Reg Ind Counsellor.

Address: Genevieve Picquart, 117, Lansdowne Place, Hove, Sussex, BN3 1FP. (Wheelchair access). *Tel*: 01273 730520. *Fax:* 01273 206508. *E-mail:* www.picquart.co.uk May 2000

Pinehurst Centre

This is a centre where therapy is available; psychotherapy, hypnotherapy. For details of individual counsellors, please see under their names: Beryl Hope, Ben Mooncie and Joy Oakley.

Address: The Pinehurst Centre, 3 Avondale Road, St Leonards, TN38 0SA. *Tel*: 01424 423687. Jul 2000

Popkin, Jen

Jen is a general counsellor, hypnotherapist and counselling supervisor. She deals with abuse, alcohol abuse, addictions, eating disorders, relationship problems, divorce recovery, stress management and critical incident debriefing. Jen works with individuals, couples, young people, groups and organisations. Her clientele has included those needing wheelchair access, people with learning disabilities and victims of crime and violence. She is in ongoing supervision herself. Her theoretical approach is eclectic and integrative.

Jen also works at the Springfield Centre which "provides a holistic service and training, including the counselling therapy, massage, reflexology, healing and aromatherapy. Anyone can make an initial enquiry at the telephone number given below. Hours and fees are negotiated individually with the client. Early appointments can be made to suit some who go to work (e.g. 8.00am), evenings and occasional weekends. Jen's fees are £15 - £25 per session and are negotiable for non-earning clients.

Qualifications: include MSc Couns (London); Dip Hypnotherapy (NAHP); MA (Education). Code of Ethics: BAC.

Address: Jen Popkin, The Springfield Centre, 4, Springfield Rd, St Leonards, Sussex, TN38 0TU. (There is wheelchair access). *Tel*: 01424 428470. May 2000

Powe, Roger

Roger is a general counsellor. He counsels bereavement, stress, relationship problems and deals with sex, work and educational related issues. He counsels mostly long-term. Roger works with individuals and is in personal therapy and ongoing supervision himself. His clients include young people, executives and managers; in fact anyone. He has a psychodynamic theoretical approach. Roger's fees are £20 per session with a sliding scale for the low-waged.

Qualifications: include BAC AccC; MA; BEd; Dip Humanities (London); Adv Dip Couns (Northbrook Coll.). Code of Ethics: BAC. Registration: UKRC Reg Ind Counsellor.

Address: Roger Powe, 8, Preston Lodge, 10, Little Preston Street, Brighton, Sussex, BN1 2HQ. *Tel:* 01273 726398. May 2000

Rae, Frances

Frances is trained to offer counselling help to couples and families as well as to individuals. Her approach invites clients to look at significant relationships and beliefs - past, present and future. She offers both short and long term work in response to clients' needs. She is a member of UKCP (United Kingdom Council for Psychotherapy).

Qualifications: BA in Psychology & Philosophy; PCGE; DST. Helping couples, individuals and families.

Address: Frances Rae, The Counselling Partnership, 21, Court Road, Tunbridge Wells, Kent. TN4 8EB. *Tel*: 01892 543025. May 2000

Redsull, Hazel

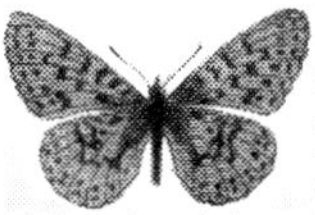

Hazel is an art psychotherapist with many years' experience of an eclectic practice, working with adults, children and adolescents. She is at ease working with art drama play and traditional verbal therapies. As a visiting lecturer at Goldsmiths College she can also offer experimental workshop training days to work groups of any profession. Bereavement and post trauma work also forms part of her practice. *Qualifications*: Registered Art Therapist of BAAT; SRAT (A).

Address: Gatehouse Therapy Centre, Reeves Gatehouse, Staplecross Road, Northiam, Sussex, TN31 6JN. *Tel*: 01580 831751. *Fax:* 01580 830964. There is wheelchair access with toilet facilities. The Gatehouse is situated in beautiful Wealden countryside and is an ideal setting for professional training days. Fees are negotiable. Jun 2000

Richardson, Madeleine

Madeleine is a psychotherapist, and counselling supervisor. She deals with abuse, anxiety, phobias, stress and trauma. She counsels identity and relationship problems, sex-related and sexuality issues. She works with individuals and couples, organisations and includes all. Her clientele includes carers, and the helping and caring professionals. She is in personal therapy and ongoing supervision. Her theoretical approach is integrative, humanistic, systemic, behavioural and psychodynamic. Madeleine's fees are £40 per session. Madeleine is a member of the Beech Group (see separate entry).

Qualifications: include BAC AccC; BASMT Acc; NMGC Acc; Sexual Therapist; Parks Inner Child Therapist; Memb ASSP; Qualified Family Mediator. Code of Ethics: BAC, BASMT, BABCP. Registration: UKRC Reg Ind Counsellor, UKCP Reg Psychotherapist.

Address: Madeleine Richardson, The Beech Group, 221, Preston Road, Brighton, Sussex, BN1 6SA. *Answerphone:* 01273 504385. May 2000

Rignell, John

John deals with general counselling, psychotherapy and short-term counselling. He works with individuals and his clientele includes helping and caring professionals, young people, minorities, and men. John has ongoing personal therapy and supervision himself. His theoretical approach is psychodynamic. John's fees are £15-30 per session.

Qualifications: include BAC AccC; PG Dip Dramatherapy; Dip Adv Psychodynamic Couns (WPF1994); Memb IPC; Psychoanalytic Psychotherapy. Code of Ethics: BAC. Registration: UKRC Reg Ind Counsellor.

Address: John Rignell, 4, Temple Gardens, Brighton, Sussex, BN1 3AE. *Tel*: 01273 204314. May 2000

Rock Clinic Association

The Rock Clinic Association provides good quality orthodox complementary and psychological medicine and therapy throughout East Sussex. They offer low cost and affordable counselling to those who cannot afford to pay privately or cannot wait for NHS treatment. *Contact:* Melanie Withers. Registered Charity No. 1057328.

Address: Rock Clinic Association, 270, Eastern Road, Brighton, BN2 5TA, East Sussex. *Tel:* 01273 621841. *E-mail:* therock@pavilion.co.uk *Website:* www.pavilion.co.uk/the-rock-clinic Jun 2000

Rock, Gillian

Gillian is a general counsellor a nd counselling supervisor. She deals with abuse, bereavement, depression, stress and relationship problems. She works with individuals, couples and groups. She offers both short and long-term counselling. She has ongoing personal therapy and supervision herself. Gillian's theoretical approach is psychodynamic and integrative. Her fees are £20 - £30 per session and are agreed at assessment.

Qualifications: BAC AccC; dip Couns (Crawley 1994); Cert Acc Cruse Bereavement Care 1994; Cruse Supervisor's Cert. 1995; Post Qual Cert Psychodynamic couns (sussex 1997); Post Qual Cert Personal Development in Clinical Supervision (Sussex 1999). Code of Ethics: BAC Registered Practitioner. UKRC Reg Ind Counsellor.

Address: Gillian Rock, 61b, Beaconsfield Villas, Brighton, Sussex, BN1 6HB. *Tel:* 01273 502736 or 01273 502900 (answerphone only). Jun 2000

Russell, Nina

Analytical Psychologist (Jungian), The British Assoc. of Psychotherapists.

Address: Mrs Nina P. Russell, 46, Elizbaeth Avenue, Hove, East Sussex, BN3 6WG. *Tel:* 01273 507555. 5798 Jun 2000

Sanders, Peter

Peter has a private practice offering psychotherapy and counselling for individuals, groups, couples and families using transactional analysis. He offers tuition, and he is also a counselling supervisor. He gives staff support for teams in caring agencies, training and nurturing events. Hours: daytime, some evenings, occasional weekends. Home visits as an alternative.

Peter Sanders is on the register of the United Kingdom Council for Psychotherapy as a Transactional Analyst with clinical speciality, i.e. Psychotherapist within the Integrative/Humanistic ethical codes. There is no wheelchair access, but home visits are offered. Peter's fees are standard rate of £35 per hour, with no concessions; group £20 per 2-hour; couples £45 per hour; organisation work £50 per hour.

Qualifications: BA Honours; CQSW; DipSW; CTA. He is registered with the UK Council for Psychotherapy.

Address: Peter Sanders, Midsummer House, 66, St Helen's Park Road, Hastings, East Sussex, TN34 2JJ. *Tel*: 01424 420615. *E-mail*: ph.sanders@talk21.com May 2000

Schueppert, Deirdre

See under Tunbridge Wells Counselling Centre. May 2000 0

Short, Nigel

Nigel is a cognitive behavioural psychotherapist. He offers therapy to people experiencing personal distress, particularly those with anxiety related difficulties e.g. phobias, depression, post-traumatic stress disorder, obsessive and compulsive problems, chronic fatigue syndrome. He has ongoing clinical supervision. Nigel's fees are £55 per session.

Qualifications: BSc (Hons. Nurs.); BsC (Hons. CBT); RGN; RMN; PGCE; Accredited UKCP Psychotherapist.

Address: 34, Emmanuel Road, Hastings, Sussex, TN34 3LB. *Tel:* 01424 444951. 5409 May 2000

Sidhu, Frankie

Frankie is a general counsellor, psychotherapist, counselling supervisor and tutor. Areas of speciality include addiction, anxiety, phobias, ME, bereavement, relationships, parenting, personal growth and meaning, lesbian gay issues around coming out and identity. Frankie's clients include students and trainees, people working in the helping professions and people who feel that there *must* be more to life! She works with individuals and groups. Frankie is in personal therapy and professional supervision herself. Her theoretical model is psychosynthesis which has a transpersonal perspective and her Brighton practice is 'Gay Affirmative'. Fees are £25 - £40 per one hour session.

Qualifications: Diploma Psychosynthesis Counselling & Therapy (PET); Advanced Diploma Psychosynthesis Psythotherapy (PET); Cert. Counselling Supervision (Cascade). Frankie Sidhu is in the practitioners' register of United Kingdom Council for Psychotherapy, within the Association of Accredited Psychospiritual Psychotherapists and British Association of Counselling ethical codes.

Address: Mrs Frankie Sidhu, Preston Circus, Brighton, East Sussex. *Tel:* 01273 603896. Telephone for a free half-hour initial meeting. May 2000

Simanowitz, Val

Val is a general counsellor and counselling supervisor. She deals with anxiety, phobias, depression, eating disorders, inter-cultural issues and personal growth. She works with individuals and couples and anyone who needs counselling. Val's clientele includes helping and caring professionals, students and trainees, oppressed groups such as refugees, and women. She has ongoing therapy and supervision herself. Her theoretical approach is person-centred and integrative. Val's fees are £25 per session, but with a sliding scale.

Qualifications: these include BAC. AccC; BA (Hons); MA; Dip Couns (E. Lon. Univ. 1977); Cert Supervision (Maudsley 1993); Memb AHPP. Code of Ethics: BAC. Registration: UKRC Reg Ind Counsellors.

Address: Val Simanowitz, 2, High Pastures, Graywood, East Hoathley, Lewes, East Sussex, BN8 6QT. *Tel*: 0182 587 2524. May 2000

Stedman, John

John is a general counsellor, trained psychoanalytic psychotherapist and counselling supervisor. He deals with relationship and sex-related problems and bereavement counselling. He counsels individuals and his clientele includes helping and caring professionals, religious groups and other minorities. His theoretical approach is psychodynamic and eclectic. John's fees are £25-30 per session, but are dependent on income. *Qualifications*: these include Dip Theology (London); trained Psychoanalytic Psychother-apist (LCIP); Memb BCP APPNHS; BAC.

Address: John Stedman, Lincoln Centre & Institute for Psychotherapy, 22, Little Western Street, Hove, Sussex, BN3 1AG. *Tel*: 01273 739668. Jun 2000

Stehle, Peter

Peter is an existential psychotherapist and counselling psychologist. *Qualifications:* AdvDipExPsych, MA, BA, BSc. Registered Psyotherapist (UKCP) and Counselling Psychologist.

Address: 2, Wickham Manor Cottage, Pannel Lane, Winchelsea, East Sussex, TN36 4AG. *Tel:* 01797 227009. *E-mail:* fp.stehle@talk21.com May 2000

Stockdale, Mel

He describes himself as providing "Individual counselling/psychotherapy for a wide range of personal problems". He provides an eclectic combination of Rogerian, cognitive/behavioural, & hypnotherapeutic approaches. He can use hypnotherapy if appropriate and with the client's permission. In addition, Mel can provide counselling for occupational choice and work related problems.

A man of mature years, Mel Stockdale is a Chartered Psychologist with NHS experience of clinical psychology as well as in counselling and hypnotherapy. He is married with three children and three grandchildren. Clients may contact Mel direct or through the professional services Hours: The service is provided during office hours. Fees are arranged individually with the client - reduced fees may be available. Private clients are seen at Mel's home in Robertsbridge. There is no wheelchair access. Mel's fees are currently £30 per 50 minutes session.

Qualifications: Degrees in psychology BA, & theology BD; Career Guidance Dip.CG; Hypnosis & Psychotherapy, DHP; & Advanced Counselling, Dip.Couns.; Chartered Psychologist, C.Psychol; Member of British Society for Experimental & Clinical Hypnosis, MBSECH.

Address: Mel Stockdale, 13, Mill Rise, Robertsbridge, East Sussex, TN32 5EF. *Tel*: 01580 881857. May 2000

Suss, Lawrence

Lawrence is a counsellor, psychotherapist and analyst and also provides counselling supervision. He deals with relationship and trauma counselling and personal growth. He counsels on both a short-term and long-term timespan with individuals, couples and groups. His clients include students, helping and caring professionals and he counsels both men and women. Lawrence's theoretical approach is psychodynamic, analytic and CAT. His fees are £35 but are negotiable.

Qualifications: include BAC AccC; BSc; DMS; Dip Couns (Brighton1994); Brief Psychotherapy (CAT); and Training in Marital, Gestalt, Psychoanalytic Psychotherapy (AGIP). Codes of Ethics: BAC, AGIP, ACAT. Registration: UKRC Reg Ind Counsellors. UKCP registered psychoanalytic psychotherapist.

Address: Lawrence Suss, 61b, Beaconsfield Villas, Brighton, Sussex, BN1 6HB. *Tel*: 01273 508688 / 502900. May 2000

Sweeting, Gina

Gina is a member of the Beech Group. Please see under 'Beech'.

Taylor, Margaret

Margaret is a State Registered Art Therapist with 13 years' experience in the following areas of clinical practice within the NHS: Forensic Psychiatry, Adult General Psychiatry, Learning Disabilities and Care of the Elderly. *Qualifications:* Dip. A.T., R.A.Th.

Contact address: Sussex Autistic Community Trust, Unit C, The Roebuck Centre, Roebuck Street, Hastings, TN34 3BB, East Sussex. *Tel*: 01424 722516. May 2000

Thomas, Richard

Qualifications: MA Dip Couns. Psychotherapy and counselling; Post. Grad. Dip. in Relationship and psychosexual therapy. NHS clinical experience. Individual, couples, relationships. Stress management courses.

Address: Richard Thomas, 14, Wickham Avenue, Bexhill, Sussex, TN39 3EN. *Tel*: Freephone 0800 731 3168 (24 hour answerphone). Jul 2000

Thomson, Kay

Qualified counsellor and therapist providing a private counselling service to people who are experiencing difficulties in their life for which they feel therapeutic help might be the answer. Particular experience in working with adults who have been abused in their childhoods. Private supervision service to counsellors. Fees: Initial consultation free of charge; then a standard fee of £30 per one hour session.

Qualifications: Include Dip. Counselling, (1992); MA Counselling Psychology and Family Therapy training (1995); Certificate in Person Centred Art Therapy (1999). Kay Thomson is included on the Registration of Supervisors for the PG Diploma counselling (Univ Brighton). MBr Assoc of Couns. Code of Ethics: BAC.

Address: Kay Thomson, 125, Old London Road, Hastings, East Sussex, TN35 5LY. *Tel*: 01424 440016. Jul 2000

Tredgold, Clare

Psychoanalytic Psychotherapist, London Centre for Psychotherapy.

Address: Mrs Clare Tredgold, 13, Florence Road, Brighton, BN1 6DL. *Tel:* 01273 502112. 5798

Tunbridge Wells Centre

Offers professional counselling to individuals or couples who are experiencing personal relationship or family problems.The service is not free although there is a flexible scale of fees. Most of the work is long-term, with individuals. Clients are invited to an initial assessment interview and subsequently offered counselling, once a week, if it is felt to be appropriate. If clients are using drink/drugs, the psychodynamic model of counselling that is used would not be appropriate.

All the counsellors are volunteers, but have been through or are receiving training to diploma level or higher, and all attend weekly supervision.

Tunbridge Wells Counselling Centre is part of a national network of counselling centres, affiliated to the Westminster Pastoral Foundation based at Kensington.

Head of Centre: Dr Marie Botha; Head of counselling: Mrs Deirdre Schueppert; Head of training: Mrs Sarah Halliwell; Couples counsellor: Michael Montier; Administrator: Marilyn Foster. See individual entries in this chapter.

Address: Tunbridge Wells Counselling Centre, St George's Centre, 7, Chilston Road, Tunbridge Wells, Kent, TN4 9LP. *Tel:* 01892 548750.
E-mail: twcccounselling@ukonline.co.uk May 2000

Tyndale, Anne

Psychoanalytic Psychotherapist, The British Assoc. of Psychotherapists. *Address:* Mrs Anne Tyndale, 18, Montpelier Crescent, Brighton, BN1 3JF, East Sussex. *Tel:* 01273 775956. 5798 Jun 2000

Ward, George

Psychoanalytic Psychotherapist, The Lincoln Clinic & Centre for Psychotherapy. *Qualifications:* C. Psychol.
Address: Mr George W. Ward, The Lodge, Surrenden Park, Brighton, BN1 6XA. *Tel:* 01273 884270.

Head of Personal Counselling & Psychotherapy, University of Brighton.

Address: Mr George W. Ward, Patcham House, Park Street, Falmer, Brighton, BN1 9PH. *Tel:* 01273 642853. *E-mail:* gwward@bton.ac.uk 5798 Jun 2000

Wilson, Andrew

Counsellor and member of The Beech Group. Please see under 'Beech'. May 2000

Withers, Melanie

Melanie is a general counsellor, psychotherapist and counselling supervisor. She deals with eating disorders, anxiety, phobias, stress, bereavement and relationship issues. She counsels both long-term and short-term. She works with individuals, couples and groups. She also speaks French as an alternative language. Her clientele includes students, and helping and caring professionals and covers both genders. Her theoretical approach is psychodynamic. Melanie's fees are £20-30 per session.

Qualifications: include BAC AccC; BA; PGCE; PG Dip Couns; MA Couns Psychol; MA Supervision; Solution Focused Brief Therapy (WPF); Full Memb Brighton Assoc of Psychodynamic Couns. Code of Ethics: BAC. Registration: BAPPS (UKCP) Registered supervisor. UKRC Reg Ind Counsellor.

Address: Melanie Withers, The Rock Clinic, 270, Eastern Rd, Brighton, Sussex, BN2 5TA. *Tel*: 01273 621841. May 2000

Withers, Robert

Analyst (Jungian), Society of Analytical Psychology. Robert is a co-director of The Rock Clinic (see separate entry).

Address: Robert J. Withers, The Rock Clinic, 270, Eastern Road, Brighton, BN2 5TA. *Tel:* 01273 621841. 5798 Jun 2000

Counsellors By Town

Counsellors & therapists listed by location. For further information about an individual counsellor, please see 'Counsellors & Therapists' page 188.

Battle
Sue Cook; Mel Stockdale.

Bexhill
Anthony Anderson; Steve Clifford; Lorna Couldrick; Christine Coxhead; Prue Doherty.

Brighton & Hove
Gail Alexander; June Broadhurst; Susan Chiswell Jones; Daryl Cohen; Sue Cottrell; Jenny Deadman; Jessica Fox; Eogain Gallagher; Betty Gilbert; Francoise Hutton; Leslie Ironside; Lynn Jackson; Wendy Lidster; Barbara Lloyd; Graham Molyneux; Paul Morgan; Edna Murdoch; Frances Neilson; Genieve Picquart; Roger Powe; Madeleine Richardson; John Rignall; Gillian Rock; Nina Russell; Frankie Sidhu; John Stedman; Lawrence Suss; Clare Tredgold; Anne Tynedale; George Ward; Melanie Withers; Robert Withers.

Crowborough
Rosemary Dixon-Nuttall.

Eastbourne
Sandy Adey; Joy Cobban; Richard Morgan-Jones.

Hastings & St Leonards
Sandy Adey; Counselling Centre; Simon Howell; Francesca Inskipp; Mary Jenkins; Pauline Mackay-Danton; Sally McLauglin; Pinehurst Centre; Beryl Hope; Hugh Maxwell; Sue Michaelson; Ben Mooncie; Joy Oakley; Jen Popkin; Peter Saunders; Nigel Short; Margaret Taylor; Kay Thompson.

Lewes
Michael Bulman; Philipa Cannan; Jennifer Leeburn; Peter Masani; Jean Mulvey; Val Simanowitz.

Rye
Jill Halpin.

Tunbridge Wells
Dr Marie Botha; Val Cunningham.

Uckfield
Monika Jephcott.

Wadhurst
Carol Geer; Catherine Kaplinsky.

Westfield
Elli Buffery.

Winchelsea
Peter Stehle.

Crises & Emergencies

Crisis Card
A small card, issued by Mental Health Services, Hastings & Rother. It is intended that people suffering from a mental illness may carry around with them a Crisis Card. The wording on the card is as shown, below. [6052 Oct 99]

Local Organisations

Ambulance Service
Phone '999' and ask for an ambulance.

Weekend Crisis Line
Hastings & Rother Mental Health Weekend Crisis Telephone Line. A confidential telephone advice line available at weekends and Bank Holidays, operated by a psychiatric nurse. This service offers a chance to discuss any concerns about mental health problems. Contact is made with other services only if the caller wishes. An answerphone system is in operation and calls will be returned as soon as possible. Anyone may telephone. *Contact Name*: Sarah Tindall.

Hours: Weekends and Bank Holidays 9.00am to 5.00pm. *Address*: Mental Health Weekend Crisis Telephone Line, Conquest Hospital, The Ridge, Hastings, East Sussex. *Tel:* 01424 758057. [6056 Jul 2000]

Crisis Response Service
'We work to provide the community with an assessment and treatment service that will attempt to respond within 4 hours, with priorities given to emergency cases. We offer this to anyone of 16 years (if they have left school), up to 65 years of age who, in the opinion of a health service professional* is suffering from a mental health crisis.

We aim to provide an alternative to treatment in hospital and to enable the individ-

Crisis Card

For use if:
Name: ....
Address: ....
is involved in a MENTAL HEALTH EMERGENCY. **Important:** If I appear to be experiencing Mental Health difficulties that require decisions to be taken either against my wishes or in the absence of my agreement, then I request the following actions to be taken:
(A) That my nominee, below, be contacted immediately; informed of what is happening and requested to attend as a matter of urgency.

My nominee is:
Name: ....
Address: ....
....
Tel: ....

(B) That the following information be taken into account:
....
....
....
....

My GP/Doctor is: ....
....
Tel. No: ....

My Consultant is: ....
....
Tel. No: ....

My medication is: ....
....
....
Signed: ....
Date: ....

ual, where possible, to remain in their own environment. We work with clients for up to 3 weeks, providing a needs-led approach, ensuring the development of client participation, liaising with other services in an efficient and effective way.

Contact: Matt Fribbens, Team Manager. The team consists of a Consultant Psychiatrist, a Senior Clinical Medical Officer and a Staff Grade Psychiatrist, 6 qualified Psychiatric Nurses and a Community Support Worker and a qualified social worker.

Address: Crisis Response Service, Woodlands, Conquest Hospital, 729, The Ridge, St Leonards-on-Sea, East Sussex, TN37 7RD. *Tel:* 01424 757075 or 01424 757076. *Fax:* 01424 758901. [Jun 2000]

Helplines

Eastbourne Mental Health Helpline
Out of office hours: *Tel*: 01273 320202 Emergency Duty Service). [Jul 2000]

Mental Health Helpline
Tel: 0345 697590, 6pm to midnight, daily. [Jul 2000]

Hospital A & E Departments

'A & E' means 'Accident & Emergency'.

Brighton
Address: The Royal Sussex County Hospital, Eastern Road, Brighton, Sussex. *Tel*: 01273 696955. [Jul 2000]

Eastbourne
Address: Eastbourne District General Hospital, Kings Drive, Eastbourne, Sussex. *Tel*: 01323 417400. [Jul 2000]

Hastings
Address: Conquest Hospital, The Ridge, St Leonards-on-Sea, Sussex, TN37 7RD. *Tel*: 01424 755255. *Accident & Emergency Helpline* 01424 758106. [Jul 2000]

Haywards Heath
Address: Princess Royal Hospital, Lewes Road, Haywards Heath, Sussex. *Tel*: 01444 441881. [Jul 2000]

Tunbridge Wells
Address: Kent & Sussex Hospital, Mount Ephraim, Tunbridge Wells, Kent. *Tel*: 01892 526111. [Jul 2000]

Mental Health Helpline

A new service for people with mental health issues is a county-wide out of hours telephone helpline. The service is available from 6.00pm to midnight weekdays and 2.00pm at weekends.

The helpline is linked to the National Schizophrenia Fellowship (NSF) co-ordinator and is intended to complement support offered by the Samaritans. The calls are free and the numbers are 0808 808 3333 for English speakers; and 0808 800 2073 for Asian language speakers.[Jul 2000]

Police

Telephone '999' and ask for the police.

Samaritans

A listening service for any caller who is despairing, suicidal, or going through a crisis in their life. We do not give advice or offer to solve problems, but are here 24 hours a day. People can talk for as long as they need to and very often find their own solutions by talking through problems with a caring, sympathetic person. Anyone can phone or come into the Centre for a chat. *Hours*: The Centre is open to visitors from 9.30am to 9.30pm, and there is telephone help 24 hours a day.

We Listen

It doesn't matter who you are; if you're in crisis, despairing or suicidal it can make all the difference to talk about how you are feeling. Problems can get on top of anyone. Men and women. Gay and straight. Any religion and colour. Any age.

You can talk to us about anything that is troubling you; we will not judge you; we will not tell you what to do, but we will try to help you think things through; we will listen with an open mind for as long as you need.

You can speak in total confidence to one of our volunteers. They come from all walks of life and every kind of background. All are carefully trained to listen.

Address: Hastings and Rother Samaritans, 26, St. Andrews Square, Hastings, Sussex, TN34 1SR. *Tel*: 01424 436666. 6053 Jul 2000

Sanctuary Service

The Sanctuary, which is part of the larger organisation Turning Point, is a 24-hour service providing accommodation and emotional support for people who are experiencing mental health problems and feel that they have reached a crisis. Length of stay is usually 3 to 5 days. The service aims to provide a non-medical alternative to psychiatric admission for those unable to be supported in their present environment and who might otherwise be considered for hospital admission. *Contact*: Mr G. Body, manager. *Hours*: 24-hour service, but clients accepted only up until 9.00pm.

Address: Sanctuary Service, 36, Ashburnham Road, Hastings, Sussex, TN35 5JL. *Tel*: 01424 200353. *Fax*: 01424 200352. *E-mail:* sanctuary@hastings.firm.org.uk Jul 2000

Social Services

Emergency duty service outside of office hours, covering the whole of East Sussex and Brighton and Hove. *Tel:* 01273 320202. 5953 Jul 2000

National Organisations

Refuge

National crisis line. *Tel*: 0870 599 5443. Jul 2000

Samaritans

The Samaritans are available at any hour of the day or night to offer confidential emotional support to those in crisis and in danger of taking their own lives. One of their slogans is *Whatever you're going through, we'll go through it with you.* There are now over 200 branches in the UK and Eire.

Address: The Samaritans, 10, The Grove, Slough, SL1 1QP. *Tel:* 01753 532713. Website: www.samaritans.org.uk Jul 2000

Samaritans National Helpline

If you need to talk confidentially, we are available 24 hours a day, 365 days a year for the cost of a local call. *Tel*: 08457 90 90 90. *Website*: www.samaritans.org.uk Jul 2000

Further Information

Crisis Services Factsheet

George Stewart, MIND Information Unit, February 1998. Price 50p. Available from Mind Mail Order Service. *Tel*: 020 8221 9666.

Day Centres & Drop-in Centres

We are lucky to have two local day centres in Bexhill and Hastings and two local drop-in centres in St Leonards and Hastings. Find out here the difference between the two types of centre and more about the services they offer ...

Day v drop-in

To attend a day centre, one is normally referred by a health professional, but to attend a drop-in centre one simply, well, drops in. Drop-in centres are therefore more informal, providing 'open access' to anyone who wants to call ... you can come and go as you please. You'll get a warm welcome, information, support and advice. The two day centres locally are the 73a Centre in Bexhill and the Hastings Day Centre. The two drop-in centres are the Seaview Projects in St Leonards and Xtrax in Hastings.

Local Organisations

Bexhill 73a Centre

The 73a Centre is for the care and support of people living in the community who have mental health problems. The Centre is strongly committed to active participation and involvement of members in the day-to-day running and development of the centre, and is open 7 days a week. Socialising, group meetings, outings, sport, recreation and education all assist in enabling people to regain self-esteem and confidence. It is located next door to the Aldi Supermarket in London Road. *Contact:* Andrew Voyce, User representative. *Hours:* Mondays to Fridays 9am to 5pm; Saturdays & Sundays: 10.00am to 4.00p.m. There is access for the disabled.

Address: 73a Resource Centre, 73a, London Road, Bexhill, Sussex, TN39 2LB. *Tel:* 01424 213099. 5867 Jun 2000

Hastings Day Centre

The Hastings Day Centre provides day support for people aged 18-65 with long-term mental health problems. It currently serves a group of 60 people drawn mainly from Hastings and St. Leonards.

The centre fosters a warm and friendly atmosphere, encourages participation and self-expression and provides an active programme selected by centre users. *Hours:* Mondays 9.30am to 1.00pm.Tuesdays to Fridays 9.30am to 4.00pm. There is no fee, but £1.40 is charged for lunch. Transport is available within Hastings & St. Leonards for a small fee. Centre manager: Franco Di Francesco. The centre has been managed by Maca, (see below), since July 2000 and the accommodation is provided by Hastings Mind.

Address: Hastings Day Centre, 6, St. Helen's Crescent, Hastings, East Sussex, TN34 2EW. *Tel:* 01424 434886. *E-mail:* maca@hastingsdc.freeserve.co.uk Jul 2000

Maca
Please see under 'National Organisations' for more details of this charity. Maca runs the Hastings Day Centre.
Contact: Tom Gourlay. *Tel:* 01424 733900. *Mobile:* 07778 659293.
E-mail: maca.bexhill@dial.pipex.com Jul 2000

Salvation Army
Local Corps & Community Centres
Address: The Salvation Army, London Road, Bexhill-on-Sea, Sussex. *Tel*: 01424 218203. Jul 2000

Address: The Salvation Army, Hastings Citadel, St Andrews Square, Hastings, Sussex. *Tel*: 01424 426894. Jul 2000

Address: The Salvation Army, Royal Sussex Crescent, Eastbourne Old Town, Eastbourne, Sussex. *Tel*: 01323 726231. Jul 2000

Salvation Army Day Centre
Dedicated to helping all those in need without bias to age, culture, race or religion. The centre provides hot wholesome meals, advice, clothes, sleeping bags, help with accommodation, financial assistance, travel warrants, support counselling, telephone, family tracing, general advice, food parcels, days out and information on other agencies in the area. Open every day with quiz afternoons and indoor bowls on Monday afternoons.The Centre also houses a washing machine and shower facilities are provided. *Contact:* Paul Sibley, manager.

Address: Salvation Army Day Centre, Hastings Citadel, St Andrew's Square, Hastings, East Sussex, TN34 1SR. *Tel/Fax:* 01424 426894. 5867

Seaview Projects
Seaview Projects works with a range of socially excluded clients by providing a drop-in centre and housing services. The overall aim is to help clients achieve self-dependence. The Drop-in-Centre provides a supportive environment where problems can be dealt with and new skills learnt and practised. Housing Services provide short-term emergency accommodation, long-term placement and seven day a week, day and evening home support work. Seaview Projects also provides specialist help to clients with multiple needs. *Hours:* Mondays to Fridays 10.00am to 4.00pm. *Contact*: Director: John Evans; Drop-in Centre Manager: Fiona Cameron; Housing Services Manager: Mary Denning.

Address: Seaview Projects, Southwater Centre, Hatherley Road, St. Leonards-on-Sea, East Sussex, TN37 6LB. *Tel:* 01424 717981. *Fax:* 01424 722601. *E-Mail:* john@seaview,cablenet.co.uk May 2000

XTRAX
Xtrax is a young people's centre offering information, advice and support to young people aged 16-25, and also recreational facilities, entertainment, cheap food, laundry facilities and shower facilities. *Hours:* Mondays, Wednesdays, Fridays & Sundays 2.00 to 10.00pm. *Contact:* Terry Drinkwater.

Address: Xtrax, Young People's Centre, Provincial House, Havelock Road, Hastings, East Sussex, TN34 1BP. *Tel:* 01424 722524. *Fax:* 01424 204316. *E-Mail:* xtrax@tesco.net Jul 2000

National Organisations

Maca
MACA (Mental After Care Association) is 'a leading national charity with over 75 services committed to promoting quality of life for people with mental health needs and their carers.' Services provided include: a range of accommodation with support; community support services; day schemes with employment training; court diversion and other projects for people in contact with the criminal justice system. 5985

London Office
Chief executive: Gil Hitchon. *Address:* MACA, 25, Bedford Square, London, WC1B 3HW. *Tel:* 020 7436 6194. *Fax:* 020 7637 1980. *Website:* www.maca.org.uk Jul 2000

Maca South
Contact: John McKelvie. *Address:* MACA South, 94B, High Street, Epsom, Surrey, KT19 8BJ. *Tel:* 01372 722970. *Fax:* 91372 722980. *E-mail:* maca.south@dial.piper.com Jul 2000

Salvation Army

Address: The Salvation Army, 101, Newington Causeway, London, SE1 6BN. *Tel*: 020 7367 4500. *Fax*: 020 7367 4728. *Website:* www.salvation.org Jul 2000

London South East
Address: The Salvation Army, Div. HQ., 1, East Court, Enterprise Road, Maidstone, Kent, ME15 6JF. *Tel*: 01622 775000. *Fax*: 01622 775011. Jul 2000

See also these chapters ...

Mind Organisation, page 245.

Employment & Training

Unemployment is often an additional problem faced by people who have had mental health problems. Yet having a job can be very important in helping people cope in the community, especially after a period in hospital. 0534

Unemployment

Unemployment is often an additional problem faced by people who have had mental health problems. Yet having a job can be very important in helping people cope in the community, especially after a period in hospital.

Your options may range from trying the mainstream job market to voluntary work or sheltered or supported work or rehabilitation. Getting back into paid work can be difficult and your choices limited, but there is help and advice available in Hastings & Rother. 0534

Job Directory

A new job directory to help people with learning disabilities find work in East Sussex. The directory lists 30 employment projects countywide, which offer sheltered workshops, adult education, horticultural opportunities and various work preparation programmes.

Developed by the County Council's Social Services Learning Disability Services and its Employment Service, Firstbridge, the directories, are available in libraries, Citizen's Advice Bureaux and day centres.

Local Organisations

CRI

CRI is an employment, education and training outreach project, which aims to raise employment, education and training opportunities for young people aged 16 - 25 in Hastings and St Leonards.

Tel: 01424 719196. *Fax:* 01424 719012.
E-mail: eetraining@2000fsnet.co.uk 5833 May 2000

EMAS

EMAS (Employment Medical Advisory Service), offers help and advice on occupational health matters in the workplace, including mental health issues.

Address: EMAS, 3, East Grinstead House, London Road, East Grinstead, West Sussex, RH19 1RR. *Tel:* 01342 334281. May 2000

Firstbridge

Opportunities for all to be involved: users of services for disabled people; providers of those services; local employers.

Firstbridge is a partnership between the following agencies: East Sussex County Council, Workability, East Sussex Disability Association, ECAT Enterprise, Sussex Carers Services. 5494

Information service

A free phone information helpline staffed by an employment information officer. For queries on issues related to: disability employment; available services; relevant legislation; etc. An occupational therapist and independent living adviser are also available for consultation.

Address: Firstbridge Employment Services, Bell Lane, Uckfield, Sussex, TN22 1AQ. *Tel:* 01825 761811.

Helpline: 0800 0924 688[5494]

Hastings Careers Centre

Services include careers guidance; comprehensive careers/education library (free and open access for all); job/training vacancies for 16 - 17 year olds; curriculum vitae service for 16 - 17 year olds.

No charge is made for clients up to and including 19 years of age. Services may be free for other clients - contact the Careers Centre for details. Team manager: Julie Bolwell. *Hours:* Mondays to Thursdays 9am to 4.30pm; Fridays 9am to 4pm.

Address: Sussex Careers Services, First Floor, Queensbury House, Havelock Road, Hastings, East Sussex, TN34 1BP. *Tel:* 01424 425780. *Fax:* 01424 431564. *E-mail:* hastings@sussexcareers.co.uk [5846]

Hastings College

Guidance Service: Hastings College of Arts & Technology offers a Guidance Service. Prospective students can get impartial advice and guidance about education and training.

All options are discussed and help and support is offered to people who are making decisions about their next steps. This service is also offered in the community to either individuals or groups living in the Hastings and Rother areas. Contact: Jayne Ayres (guidance co-ordinator) or Sandra Brace.

Address: Hastings College of Arts & Technology, Guidance Department, Archery Road, St Leonards-on-Sea, East Sussex, TN38 0HX. *Tel:* 01424 442222, ext. 343. *Fax:* 01424 721763.

E-mail: guidance@hast [May 2000]

Students Union

Providing student services, sports and social facilities. *Contacts:* Matt Davey, President; Ms Stella Hole, Support officer. *Address:* Hastings College of Arts & Technology, Students Union, Archery Road, St Leonards-on-Sea, East Suyssex, TN38 0HX. *Tel:* 01424 420804. *Fax:* 01424 721763. [5867 Jun 2000]

School of Health & Social Studies

As part of Supportive Education, the School of Health and Social Studies runs part-time and full-time courses, day and evening, for people of all ages who are experiencing learning difficulties.

Courses take place Mondays to Fridays.There is an answerphone service available outside office hours. Enquiries should be made to Peter Suret, head of school; or Alison Russell, deputy head of school. *Address:* School of Health and Social Studies, 80, St Saviours Road, St Leonards-on-Sea, East Sussex, TN38 0AR. *Tel:* 01424 442222, ext. 416.

E-mail: suped@hcat.fsbusiness.co.uk

Website: www.hastings.ac.uk [5820]

Hastings Sheltered Workshop

Located at the Brittania Enterprise Centre, The HSW provides work activities and training in a supportive environment. It can be used by any person who has, or is currently suffering from, mental health or stress related problems. It helps to develop skills and to regain lost confidence.

The types of activities available are varied and include woodwork, horticulture, upholstery and light craft work. Enquiries can be made by any professional person involved in the person's care. *Contact:* Peter Howard, project manager.

Address: Hastings Sheltered Workshop, Britannia Enterprise Centre, Waterworks

Road, Hastings, East Sussex, TN34 1RT. *Tel:* 01424 718060. [Jun 2000]

Helpline

Helpline for employment and disability enquiries. This is a freephone helpline for people with disabilities or health problems to enquire about employment or training opportunities. It covers London and the south-east and is staffed by disability employment advisers. Times of opening: Mondays to Fridays 9 to 5pm. *Tel:* 0800 5280462. [Jul 2000]

Job Centres

The Disability Employment Advisers at job centres now run an 'Access to Work' programme and a 'Job Introduction Scheme'.

Bexhill Job Centre

Advice and help for people with disabilities who are seeking employment or training course/rehabilitation leading towards employment. You may apply direct to the Job Centre. Nigel Baker, Disability Employment Adviser. *Address:* The Job Centre, 41, St. Leonards Road, Bexhill-on-Sea, East Sussex, TN40 1HS. *Tel:* 01424 783100. *Fax:* 01424 783105. [Jul 2000]

Hastings Castle Job Centre

Contact: Nigel Baker, Disability Employment Adviser. *Address:* Employment Service Job Centre, Aquila House, Breeds Place, Hastings, East Sussex, TN34 1EG. *Tel:* 01424 784300. *Fax:* 01424 784398. [Jul 2000]

Hastings Ashdown Job Centre

Contact: Mrs Norma Longmore, Disability Employment Adviser. *Address:* Employment Service Job Centre, Ashdown House, Sedlescombe Road North, St Leonards-on-Sea, East Sussex, TN37 7EL. *Tel:* 01424 784400. *Fax:* 01424 784453. [May 2000]

Tomorrows People Trust

Helping people to find real jobs. In the last thirteen years the Trust has helped over two million people. Their aim is to get people out of the dependency culture and into the workplace, the target group being people unemployed for over six months.

Within Hastings, the Trust runs Workroute, a one-to-one guidance programme helping people back to work; and the volunteer option of New Deal, i.e. placing 18 to 25 year olds into charities. *Contacts:* Mrs Corinne Gardner, chairperson; John Page-May, co-ordinator.

Address: Tomorrows People Trust, Hanover House, 33, The Avenue, Eastbourne, East Sussex, TN34 1NY. *Tel:* 01323 411255. *Fax:* 01323 738214. [5867]

Workability

A supportive service for employment and training, helping people with mental health needs access vocational opportunities. Clients may not apply directly to Workability, but must be referred via Westwood House or other professional body.

Address: Workability, 34/35, Wellington Square, Hastings, East Sussex, TN34 1PN. *Tel:* 01424 723304. *Fax:* 01424 723305. *E-mail:* workability-hastings@pact.org.uk [5867]

National Organisations

Employment Service Direct

Job seekers' hotline; database of 300,000 vacancies for the price of a local call. *Tel:* 0845 6060 234.

Website: www.employmentservice.gov.uk [Jul 2000]

Shaw Trust

The charity, Shaw Trust, was founded in 1981 during the International Year for Disabled Persons, in the village of Shaw, specifically to meet the known needs of a small group of individuals living in that part of Wiltshire. All were severely disabled, but each one had employment capabilities. Real jobs were found with employers; the individuals thrived and their skills and self-confidence quickly grew.

The employers found an added quality in their workforce - a greater understanding and a recognition that people with a very wide range of disabilities had much to offer their colleagues in the workplace.

After sixteen years of growth, Shaw Trust is among the leaders in supporting disabled people in work throughout Great Britain.

- Shaw Trust is a charity which enables people with disabilities and mental health problems to maximise their potential in work opportunities.
- Shaw Trust is currently supporting over 2,500 people with all types of disabilities in employment.
- Shaw Trust provides rehabilitation, vocational training, work tasters and work preparation, annually assisting a further 2,500 people.
- Shaw Trust is working in partnership with over 2,000 companies to support people with disabilities in employment.
- Shaw Trust is also working in partnership with over 40 health authorities, social services departments and TECs and within a number of European initiatives.
- Shaw Trust has a network of over 200 staff covering England, Wales and Scotland.
- Shaw Trust has over 40 shops in the UK.

Address: Shaw Trust, Southern Regional Office, St Peter's Centre, Reardon Street, Wapping, London, E1W 2QH.
Tel: 020 7977 6800. *Fax:* 020 7977 6816.
Minicom: 0345697288. *E-mail:* southern.region@shaw-trust.org.uk
Website: www.shaw-trust.org.uk 6067 Jul 2000

Further Information

Providing Information

Providing Information on seeking employment and/or training after experiencing mental distress. By Kaaren Cruse. Published by MIND Information Unit. Updated Nov. 1998. £1.36. Available from Mind Mail Order Service. *Tel*: 020 8221 9666.

Surviving Working Life

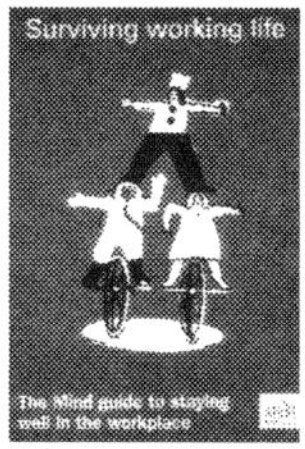

Surviving Working Life. The Mind guide to staying well in the workplace. This booklet is about staying well at work - whether you are returning to the world of work after time away with mental distress, in fear of 'going under' with work stress, or trying to maintain a healthy working life. Published by Mind, 2000. ISBN: 1-874690-91-X. 18 pages. £1.36. Available from Mind Mail Order Service. *Tel*: 020 8221 9666. 5251

See also these chapters ...

Voluntary work, page 266.

Acknowledgements
Our grateful thanks to Peter Howard of Hastings Sheltered Workshop for editorial assistance with this chapter.

Housing

Living in unsuitable accommodation can be an additional problem faced by people with mental health problems. You may want to live independently in your own house or flat, have some independence and some support, or you may choose a residential home or hostel. [5224]

Homelessness

Under the Housing Act 1996, all councils have a legal duty to provide accommodation for up to two years for people in priority need who are homeless. People with mental health problems may be classed as 'vulnerable' and therefore in priority need. If you fit these criteria you will need a letter from your doctor or CPN to support your claim. [0534]

Local Organisations

Citizens' Advice Bureaux

CABs hold lists of housing associations and housing co-operatives in this area. See the section 'Citizens' Advice Bureaux', in the 'Advice' chapter, page 150.

Hastings Borough Council

Hastings Borough Council Housing Services. Advice and assistance on housing matters. There are two departments: 'Housing renewal' and 'Housing needs'.

'Housing Renewal' deals with disrepair of property, enforcement and grants.

'Housing needs' deals with the waiting list for Housing Associations and homelessness and advice. The housing advice and tenancy relations officers deal with disputes involving the landlords such as harassment or interfering with quiet enjoyment.

Anyone can make an enquiry by telephone or in person. Advice interviews are by prior appointment either at the office or elsewhere if preferred. The advice is free.

Advice interviews are generally by appointment, but some issues can be dealt with immediately on enquiry. Office hours are Mondays to Thursdays, 8.45 am to 5.00 pm, and Fridays 8.45 am to 4.30 pm. *Contact:* Karen Sedgewick, Housing Policy & Resources Manager.

Address: Hastings Borough Council Housing Services Department, Jackson Hall, Portland Place, Hastings, East Sussex TN34 1QN. *Tel:* 01424 781212; 781066. *Fax:* 01424 781305. *Minicom:* 01424 781755. *E-mail:* ksedgwick@hastings.gov.uk [Jul 2000]

Hastings Community Housing

The Hastings Community Housing Association (HCHA) provides shared housing for single persons between the ages of 16-25 years, with support, move-on accommodation for single persons, plus accommodation for small families.

Anyone may apply, either direct to the HCHA or through another agency. The office hours are Monday to Friday, 9.00 am to 5.00 pm. Some flats and houses are available for disabled applicants.

There is a shared housing project for young women. The HCHA is not specifically targeted at clients with mental health problems, but the waiting list is open to all applicants. *Contact:* Christine McPherson.

Address: Hastings Community Housing Association, 16, Havelock Road, Hastings, East Sussex, TN34 1BP. *Tel:* 01424 445354. *Fax:* 01424 420543. May 2000

Hastings Furniture Service

This registered charity (No. 1003257) is run entirely to serve the needs of the disadvantaged; that is, the elderly and infirm, the unemployed, the homeless and single parents. Its aims are to provide good quality, clean, used furniture and other essential household goods at low affordable prices to those who have no other means of furnishing their accommodation. Contact Name: Nick Bellis and David Newstead. *Office hours:* of Hastings Furniture Service are Mondays to Fridays 9.30 am to 4.30 pm.

Vouchers

The prices of the furniture on offer are generally well below normal trade prices.To apply, you must be in receipt of State Benefit and you must obtain a 'referral voucher'. These vouchers can be obtained from any one of the following three agencies: Age Concern, HARC and the CAB.

Age Concern

For the aged only. *Address:* 48, Cambridge Gardens, Hastings. *Tel:* 01424 426162;

HARC

For all age groups. *Address: HARC,* 8, CambridgeRoad, Hasting. *Tel:* 01424 428375;

CAB, Hastings.

For all age groups. *Address:* CAB, 24, Cornwallis Terrace, Hastings. *Tel:* 01424 430400;

CAB, Bexhill

For all age groups. *Address:* CAB, 38, Sackville Road, Bexhill. Tel: 01424 215055.

Address: Hastings Furniture Service Ltd., 6-10, Dorset Place, Hastings, East Sussex, TN34 1GL. *Tel:* 01424 446335. May 2000

Moat Care and Repair

This is a home improvement agency, providing elderly, disabled and other householders with advice and assistance to carry out building repairs or adaptations. Anyone may apply.

"Moat Care & Repair aims to maximise people's opportunities to remain in their own homes with greater independence and increased comfort and security. We can help with anything from a minor repair to a major adaptation. We will try to help with anything that will make you more comfortable and secure in your own home.

We can provide you with the following: a visit to your home to discuss any repairs or adaptations you need; discuss funding for the work and help you to apply for any grants or loans that may be available; liaise with the local authority or social services where necessary; help you find a suitable builder and supervise the works; give you support and practical help before, during and after the work is completed."

Moat Care & Repair is an Industrial & Provident Society with charitable aims. It is a member of the Moat Housing Group. Office hours are Monday to Friday 9.00 am to 5.00 pm. *Contacts:* Ann Smith and Myra Hopkins.

Address: Moat Care and Repair, Ground floor, 7, Havelock Road, Hastings, East Sussex, TN34 1BP. *Tel:* 01424 721992. *Fax:* 01424 461702. *E-mail:* info@moat.co.uk May 2000

Mental Health Accommodation

This agency provides accommodation in the community for adults with long term mental health problems, and continues to support clients in housing matters. Referrals are accepted from any source, but prospective clients are subject to an NHS and Community Care Act assessment. Contact: John Banks, Manager.

Hours: Mondays to Thursdays: 9.00am to 5.00 pm. Fridays: 9.00am to 4.30 pm.

Address: Mental Health Accommodation Team, ESCC Social Services Department, 8, London Road, Bexhill-on-Sea, East Sussex, TN39 4JU. Tel: 01424 730512. *Fax:* 01424 423349. Jul 2000

Orbit Housing Association

The provision of affordable social housing of good quality. Direct applications are accepted for bedsits/one beds. *Contact:* Mrs Carol Lord. *Office hours:* Mondays to Fridays: 9.00am to 5.00pm.

Address: Orbit Housing Association, 1-3, The Oaks, Little Ridge Avenue, St. Leonards-on-Sea, East Sussex TN37 7UW. *Tel:* 01424 757700. *Fax:* 01424 756967. Jul 2000

Rother District Council

Address: Rother District Council, Town Hall, Bexhill-on-Sea, East Sussex, TN39 3KX. *Tel*: 01424 787878. *Hours*: Mondays to Fridays 8.30am to 4.30pm. *Information Helpline (Freephone)*: 0800 393964. Jul 2000

Seaview Projects

Seaview exists to help any person suffering from any form of deprivation, particularly those with mental health problems. Seaview Projects provides the following to anyone over 16 years of age: a drop in centre; an accommodation support service and a health care programme.

Anyone may apply, in person or by telephone. There is a nominal charge for tea, coffee and meals. Volunteer help is welcome. *Contact:* John Evans. *Office hours:* Mondays to Fridays 10.00am to 4.00pm.

Address: Southwater Centre, Hatherley Road, St. Leonards-on-Sea, East Sussex, TN37 6LB. *Tel:* 01424 717981. *Answerphone/Fax:* 01424 722601. Jul 2000

SHAH Housing Aid Centre

"SHAH provides a free, independent and comprehensive Housing Aid Service. That service encompasses three distinct elements:

Advice and Information: Practical information and advice on housing rights along with sources of further help and details of services other local agencies provide.

Accommodation: Practical help and assistance in finding and keeping a home.

Advocacy and Representation:
'Representing the client, such as negotiating with a local authority or landlord, or representation in Tribunals and in Court.' [Quotation taken from SHAH's website].

SHAH is a part of Shelter's national housing aid network, offering free independent and confidential legal advice, information and services for all housing related concerns. SHAH is a registered charity. It is grant-aided by Hastings Borough Council, Rother District Council, Shelter and by public donations. *Contact:* Richard Lynch. Accommodation co-ordinator: Marie Lapierre.

Office hours: are Mondays, Tuesdays and Thursdays: 10.00am to 1.00pm & 2.00 to 5.00pm; Wednesdays and Fridays: 10.00am to 1.00pm (appointments only: 2.00 to 5.00pm).

Address: SHAH Housing Aid Centre, 48, Cambridge Gardens, Hastings, East Sussex TN34 1EN. *Tel:* 01424 438075. *Website:* www.shah-hastings.demon.co.uk May 2000

Youth Accommodation Support

The Youth Accommodation Support project exists to support young people aged 16-25 in securing and maintaining tenancies. It is managed by SARO (Sussex Association for the Rehabilitation of Offenders), funded by Lottery and employs two full-time staff. The project is office-based but also offers an outreach service to both individuals, and other organisations.

The project offers information, advice, advocacy and support to its clients on (but not exclusively) housing and related matters. It also networks and 'jointworks' with many other service providers to ensure an 'holistic' approach. *Contacts:* Ms Susan Vaughan, Project leader; Ms Lorraine Roberts, Project worker.

Address: Youth Accommodation Support Project, 45, Cambridge Road, Hastings, Sussex, TN34 1DT. *Tel:* 01424 423344. *Fax:* 01424 429989. *E-mail:* yasproject@saro61.freeserve.co.uk [5867]

1066 Housing Association

The major landlord in Hastings & St Leonards, with around 1 in 8 local people living in their properties. They actively support 17 local residents' associations, which meet together as the Tenants Consultative Group.

1066 HA is a community-owned voluntary organisation and works in partnership with residents and community groups and many other organisations, to develop and support community and regeneration projects. They are the holders of a Charter Mark and the 1998 Participation into Practice Award.

Contact: Mr Robin Deane, Tenant Liaison Manager. *Tel:* 01424 781291. *Fax:* 01424 781255; Mr Gary Storer, Residents Association Information & Training.

Address: 1066 Housing Association, Queensbury House, Havelock Road, Hastings, East Sussex, TN34 1W4. [5867]

National Organisations

Shelterline

Shelterline is a free national 24-hour helpline for all housing problems.

Address: Shelter, 88, Old Street, London, EC1V 9HU. *Tel:* 020 7505 2000. Shelterline: 0808 800 4444, (calls are free). *Website:* www.shelter.org.uk [July 2000]

Warden Housing Association

WHA owns over 8,000 homes across the south of England and is part of the Home Group. WHA has 53 flats/maisonettes to rent in Hastings. *Contact:* Mrs Glynis Gatenby, Senior Housing Officer.

Office hours: are Mondays to Thursday 9am to 5pm; Fridays: 9am to 5pm.

Address: Warden Housing Association Limited, 3, Cantelupe Mews, Cantelupe Road, East Grinstead, West Sussex, RH19 3BG. *Tel:* 01342 301750. *Fax:* 01342 301650. [May 2000]

Head office is in London: *Tel:* 020 8868 9000. *Contact:* Jacky Kissai, public relations officer. [July 2000]

Further Information

Emergency Housing

Factsheet by Kaaren Cruse. Published by Mind, £0.50. Available from Mind, 020 8221 9666.

Housing Advice

Factsheet by Kaaren Cruse. Published by Mind, April 1997, £1.36. Available from Mind, tel: 020 8221 9666.

Acknowledgements
Our grateful thanks to Karen Sedgewick, Housing Policy & Resources Manager, Hastings Borough Council, for editorial assistance with this chapter.

Information

Local Organisations

Hastings Information Centre

Open 7 days a week for both resident and visitor services. *Contact:* Marilyn Wrench, manager.

Address: Hastings Information Centre, Queen's Square, Priory Meadow, Hastings, East Sussex, TN34 1TL. *Tel:* 01424 781111. *Fax:* 01424 781186. *E-mail:* hic-info@hastings.gov.uk 5878

Hastings Community News

4-page newsletter, edited by Katy Burbridge. Copy for this publication should be submitted by the 14th of each month. Katy also maintains a database of local organisations and holds a range of directories and information resources.

Tel: 01424 444010 (main office and general enquiries). *Fax:* 01424 432877. *E-mail:* infoworker@hva.k-web.co.uk Jul 2000

Health Promotion

East Sussex Brighton & Hove Health Authority Health Promotion Department. Please see main entry under 'Health Authorities' page 321.

Mental Health Information Forum

The MHIF is a group of individual workers from the voluntary, statutory and private sectors who are interested in mental health services locally. The forum was launched in 1998 and meets four times a year. As it develops, the group hopes to influence the way mental health services are provided locally. The chair of the MHIF is John Evans.

Address: Seaview Project, Southwater Centre, South-water Road, St Leonards-on-Sea, East Sussex. *Tel:* 01424 717981. 5048

Social Services Info Line

Started 1993; provides information about services to children and families, older people, people with disabilities and much more. *Hours:* Mondays to Thursdays 8.30am to 5pm; Fridays 8.30am to 4.30pm. *Tel:* 0845 601 0664. *Fax:* 01424 201946. *E-mail:* information.line@eastsussexc.c.gov.uk *Website:* www.eastsussexcc.gov.uk/soc 5953 Jun 2000

National Organisations

Healthline

Previously known as the Health Information Service, Healthline is a free confidential telephone information service which provides information on health topics and services to the general public. The service was set up in 1984 by the College of Health.

Pre-recorded tapes

The Healthline service is intended for anyone who wants to know more about a particular medical condition or is simply looking for advice on how to keep healthy. It also helps people who are uncertain whether to visit their doctor about a specific problem or who want to understand more about their own illness either before or after a medical consultation. The information is provided in the form of pre-recorded taped messages, most of which last between two and six minutes. The scripts for each tape are checked by experts in the particular field and then given final approval by the College's Chief Medical Consultant before being recorded by a professional actor or actress.

Healthline library

There are now over 500 tapes in the Healthline library covering a wide variety of topics such as cancer, homoeopathy, measles and nervous breakdown. The tapes include information about symptoms and, where appropriate, they outline the various methods of treatment available. They also state clearly when you should consult a doctor about a particular problem and, wherever possible, they include details of organisations and self-help groups you can contact.

Healthlines operators

It is important to know that the Healthline operators who play you the tapes are not medically trained so cannot give you any kind of medical advice themselves; but they do have access to certain information about clinics and services, which may be helpful to you. It is a good idea to have a pen and paper handy to note down any useful information and the names and addresses of organisations you may wish to contact.

Directory

The Healthline Service is available in several of the Regional Health Information Services on 0800 66 55 44. Most services are staffed between the hours of 10am and 5pm and some are open until 7pm. Outside these hours you can still listen to a tape provided you have a tone phone and a directory of the tapes available. If you do not have a tone phone you will have to call during operator hours. If you do not have a directory and would like one please ask the operator to send you a copy, or leave a meassage on the answerphone together with your name and address. You can also listen to a selection of Healthline tapes via NHS Direct Online at www.nhsdirect.nhs.uk

Examples of available tapes

- Anxiety: acute anxiety & panic attacks (026);
- Bed-wetting (031);
- Community services available on leaving hospital (050);
- Huntington's disease (413);
- Insomnia (206);
- ME (myalgic encephalomyelitis) (257);
- Motor neurone disease (347);
- Nervous breakdown (090);
- Pain clinics (174);
- Seasonal affective disorder syndrome (SADS) (368);
- Stammering (051);
- Vertigo (365);
- Community services available on leaving hospital (803 in Bengali-Sylheti dialect);
- Community services available on leaving hospital (903 in Urdu).

Address: College of Health, St Margaret's House, 21, Old Ford Road, London, E2 9PL. *Tel:* 020 8983 1225. *Fax:* 020 8983 1553. *Healthline:* 0800 66 55 44 [6002]

Talking Life

Publisher and supplier of audio cassette self-help health programmes. The tapes provide 'a support group in your own living room'. Examples are:

Coping with depression	£8.50
Coping with pain	£8.50
Coping with back pain	£8.50
Coping with tranquiliser addiction	£8.50
Coping with asthma	£8.50
Coping with anxiety	£8.50
Children's sleep problems	£8.50
Coping with sleep problems	£8.50
Coping with bereavement	£8.50

Address: Talking Life, PO Box 1, Wirral, Cheshire, CH47 7DD. *Tel:* 0151 632 0662. *Fax:* 0151 632 1206. *Website:* www.talkinglife.co.uk [5424]

Acknowledgements
Our grateful thanks to Barbara Hardcastle of Health Promotion for editorial assistance with this chapter.

Insurance

People with a mental health problem often face difficulties when trying to get insurance cover. At least a few organisations have begun to address this problem.

Life assurance

For advice on this subject, please call David Young of the J Rothschild Partnership, see below.

Travel insurance

The Manic Depression Fellowship offers travel insurance via arrangements with Burrows Keith Group Insurance Brokers and Folgate Insurance Company. The cover is available at present only to members of the Manic Depression Fellowship, but this may change, see 'Burrows Keith', below.

At the time of writing the annual premium for worldwide annual cover is £95. Further details from the MDF national office: 020 7793 2600. Mike Calver is the contact. The MDF publishes a pre-travel health check guide, which contains useful information on medication, what to do if ill overseas, and jet lag. 5068 Jul 2000

National Organisations

Burrows Keith Group

This insurance broker currently has an exclusive travel scheme on behalf of all members of the Manic Depression Fellowship. However, it is considering extending the arrangement to *anyone* with a mental illness. For further details of the latest position please contact Barbara Frost at Burrows.

Address: Burrows Keith Group Ltd, Canterbury House, 2-6, Sydenham Road, Croydon, CRO 9XE. *Tel:* 020 8681 2314. *Fax:* 020 8681 2471. *E-mail:* enquiries@burrowskeith.co.uk *Website:* www.burrowskeith.co.uk 6085 Jul 2000

J Rothschild Partnership

David Young has been actively involved in working with the Manic Depression Fellowship including having been chairman of the MDF Council. He has managed to help a number of members already in the area of life assurance. He is happy to help *anyone* with a mental health problem who is experiencing difficulty with life assurance and related financial matters. 5067 Jul 2000

Address: J Rothschild Partnership, Beech House, Brotherswood Court, Great Park Road, Bradley Stoke, Bristol, BS32 4QW. *Tel:* 01454 618700. *Fax:* 01454 619694. *E-mail:* david.young@tjrp.net August 2000

Further Information

Insurance Cover

Insurance Cover for people who have Mental Health Problems. By Dawn Pelle. Legal Department, Mind. July 1996. Price £0.20. Available from Mind Mail Order Service. *Tel:* 020 8221 9666.

Legal matters

Peope with mental health problems who find themselves in trouble with the law are particularly vulnerable and in need of special help. Some of that help is detailed here.

Legacies

Legacies are an extremely important source of funds, without which Hastings Mind could not continue some of its vital work. If you would like to include us in your will, please contact us. We would be delighted to provide further information.

Address: Hastings Mind, St Peter's Place, 33, St Peter's Road, St Leonards-on-Sea, East Sussex, TN37 6JQ. *Tel:* 01424 439599. [Jul 2000]

Wills

Mind publishes two free guides to will making.

Find Peace of Mind, includes a chart to help you take stock of your financial affairs and plan for the future. There is also a special section dealing with making a will for people with mental health problems.

Making Provision, explains how to

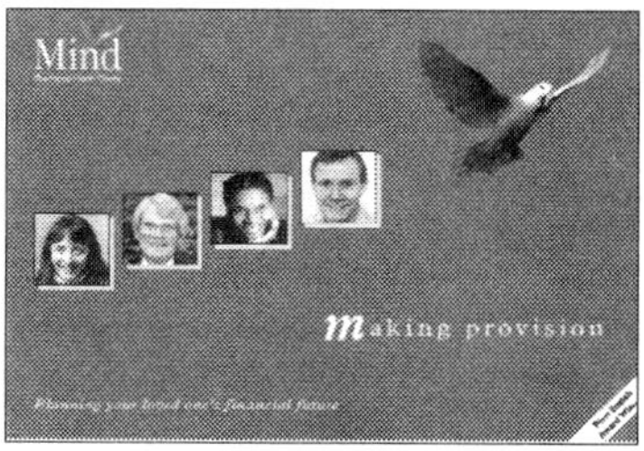

plan the financial future of a loved one who has mental health problems, and includes a section on how to protect entitlement to state funded care and benefits.

To obtain copies of these publications, write to the Legacy Officer, Mind, Freepost (WD2336), 15-19, Broadway, London, E15 4BQ. [5407, 5470, 5471]

The Mental Health Foundation also publishes a guide to will making entitled 'Guide to Making a Will'. To order your free copy simply telephone 020 7535 7430. [6028]

Local Organisations

Hastings Magistrates Court

Clerk's office open Mondays to Fridays 9.15am to 4.30pm. *Address:* Hastings & Rother Magistrates Court, Law Courts, Bohemia Road, Hastings, Sussex, TN34 1ND. *Tel:* 01424 437644. *Fax:* 01424 429878. [Jul 2000]

County Court

Open Mondays to Fridays 10am to 4pm. *Address:* Hastings County Court, Law Courts, Bohemia Road, Hastings, Sussex, TN34 1QX. *Tel:* 01424 435128. *Fax:* 01424 421585. [Jul 2000]

Court Assessment Scheme

The Court Assessment Scheme's function is to provide information to the Criminal Justice System (including the Prosecution, Defence and Probation) regarding those people referred either by the Police, the Court, Probation or Bail Information. Its function is to provide information to the courts regarding the mental health of those people it represents.

Enquiries would normally be made through a Defence Solicitor or Probabtion Officer.

Hours: Mondays to Fridays: 8.00am to 4.00pm. *Contact:* Martin Corfe, Community Mental Health Nurse; Court Assessment & Diversion Scheme Co-ordinator.

Address: Court Assessment Scheme, Ashen Hill, The Drive, Hellingly, Hailsham, East Sussex, BN27 4ER. *Direct dial:* 01323 444172. *Tel:* 01323 440022. *Fax:* 01323 847822. Jun 2000

Forensic Psychiatry Services

These are specifically for individuals who are mentally unwell and who come into trouble with the law. Dr Gregory Weppner is the consultant forensic psychiatrist. Russell Hackett is the senior manager.

Address: Forensic Psychiatry Services, Ashen Hill, The Drive, Hellingly, Hailsham, Sussex, BN27 4ER. *Tel:* 01323 440022; *fax:* 01323 847822. Jun 2000

Get It While You Can

Anyone involved in the criminal justice system who has substance misuse or related problems may apply to GIWYCP. For more information about this project, please see the entry on page 136.

Heringtons Solicitors

A local firm of solicitors, Heringtons, has three specialist mental health lawyers, David Harding, Russell Parkes and Pippa Sadhra. David Harding and Russell Parkes are on the Law Society Mental Health Review Tribunal, (a panel for solicitors and experts in this field) and Pippa Sadhra is shortly to be appointed to this panel.

David Harding is part-time president of the Mental Health Review Tribunal and his work includes not only representation of clients at tribunals, but work with the elderly in matters involving the Court of Protection and powers of attorney. The practice has offices in Battle, Eastbourne, Rye and St Leonards.

Address: Heringtons Solicitors, 84, Battle Road, St Leonards, Sussex. *Tel:* 01424 434192. *Fax:* 01424 444824. 6017 Jul 2000

Special Assessment Service

There are two units: a 20-bed medium secure unit and a low secure unit which provides assessment and rehabilitation for mentally disordered offenders and patients who need treatment in conditions of low security, if necessary over an extended period of time. Enquiries would normally be made via mental health professionals or the Criminal Justice System. Duncan Barton is the team leader.

Address: Special Assessment Service, Ashen Hill, The Drive, Hellingly, Hailsham, East Sussex, BN27 4ER. *Tel:* 01323 440022. *Fax:* 01323 847822. Jun 2000

National Organisations

Legal advice line, (Mind)

Mind has a national legal advice line open Mondays, Wednesdays and Fridays from 2 to 4.30pm. *Tel:* 020 8519 2122. Aug 2000

Legal advice line, (MDF)

The Manic Depression Fellowship offers its members a free legal advice service which operates 24 hours a day, 365 days a year. The most popular requests are for advice on State Benefit and employment, followed by debt and personal injury, but many other subjects are covered.

Address: Manic Depression Fellowship, Castle Works, 21, St George's Road, London, SE1 6ES. *Tel:* 020 7793 2600. *Fax:* 020 7793 2639. *E-mail:* mdf@mdf.org.uk 5067 Jul 2000

Matthew Trust

The Mathew Trust is a national mental health and penal reform charity. It is a grant making trust. It also helps victims of aggression (mainly women). Grants, however, are only given when all other sources of funding have been exhausted and its resources are therefore limited to mental health. *Contact:* Jean Bailie.

Address: Matthew Trust, PO Box 604, London, SW6 3AG. *Tel:* 020 7736 5976; Fax: 020 7731 6961. *E-mail:* matthewtrust@ukonline.co.uk *Website:* www.matthew-trust.org May 2000

Further Information

Legal Dictionary

The *Mind Psychiatric Legal Dictionary* is written by Richard Hallmark. Hundreds of definitions and a list of useful addresses. Published by Mind, 1997. ISBN 1-874690-55-3, 112 pages, £4.99. Available from Mind Mail Order, 020 8221 9666.

Legal Rights & Mental Health

The Mind manual. A comprehensive guide to mental health law which covers legal rights in the community and hospital. Each chapter includes sources of law and guidance, further reading and useful addresses. The information is updated three times a year. Published by Mind, 1996. ISBN 1-874690-60-X. £50. Subscriptions to updates: £25 per year. Available from Mind Mail Order, 020 8221 9666.

Criminal Justice System

'Mental illness and the criminal justice system' is available from the National Schizophrenia Fellowship. *Address:* 30, Tabernacle Street, London, EC2A 4DD. *Tel:* 020 7330 9100.

Acknowledgements
Our grateful thanks to David Harding of Heringtons Solicitors for editorial assistance with this chapter.

Media issues

If you see something on television, hear a radio programme, read an article in a publication, or see an advertisement that you feel misrepresents people suffering from mental health problems, you *can* complain about it.

About media issues

Mental illness is seldom fairly presented in the media, often conveying a very negative image of people suffering from mental health problems.

If you see something on television, hear a radio programme, read an article in a publication, or see an advertisement that you feel misrepresents people suffering from mental health problems, you can complain about it.

To do so, please contact the appropriate Watchdog organisation. You'll find details of how to get in touch in the section listed below under the heading: 'National Organisations'.

For complaints about advertisements, contact The Advertising Standards Authority. For television, try the Broadcasting Complaints Commission, the Broadcasting Standards Council, or the Independent Television Commission (also see separate heading for BBC television).

For newspapers and magazines, contact the Press Complaints Commission. For radio, contact the Radio Authority, or the National Viewers' and Listeners' Association (see also separate heading for BBC radio). For local media it is probably best to contact the editor direct in the case of a newspaper or magazine, and the senior producer if radio or television.

You can help reduce the stigma still attached to mental illness by raising awareness of inaccuracies in the way mental health issues are portrayed by the media.

Effects of stigma

The effects of the stigma of mental illness are all pervasive:

- Although 1 in 4 of the UK adult population will experience some form of mental health problem in any year, the associated stigma means many will be too embarrassed to seek help.
- Stigma adds to the sense of shame and distress felt by many sufferers, their carers, families and friends.
- Stigma makes it hard for people to gain employment or return to work after an episode of mental illness.
- Stigma makes it more difficult for people with mental health problems to form friendships and close relationships. [5346]

Code of practice

Please see under 'Press Complaints Commission', page 228.

How to make a complaint

Remember to specify the date and time of the programme, and of course, its name.

Try to give concise and solid reasons why you think the programme fell short of accepted standards. Do not be abusive - it does not help your cause. Keep a copy of your letter, and, where important, proof of posting. If possible, keep a recording of the programme or a transcript.

Complaints should be made as soon as possible after the offending article/broadcast. Letters to editors should be clearly marked 'for publication' or 'not for publication' so your wishes are clear.

Thank you
Remember, too, that if you do feel a particular story or item has been accurately and sensitively covered, you could write and say so. We all like to be praised.

Local Organisations

Arrow FM
Address: Mike Buxton, News Manager, 107.8 Arrow FM, Priory Meadow Shopping Centre, Queens Square, Hastings, East Sussex, TN34 1PJ. *Tel:* 01424 461177. *Fax:* 01424 422662.
E-mail: info@arrowfm.co.uk
Website: www.arrowfm.co.uk May 2000

Bexhill Observer
Address: The Editor, Bexhill Observer, 18, Sackville Road, Bexhill-on-Sea, East Sussex, TN39 3JL. *Tel:* 01424 730555. *Fax:* 01424 730832. *E-mail:* observer@go-free.co.uk Jul 2000

Evening Argus
Address: The Editor, Evening Argus, Crowhurst Road, Brighton, BN1 8AR. *Tel*: 01273 544544. *Fax:* 01273 505703. Jul 2000

Hastings & St Leonards Observer
Address: The Editor, Hastings & St Leonards Observer, Woods House, Telford Road, St. Leonards, Sussex, TN38 9LZ. *Tel*: 01424 854242. *Fax*: 01424 854284.
E-mail: observer@go-free.co.uk Jul 2000

Hospital Radio Hastings
Address: Hospital Radio Hastings, Conquest Hospital, The Ridge, St Leonards-on-Sea, East Sussex, TN37 7RD. *Tel*: 01424 756666. May 2000

Rye & Battle Observer
Address: The Editor, Rye & Battle Observer, Woods House, Telford Road, St. Leonards, Sussex, TN38 9LZ. *Tel*: 01424 854242. *Fax:* 01424 852850. *E-mail:* observer@go-free.co.uk Jul 2000

National Authorities

Advertising Standards Authority
For complaints about newspaper and magazine advertisements. *Address:* Advertising Standards Authority, 2, Torrington Place, London, WC1E 7HW. *Tel:* 020 7580 5555. *Fax:* 0207 7631 3051.
Website: www.asa.org.uk Jul 2000

British Board of Film Classification
For complaints about film and video classifications. *Address:* The British Board of Film Classification, 3, Soho Square, London, W1V 6HD. *Tel:* 020 7439 7961. *Fax:* 020 7287 0141. Website: www.bbfc.co.uk May 2000

Broadcasting Standards Commission
Covering all of the UK, the Commission considers two types of complaints: standards and fairness. It has the power to require recordings of broadcast material and written statements. It may also hold hearings. Its decisions are published regularly and broadcasters must report any action they have taken as a result. Additionally, the Commission can require broadcasters to publish summaries of its decisions on-air and in a newspaper or magazine.

Chairman: Lord Howe of Cheltenham, CBE; Director: Stephen Whittle; Deputy Director: Norman McLean.

Address: Broadcasting Standards Commission, 7, The Sanctuary, London, SW1P 3JS. *Tel:* 020 7808 1000. *Fax:* 020 7233 0397. *E-mail:* bsc.org.uk *Website:* www.bsc.org.uk May 2000

Department of Culture, Media & Sport
The government department responsible

for broadcasting. *Address:* Dept of Culture, Media & Sport, 2-4, Cockspur Street, London, SW1Y 5DH. *Tel:* 020 7211 6000. *E-mail:* enquiries@culture.gov.uk
Website: www.culture.gov.uk [May 2000]

Independent Television Commission
For complaints about ITV, C4, C5 and licensed cable or satellite. *Address:* Independent Television Commission, 33, Foley Street, London, W1P 7LB. *Tel:* 020 7580 5555. *Fax:* 020 7306 7800. [May 2000]

Internet Watch Foundation
For complaints about the Internet. *Address:* Internet Watch Foundation, East View, 5, Coles Lane, Oakington, Cambridge, CB4 5BA. *Tel:* 01223 237700. *Fax:* 01223 235870. *E-mail:* 01223 235870. *Website:* www.internetwatch.org.uk [May 20000]

National Viewers' & Listeners' Assn
National Viewers' & Listeners' Association. The NVALA recommends that all complaints about programme content be made to the Broadcasting Standards Commission. *It is important that viewers and listeners write because statistics on complaints received are published annually.* Director: John C. Beyer. *Address*: National Viewers' & Listeners' Association, 3, Willow House, Kennington Road, Ashford, Kent, TN24 0NR. *Tel:* 01233 633936. *Fax:* 01233 633836.
E-mail: info@nvala,org [5581]

Press Complaints Commission
Chairman: Lord Wakeham; *Director:* Guy Black; *Public Relations Officer:* Luke Chauveau. The Press Complaints Commission is an independent body founded to oversee self-regulation of the press. They deal with complaints by the public about contents and conduct of British newspapers and magazines and advise editors on journalistic ethics. Complaints must be about the failure of newspapers or magazines to follow the letter or spirit of a Code of Practice, drafted by the newspaper and magazine editors, adopted by the industry and supervised by the Commission. [May 2000]

Paragraph 13, 'Discrimination', of the *Code of Practice* published by the Press Complaints Commission states:

i) The press must avoid prejudicial or pejorative reference to a person's race, colour, religion, sex or sexual orientation or to any physical or mental illness or disability.

ii) It must avoid publishing details of a person's race, colour, religion, sexual orientation, physical or mental illness or disability unless these are directly relevant to the story.

Address: Press Complaints Commission, 1, Salisbury Square, London EC4Y 8JB. *Tel:* 020 7353 1248. *Fax:* 020 7353 8355. Telephone for the deaf & hard of hearing, *Tel:* 020 7583 2264. *E-mail:* pcc@pcc.org.uk
Website: www.pcc.org.uk [5411]

Radio Authority
The Radio Authority licenses and regulates all independent radio services. It has three main tasks, i.e. to plan frequencies, appoint licensees with a view to broadening listener choice, and to regulate programming and advertising. It is required, after consultation, to publish codes to which its licenses must adhere.

Address: Radio Authority, Holbrook House, 14, Great Queen Street, London, WC2B 5DG. *Tel*: 020 7430 2724. *Fax*: 020 7405 7062.
E-mail: info@radioauthority.org.uk
Website: www.radioauthority.org.uk [May 2000]

BBC Television & Radio

Programme Complaints Unit
If you believe there has been a serious breach of BBC programme standards, contact this office. *Address:* Head of Programme Complaints, BBC, Broadcasting House, Portland Place,

London, W1A 1AA. *Tel*: 020 7580 4468. Jul 2000

Feedback
Address: Feedback, PO Box 2100, London, W1A 1QT. *Tel*: 020 7436 0555. *Public phon-in:* 08700 100 400. *E-mail:* feedback@bbc.co.uk Jul 2000

Points of View
The address to write to is Points of View, BBC TV, London, W12 7TS. *Tel*: 020 8811 1050. *E-mail*: pov@bbc.co.uk Jul 2000

Promises
A *Statement of Promises* is published annually by the BBC. The 1999-2000 statement says "Where the complaint is justified, we apologise; explain what happened, and tell you what we propose to do to avoid the same thing happening again."

The BBC has undertaken to acknowledge serious complaints on receipt and to give a full response within 20 working days, or 35 days for a complex matter.

BBC Information
If you have a query or comment about BBC programmes, BBC Information operates 24 hours a day, seven days a week. *Address:* BBC Information, PO BOX 1116, Belfast, BT2 7AJ. *Tel:* 08700 100 222. *Fax:* 028 9032 6453. 5581

Radio 4
'Today' programme: Richard Hannaford, health correspondent. 020 8743 8000. Jul 2000

Radio Information Office
Radio Information Office open 7.30 am to 9 pm. *Tel*: 0870 0100 222. Jul 2000

TV Information Office
Open 8am to midnight. *Tel:* 0208 743 8000. Jul 2000

Viewers & Listeners
Viewers' and listeners' complaints to BBC Information. 8am to midnight. *Tel:* 0870 0100 222. *E-mail:* vlc@bbc.co.uk Jul 2000

Independent Television

Anglia Television
Address: Anglia Television Ltd., Anglia House, Norwich, NR1 3JG. *Tel:* 01603 615151. *Fax:* 01603 631032.
E-mail: angliatv@angliatv.co.uk
Website: www.anglia.tv.co.uk Feb 2000

Border Television
Address: Border Television plc, The Television Centre, Carlisle, CA1 3NT. *Tel:* 01228 525101. Fax: 01228 541384.
E-mail: ian@border-tv.com
Website: www.border-tv.com Feb 2000

Cable Television
Address: Cable Television, Programme Complaints Division, Independent Television Commission (ITC), 33, Foley Street, London, W1P 7LB. *Tel:* 020 7255 3000. *Fax:* 020 7306 7800.
E-mail: publicaffairs@itc.org.uk
Website: 222.itc.org.uk Feb 2000

Carlton Television
Address: Carlton Television, 101, St Martin's Lane, London, WC2N 4AZ. *Tel:* 020 7240 4000. *Fax:* 020 7240 4171.
E-mail: dutyoffice@carltontv.co.uk
Website: www.carltontv.co.uk Feb 2000

Central Broadcasting
Address: Central Broadcasting, Central Court, Gas Street, Birmingham, B1 2JT. *Tel:* 0121 643 9898. *Fax:* 0121 634 4740.
Website: www.centraltv.co.uk Feb 2000

Channel 4 Television Corporation
Address: Channel 4 Television Corporation, 124, Horseferry Road, London, SW1P 2TX. *Tel:* 020 7396 4444. *Fax:* 020 7306 8347.
E-mail: viewer_enqs@channel4.co.uk
Website: www.channel4.com Feb 2000

Channel 5 Broadcasting Ltd
Address: Channel 5 Broadcasting Ltd., 22, Long Acre, London, WC2E 9LY. *Tel:* 020 7550 5555. *Fax:* 020 7550 5678. *E-mail:*

dutyoffice@channel5.co.uk
Website: www.channel5.co.uk Feb 2000

Channel Television Ltd
Address: Channel Television Ltd., Television Centre, St. Helier, Jersey, Channel Islands, JE1 3ZD. *Tel:* 01534 816816. *Fax:* 01534 816817. *E-mail:* broadcast@channeltv.co.uk *Website:* www.channeltv.co.uk Feb 2000

GMTV Ltd
Address: The London Television Centre, Upper Ground, London, SE1 9TT. *Tel:* 020 7827 7000. *Fax:* 020 7827 7001.
E-mail: talk2us@gmtv.co.uk Jul 2000

Grampian Television Ltd
Address: Grampian Television Ltd., Queen's Cross, Aberdeen, AB15 2XJ. *Tel:* 01224 846846. *Fax:* 01224 846800.
E-mail: gtv@grampiantv.co.uk
Website: scottishmediagroup.com Feb 2000

Granada Television Ltd
Address: Granada Television Ltd., Quay Street, Manchester, M60 9EA. *Tel:* 0161 832 7211. *Fax:* 0161 827 2180.
Website: www.granadatv.co.uk Feb 2000

HTV Wales
Address: HTV Wales, The Television Centre, Culverhouse Cross, Cardiff, CF5 6XJ. *Tel:* 029 2059 0590. *Fax:* 029 2059 7183.
E-mail: htv@htv.co.uk Feb 2000

HTV West
Address: HTV West, The Television Centre, Bath Road, Bristol, BS4 3HG. *Tel:* 0117 972 2722. *Fax:* 0117 972 2400.
Website: www.htv.co.uk Feb 2000

Independent Television News Ltd (ITN)
Address: Independent Television News Ltd (ITN), 200, Gray's Inn Road, London, WC1X 8XZ. *Tel:* 020 7833 3000. *Fax:* 020 7430 4228. *E-mail:* viewer.liaison@itn.co.uk Jul 2000
Website: www.itn.co.uk Feb 2000

London Weekend Television Ltd
Address: London Weekend Television Ltd., The London Television Centre, Upper Ground, London, SE1 9LT. *Tel:* 020 7620 1620. *Fax:* 020 7621 1290. *E-mail:* viewers@lwt.co.uk *Website:* www.lwt.co.uk Feb 2000

Meridian Broadcasting Ltd
Address: Meridian Broadcasting Ltd., Television Centre, Southampton, SO14 0PZ. *Tel:* 023 8022 2555. *Fax:* 023 8033 5050.
E-mail: dutyoffice@meridiantv.com
Website: www.meridian.tv.co.uk Feb 2000

OnDigital
Address: 346, Queenstown Road, London, SW8 4NE. *Tel:* 020 7819 8000. *Fax:* 020 7810 8100. *Website:* www.ondigital.co.uk Feb 2000

S4C
Address: Parc Busnes Ty Glas, Llanishen/Llanisien, Cardiff/Caerdydd, CF4 5DU. *Tel:* 029 2074 1458. *Fax:* 029 2075 1457. *E-mail:* s4c@s4c.co.uk
Website: www.s4c.co.uk Feb 2000

Scottish Television Ltd
Address: Scottish Television Ltd., Cowcaddens, Glasgow, G2 3PR. *Tel:* 0141 300 3000. *Fax:* 0141 300 3030. *Website:* www.scottishmediagroup.com Feb 2000

SKY
Address: British Sky Broadcasting Ltd (SKY), 6, Centaurs Business Park, Grant Way, Isleworth, TW7 5QD. *Tel:* 020 7705 3000. *Fax:* 020 7705 3030. E-*mail:* feedback@sky.co.uk *Website:* www.sky.co.uk (*Also covers Sky digital broadcasts*). Feb 2000

Tyne Tees Television Ltd
Address: Tyne Tees Television Ltd., The Television Centre, City Road, Newcastle upon Tyne, NE1 2AL. *Tel:* 0191 261 0181. *Fax:* 0191 261 2302.
E-mail: tyne.tees@granadamedia.com Feb 2000

Ulster Television plc
Address: Ulster Television plc, Havelock House, Ormeau Road, Belfast, BT7 1EB. *Tel:* 028 9032 8122. *Fax:* 028 9024 6695.

E-mail: info@utv.live.com
Website: www.utvlive.com Feb 2000

Westcountry Television Ltd
Address: Westcountry Television Ltd., Langage Science Park, Plymouth, PL7 5BQ. *Tel:* 01752 333333. *Fax:* 01752 333444. *E-mail:* info@westcountry.co.uk Feb 2000

Yorkshire Television Ltd
Address: Yorkshire Television Ltd., The Television Centre, Leeds, LS3 1JS. *Tel:* 0113 243 8283. *Fax:* 0113 244 5107. Feb 2000

National Newspapers

Daily Express
Address: The Editor, Daily Express, Ludgate House, 245, Blackfriars Road, London, SE1 9UX. *Tel*: 020 7928 8000. *Fax:* 020 7633 0244. *Website:* www.expressnewspapers.co.uk Jul 2000

Daily Mail
Address: The Editor, Daily Mail, Northcliffe House, 2, Derry Street, London, W8 5TT. *Tel*: 020 7938 6000. *Fax*: 020 7937 4463. *E-mail*: news@daily-mail.co.uk Jul 2000

Daily Mirror
Address: The Editor, Daily Mirror, 1, Canada Square, Canary Wharf, London, E14 5AP. *Tel*: 020 7510 3000. *Fax*: 020 7293 2435. Jul 2000

Daily Telegraph
'Health and well-being' by Dr Sarah Brewer:
(e-mail: drsarah@bizonline.co.uk). *Address:* The Editor, Daily Telegraph, 1, Canada Sq. Canary Wharf, London, E14 5DT. *Tel:* 020 7538 5000. *Fax:* 020 7513 2508. Jul 2000

Evening Standard
Address: The Editor, Evening Standard, Northcliffe House, 2, Derry Street, London, W8 5TT. *Tel*: 020 7937 3193. Jul 2000

Financial Times
Address: The Editor, Financial Times, 1, Southwark Bridge, London, SE1 9HL. *Tel*: 020 7873 3000. *Fax*: 020 7873 3076. Jul 2000

Guardian
Address: The Editor, The Guardian, 119, Farringdon Road, London, EC1R 3ER. *Tel*: 020 7278 2332. *Fax:* 020 7837 2114. Jul 2000

Independent
Address: The Editor,The Independent, 1, Canada Square, Canary Wharf, London, E14 5DL. *Tel*: 020 7293 2000. *Fax*: 020 7293 2047. Jul 2000

Mail on Sunday
Address: The Editor, The Mail on Sunday, Northcliffe House, 2, Derry Street, London, W8 5TT. *Tel*: 020 7938 6000. *Fax*: 020 7937 7896. Jul 2000

News of the World
Address: The Editor, News of the World, 1, Virginia Street, London, E1 9XR. *Tel*: 020 7782 4000. *Fax*: 020 7583 9504. Jul 2000

Sun
Address: The Editor, The Sun, 1, Virginia Street, London E1 9XP. Tel: 020 7782 4000. Fax: 020 7782 5606. Jul 2000

Sunday Telegraph
Address: The Editor, The Sunday Telegraph, 1, Canada Square, Canary Wharf, London, E14 5DT. *Tel:* 020 7538 5000. *Fax:* 020 7538 6242. *Website:* www.telegraph.co.uk Jul 2000

Sunday Times
Address: The Editor, The Sunday Times, Times Newspapers, PO Box 495, 1, Pennington Street, London, E1 9XW. *Tel*: 020 7782 5000. *Fax*: 020 7782 5542. Jul 2000

Times
Address: The Editor, 1, Pennington Street, London, E98 1TT. *Tel:* 020 7782 5000. May 2000

National Organisations

Mental Health Media

An organisation offering one day practical media skills training courses for mental health workers, service users and survivors. "Can help you change the media agenda. With the right skills you can promote your services and show mental health issues in a more positive light."

Contact: Beate Kubitz, Head of Training and Communications: *Address:* Mental Health Media, The Resource Centre, 356 Holloway Road, London, N7 6PA. *Tel:* 020 7700 8171. *Fax:* 020 7686 0959. *Website:* www.mhmedia.com [5097 Jul 2000]

Further Information

Code of Practice

The Press Standards Board for Finance publishes a free 'Code of Practice' for newspaper and magazine publishing in the UK.

Address: The Press Standards Board of Finance Ltd., 30, George Square, Glasgow, G2 1EG. [5349]

Media Resources Pack

A free set of guidelines to mental health reporting is available from the Health Promotion Office. *Address*: Hastings & Rother Health Promotion office, ESBH-HA, 3rd floor, Hanover House, Marine Court, St Leonards-on-Sea, East Sussex, TN38 0DX. *Tel*: 01424 441933. [5346]

Mental Health in the Media

The National Union of Journalists publishes a free practical guide for journalists and broadcasters entitled 'Mental Health in the Media'. *Address*: Scottish Association for Mental Health, Atlantic House, 38, Gardner's Crescent, Edinburgh, EH3 8DQ. *Tel*: 031 229 9687. [5348]

Suicide

A media guidlines booklet (20 pages) entitled 'Media Guidelines on the portrayal of suicide' is available from the Samaritans.

Address: The Samaritans, 10, The Grove, Slough, SL1 1QP. *Tel*: 01753 532713. *E-mail*: e.borton@samaritans.org.uk. [5347]

Acknowledgements

Our grateful thanks to Madeleine Mayhew of the Communications Department, East Sussex, Brighton & Hove Health Authority, for editorial assistance with this chapter.

Medication

Today, psychiatrists have a whole cornucopia of magic pills which they can prescribe to alleviate mental distress. Here the various common medications are described together with a simple explanation of how they are thought to work. The issue of side-effects is not overlooked.

Antibiotics

Antibiotics are important medicines. They help us fight infection that are caused by bacteria. So we need to look after them. Bacteria are clever; they adapt and find ways to survive the effects of an antibiotic. They become antibiotic resistant so that the antibiotic no longer works. The more we use an antibiotic, the more likely it is that the bacteria will become resistant to it. And the problem is getting more common. So what can we do?

Here is the NHS News five-point plan:

1. Do not take antibiotics when they are not needed. Many infections get better just as quickly without antibiotics.
2. Remember antibiotics do not work on coughs and colds. Try other medicines instead such as paracetemol or a cold remedy - ask your high street pharmacist.
3. Do not expect your GP to prescribe antibiotics for you or your family. Antibiotics do not work against viruses.
4. If you are given antibiotics, take the whole course unless your pharmacist or GP advises otherwise. Antibiotic resistance is more likely if you take antibiotics just when you remember or in too low a dose.
5. Antibiotics are life-savers for infections such as meningitis, a kidney infection or pneumonia. By not using them unnecessarily, they are more likely to work when we need them.

Remember, if you are worried, ask your pharmacist or GP for advice. [5095]

Anti-depressants

There are two main types. There is an older group of drugs that have been available on prescription for over twenty years. These are called tricyclic anti-depressants and include amitriptyline (Tryptisol), imipramine (Tofranil) and dothiepin (Prothiaden).

In the last ten years newer drugs have been introduced which seem to work just as well, but tend to have fewer side effects. These include lofepramine (Gamanil) and fluoxetine (Prozac).

MAOIs

Another group, the monoamine oxidase inhibitors (MAOIs), is occasionally used for depression that has not responded to other treatments. Patients have to avoid certain foods when taking these and will be given a special card by the doctor or pharmacist. As well as being used to relieve depression, they are frequently used in general medicine to relieve unusual or persistent pain that may not have responded to other treatments.

Side effects

Anti-depressants are not addictive; the main side effects of the older (tricyclic) anti-depressants are drowsiness, dry mouth and constipation. These are uncommon with the newer ones, which may produce restlessness and loss of appetite. In general any side effects are much worse at the beginning of treatment and get better after a few days, even if the dose stays the same.

Lower doses

Side effects are less noticeable when lower doses are used, so a low dose is often recommended at first, increasing after a few days to the full dosage. If you are concerned about side effects, please mention this to the doctor before the prescription is given, as this may affect the choice of drug. In regular dosage the old anti-depressants can stimulate the appetite so that you eat more and gain weight. This may be a good thing, but only if you are underweight when you start.

How long is a course of treatment?

Taken regularly, anti-depressants will start to lift the feeling and symptoms of depression within two to four weeks. The same delay is shown when anti-depressants are used to treat anxiety, phobias and panic. It is important to try to continue the course of treatment in the early stages even if you have some of the side effects mentioned above; it is better to continue treatment at a lower dose than to give up altogether.

For a few people with many episodes of depression, it is recommended that treatment with anti-depressants is continued for many months or years. It is more common to continue for 3 to 4 months after the symptoms are relieved, before reducing the tablets over a few weeks, before stopping them. 5228

Anti-psychotic drugs

Examples are Largactil, Stelazine, Haldol. Sometimes called 'major tranquilisers', these drugs are usually given to people with severe problems such as delusions and hallucinations and manic or disturbed behaviour. They are designed to suppress these distressing symptoms, but can have side effects, which include weight gain, blurred vision, restlessness and involuntary movements of the face and body. Side effects can be related to dosage, so if you are prescribed anti-psychotic drugs, it is important to have your treatment reviewed regularly. They can be given as tablets or injections. 0534

Depot injections

Depot injections are forms of medication injected into muscle so that they are absorbed slowly. The drugs described here are called 'anti-psychotic' because they treat the symptoms commonly found in types of illness such as schizophrenia and manic depression. The drugs are the same as those taken by mouth for these conditions.

Why are they used?

The main advantage of depot anti-psychotic medications is that they have to be given only once every week or every few weeks, while tablets need to be taken at least every day. For people who have difficulty remembering to take tablets regularly, injections may be a better way to take the right dose of medication. This is especially important for people who become unwell very quickly if they go without medication for even a short time.

How can they help?
If you have had difficulties such as interference with your thoughts, hearing voices, seeing visions, or feeling fearful and suspicious of other people, and if your doctor has made a diagnosis of schizophrenia, manic depression or another type of illness, then it is likely that you will be recommended to take an anti-psychotic drug either by mouth or by injection. Research has shown that most people with a diagnosis of schizophrenia, for example, are very much more likely to stay well and not relapse if they continue to take regular doses of anti-psychotic medication.

How are they given?
When your doctor prescribes depot injections for you, you will usually have a small 'test dose' first of all, to find out if that type of drug suits you. If there are no major side effects, then regular doses start. The injections are normally given into the muscles of the buttock, and the drug is released slowly from there over the next few weeks. You can expect the injection to be given to you in a private and comfortable room, usually by a nurse.

What are the side effects?
These injections can sometimes cause difficulties that you need to know about. Possible side effects are explained below. Only some patients get side effects, which are usually mild or temporary and respond to a reduced dose. Commonly people feel some discomfort at the injection site, especially for the first few days after each dose.

Being very similar to other drugs such as chlorpromazine (Largactil), and trifluoperazine (Stelazine) these drugs have some of the same side effects, including a tendency for you to feel restless, feeling dizzy when you get up from sitting, putting on a little weight, dryness of the mouth, blurred eyesight, and feeling stiffness in your arms, legs, neck, or mouth. This stiffness usually improves if you also take a drug such as procyclidine (Kemadrin) or orphenadrine (Disipal). In the long term there is a risk that you might develop repetitive movements in your body or face, called 'tardive dyskinesia'. For all these reasons, you can expect that your doctor will want to use the lowest effective dose of these injections to treat you. Should any of these side effects occur, bring them to the attention of your doctor or key worker.

Frequency of injecting
Most people are prescribed these injections between once a week and once every month. Your doctor will often prescribe the injections for a period of at least several months, and may recommend that you continue for several years. If this applies to you, then you can expect that the dose will be reviewed and discussed with you at regular intervals, and at least every year.

What are the names and doses?
Like other drugs, each of these injections has two different names: one is the proper name and the other is the 'trade' name which is given here. The usual range of doses suggested here is taken from the British National Formulary, a guidebook on prescribing; however, sometimes these doses are exceeded. There are several types of depot injection, and some of the most commonly used are Modecate, Depixol and Haldol.

Consent
If you are a voluntary patient, medicines can only be given to you with your consent. If you are in hospital under a section of the Mental Health Act, then sometimes you can be given these injections without your consent for the first three months of the period of detention. After this, if you do not agree to the treatment, then the hospital must ask an independent doctor from another hospital to decide whether you really need the treatment.

Precautions

The injections may make you feel slightly drowsy and you should be very careful in the amount of alcohol you drink, because this may make you even more drowsy. In particular, be cautious in driving a car or using machinery if you feel at all sleepy. Other sedative drugs, such as sleeping tablets or pills for hay fever, might have the same tendency to add to the drowsiness.

What happens if I miss an injection?

If you miss an injection you may not notice much at first. However, over the next few weeks and months the effects gradually wear off, and you may experience a worsening of your symptoms. In the longer run, you may find that you begin to feel much worse. If you have had troubling thoughts, experiences, voices or visions in the past then you may find that these begin to come back. So if you have simply missed an injection you should have another as soon as you can. But if you are not happy with taking the injection for any reason, please talk about this with your doctor before deciding to stop it.

How do I find out more about depot injections?

If you have any questions about depot injections, please arrange a time to discuss them with the doctor who you usually see for your mental health problems. 5234

Minor tranquillisers

Examples are librium, valium and mogadon. These drugs are prescribed for anxiety or agitation, or to help with sleep problems. They can be effective for the short-term relief of symptoms, but quickly become less effective and can end up producing the symptoms they are designed to relieve.

Minor tranquilisers should be prescribed for no more than two to four weeks and in special circumstances, for example to help you sleep during a crisis. After this time you can become physically and psychologically dependent on them. Their side effects include drowsiness, dizziness, apathy, increased anxiety and depression. 0534

Psychoactive drugs

Drugs which alter mood and mental state.

Side effects

See 'Tardive dyskinesia', page 238, and under 'Anti-depressants', page 233, and 'Depot injections', page 234.

Tranquillisers

Tranquillisers are commonly used drugs which, as the name suggests, calm people down. Tranquillisers are of two main types, often called major and minor tranquillisers.

Major tranquillisers

When used in high dosage, the major tranquillisers are not really used to make people feel calmer, but for the treatment of the more serious forms of mental illness such as schizophrenia and manic depressive psychosis.

However, where appropriate, illnesses can also be treated with lower doses of major tranquillisers. Chlorpromazine (Largactil) and Haloperidol (Serenace) are among the best known. In low dosage the same drugs are occasionally used to reduce anxiety. These drugs will not be discussed here in any further detail.

Minor tranquillisers

The minor tranquillisers are much more commonly prescribed and are almost always used for treating anxiety and difficulty in sleeping. Other important uses of these drugs are in reducing muscular spasm and treating some forms of epilepsy. The biggest group is called the benzodiazepines, of which diazepam (Valium) and lorazepam (Ativan) are the best known. Nitrazepam (Mogadon) and temazepam (Normison) are also used as sleeping tablets.

Side effects

The main side effects of the minor tranquillisers are drowsiness and dependence.

Drowsiness can be a problem, particularly with drugs like diazepam (Valium), which take a long time to disappear from the body. It is better not to drive or operate machinery, especially in the early days of treatment. Care should also be taken with drinking alcohol as it will increase any sleepiness produced by the medication.

Dependence is not normally a problem if the tranquillisers are taken for a few days only, but if they are taken regularly for four weeks or more, about a third of people will have increased nervousness and insomnia after stopping the drug. This can be part of a withdrawal syndrome, a physical state which is most easily relieved by taking the drug again. The withdrawal syndrome can lead to unnecessary long-term prescription.

Dependence is difficult to treat so prevention is the best course. Long-term prescription is only given under special circumstances.

How long is a course of treatment?
Because of the dependence problem, tranquillisers are only given in regular dosage for

Remember ...

Follow the instructions
Follow the instructions on the label. If you don't understand them, ask your doctor or pharmacist to explain them. Never take more than the stated dose on the label. Remember that your pharmacist will be happy to give you advice if you are not clear about anything.

Do not share your medicine
Do not share your medicine with anyone else. Do not take medicines not prescribed by your doctor. If you buy medicines 'over the counter' always check with the pharmacist that they won't interfere with medicines your doctor has prescribed. Remember to see your doctor regularly - to check that the medicines you have been prescribed are still appropriate.

Do not throw away medicines
Don't throw away unused medicines; always return them to your pharmacist. Never throw them out with the household rubbish. Don't throw away the packaging until you've finished the course.

Always drink plenty of liquid
Always drink plenty of cool liquid when taking tablets and capsules - say, a glass of water. Taking medicines 'on an empty stomach' means taking the medicine at least an hour before or two hours after a meal.

If you have trouble remembering
If you have trouble remembering when you've taken your medicine, consider getting a 'memory aid counter' or 'pill counter' from your pharmacist. These are containers with little compartments to help you to remember when to take your medication.

Storage
Keep all medicines out of the reach of children and preferably in a cool, dry place.

Side effects
If you experience any side effects, even if they seem trivial, always let your doctor know. 6065 Jul 99

a few days at a time. If given for longer, they are best taken only when required (preferably less than once a day). They begin to show their calming effects immediately and are good 'first aid' before other forms of treatment begin to work. [5228]

Tardive dyskinesia

The dictionary definition is 'A late-appearing abnormal movement, a disorder characterised by involuntary, stereotyped and rhythmic movements of the upper body and the face, most commonly tongue protrusion, rolling movements, chewing, lip-smacking, abnormal finger movements, leg-jiggling and neck, trunk and pelvis movements. It is a side effect of long-term use of anti-psychotic drugs, and once it emerges is extremely resistant to treatment'. [5093]

Katherine Darton, Information and Advice officer at Mind writes, in Jan 2000, "Not everyone who takes antipsychotics will develop tardive dyskinesia (TD). Estimates vary from 5 to 56% of people taking antipsychotics for at least three years, but the risk is higher for people on depot drugs.

Once someone has developed TD it may not go away even if they stop taking the medication, although it does in some cases. About half of patients who stop taking medication will have improvement in the symptoms, although the improvement is delayed and may take up to five years. Stopping medication is not possible for some people, and the risk of relapse or psychosis must be balanced against the risk of TD.

Another complication is that when people come off medication they may get a 'withdrawal dyskinesia', which is not necessarily the same as TD.

The new, so-called atypical antipsychotics seem to pose less of a risk of TD, and clozapine and risperidone have been found to improve it.

The risk is minimized if the lowest possible dose of medication is used. Anti-Parkinson's drugs, given for the side effects of antipsychotics, are thought to increase the risk of TD, and using low doses of antipsychotics should reduce the need for these drugs too.

Some people find that TD is improved with vitamin E, but it is not known if this would reduce the risk of TD developing." [5091, 5093]

Medications

Carbamazapine

(Tegretol) is sometimes given with, or as an alternative to, Lithium. It has its own side effects. [0534]

Chlorpromazine

Another name for Largactil; see 'Anti-psychotic drugs'.

Depixol

Proper name is Flupenthixol decanoate used for depot injections.

Diazepam

Another name for Valium. See 'Valium'.

Largactil

A major tranquilliser. See 'Tranquillisers'.

Librium

A minor tranquilliser.

Lithium

Lithium has been used as a drug since 1949. It is mainly used for treatment and prevention of mood disorders such as being low (depression) or high (mania). Lithium is prescribed in a number of preparations. There is no real difference between them. The importance is how much lithium they make available. It is important to continue with the same variety that has been prescribed for you.

When is Lithium used?

Lithium is used in treating and controlling

mood disorders like depression and mania especially when they keep coming back. It is also used to increase the effect of antidepressant drugs when these are not working enough on their own.

Lithium helps in preventing episodes of mania and depression. Even if these still occur the mood swings are usually less severe. Normally it brings about improvement quite quickly, especially in relieving depression and mania, but it may take several months or even up to two years to control mood swing.

Lithium is a safe drug, but it is important to keep blood levels within certain limits, or symptoms like shaking of the hands and legs, nausea, stomach cramps and diarrhoea may appear. These do not occur in everyone and most go away with time as the body gets used to lithium.

Taking Lithium

After the first few months, sometimes weight gain and excess urination may develop. Rarely there are problems with the thyroid gland, lithium making it less active than usual. This can be checked by your doctor using blood tests and physical examination.

Contact your doctor immediately if you get severe thirst, severe diarrhoea or vomiting, shaking of the hands and legs, muscle twitching or confusion. Some other medications, whether prescribed or over the counter, may interfere with lithium. Please check with your doctor or pharmacist before starting any new medication.

How does it act?

Lithium is believed to correct some chemical balances in brain cells which may be the underlying cause of depression or mania. The actual dose of lithium taken depends upon individual needs. Sometimes a single daily dose is enough. Mostly it is given 2 or 3 times a day. It is not an addictive drug and it is important to continue with it when you are feeling better, since suddenly stopping it may precipitate a bout of illness.

Blood tests

It is essential to have regular blood tests to check the levels of lithium in the body. At first these tests would be every week or fortnight. Later, after the levels have become stable, the frequency can be dropped to every three or four months. When you attend for the blood test, make sure that no doses have been forgotten in the past several days. The blood test is usually done 12 hours after the last dose, so that you may have to miss the morning dose.

If you have missed any doses, do not try to 'catch up' with the dose. It is important to drink plenty while on lithium. While holidaying in a hot climate try and drink more and avoid long periods in the sun. It is also important to avoid low-salt diets, heavy exercise, saunas etc.

Pregnancy

Lithium should *not* be given to pregnant women. It is important for the doctor to know if a woman patient on lithium is planning to get pregnant so that lithium can be stopped in advance.

Side effects

Like all drugs, lithium has side effects, some of which are serious, usually only when too much is being taken, and some not so serious. If lithium does not suit you or is not effective in your case, your doctor may be able to find other drugs which can be used. [5233]

Modecate

Proper name is Fluphenazine decanoate; used for depot injections.

Prozac

A drug that prolongs the action of serotonin in the brain; used as an anti-depressant. [0526]

Valium

A minor tranquilliser.

National Organisations

NICE

National Institute for Clinical Excellence. Set up by the Labour government in 1999 to advise on the use of prescribed drugs.

Further Information

Medication online

See 'Chemists' chapter, page 169, under 'Websites'.

MindinfoLine

Ten per cent of calls to Mind are about medication. Mind has launched a special service operating on Thursday mornings between 9.15 and 11.45am taking calls about psychiatric drugs. The line is manned by a pharmacist from the UK Psychiatric Pharmacy Group, based at the Maudsley Hospital. *Tel:* 020 8215 2274. [5425]

British National Formulary.

Edited by D K Mehta. Published by the British Medical Association and the Royal Pharmacological Society of Great Britain, Sept 1997. It is "intended for the guidance of medical practitioners, pharmacists, dentists, nurses, and other workers who have the necessary training and experience to interpret the information it provides."

Complete Guide to Psychiatric Drugs.

A layman's guide, 2nd edition by Ron Lacey. Published by Mind/Ebury Press, 1996, 168 pages, £9.99, ISBN 0 09 181367 0. "Mind believes that everyone either taking or involved in the use of psychiatric drugs needs to know more about them.

This revised edition of the clear and accessible guide explains the benefits, adverse effects and hazards of the complete range of pyschiatric drugs. It is designed to help people understand prescriptions, cut down the risk of dependency, get the best from their doctors and play an active part in recovery". Available from Mind Mail Order. *Tel:* 020 8221 9666.

Deprived of our Humanity

'Deprived of our humanity - the case against neuroleptic drugs'. Written by Lars Marensson, MD. Neuroleptic drugs (known as major tranquilisers) can have the effect of a lobotomy on those to whom they are prescribed long-term. In this shocking book neuroleptic survivors and doctors make their cases against the use of such drugs. Published by Les Sans Voix, 1999; ISBN 2-88462-039-7; 224 pages, £7. Available from Mind Mail Order Service, 15, Broadway, Stratford, London, E15 4BQ. *Tel:* 020 8221 9666. [5088]

Health Information Service

The HIS is a free and confidential 24-hour service. You can speak to staff during office hours, and you can listen to any of hundreds of tapes at any time, e.g: *Depression: drugs and medical treatments.* (Tape 298); *Antibiotics* (Tape 297).

Address: The College of Health, St Margaret's House, 21, Old Ford Road, London, E2 9PL. *Freephone:* 0800 66 55 44. [5367]

Medical Methods of Treatment

Written by Dr Brenda Lintner. 12-page booklet published by Sane, 1993.

Prozac Nation

By Elizabeth Wurtzel. 'The Sorrows of the rudderless children of the free-love, easy-divorce revolution. This was the generation that needed anti-depressants as a substitute for stability and family.' Published 1994.

See also ...

Chemists, page 163.
Self-management, 262.

Mental Health

What is mental health?
Mental Health: feelings of depression, anxiety or confusion are a normal response to the ups and downs of modern life. A person is described as experiencing mental health problems when such feelings are so extreme that he or she has difficulty carrying on their everyday life.

How many people have problems?
'Between 10 and 25% of the general population annually present with mental health problems. Within this figure, 2-4% will have a severe mental illness.'

What are main types of problems?
The main problems seem to be anxiety, depression, manic depression and schizophrenia. Please see separate chapters for further information on these illnesses. [1571]

Local Organisations

Mental Health Helpline
This is a county wide, out-of-hours telephone helpline for people with mental health issues. The service is available from 6pm to midnight on weekdays and from 2pm to midnight at weekends. The calls are free. Tel: 0808 808 3333, for English speakers; 0808 800 2073 for Asian language speakers. Alternatively, call 0345 697590. 6pm to midnight daily. [Jul 2000]

Mental Health Promotion
East Sussex Brighton & Hove Health Authority's Health Promotion Department has a division dedicated to the promotion of Mental Health. For details see 'Health Authorities' chapter under 'Mental Health Promotion', page 321.

National Organisations

Sainsbury Centre
The Sainsbury Centre for Mental Health aims to improve mental health services through a co-ordinated programme of research, service evaluation, service development and training.

Address: The Sainsbury Centre for Mental Health,134, Borough High Street, London, SE1 1LB. *Tel*: 020 7827 8351. *Fax:* 020 7403 9482. *Website:* www.sainsburycentre.org.uk [Jul 2000]

Mental Health Alliance
The MHA exists solely to work on the Mental Health Act Review. The co-ordinator is Margaret Pedler.

Address: Mental Health Alliance, Mind, 15-19, Broadway, London E15 4BQ. *Tel:* 020 8215 2287.
*E-mail:*mpedler@mind.org.uk [Jun 2000]

Mental Health Foundation
The MHF can seek out and provide information on a wide range of mental health topics. If you are experiencing difficulty locating information relating to a mental health issue, you may find what you are looking for by first contacting the MHF, either by letter, telephone, e-mail or through their website. Motto: 50 years of pioneering, understanding and action. *Contact:* Jowyn Jenson, Information Assistant.

The Mental Health Foundation is the UK's leading mental health and learning disabilities charity, undertaking a broad variety of research - from traditional biomedical research, to enabling and monitoring the progress of pioneering new community services, to investigating how people who are facing mental health problems manage their situation. They run a busy press and information office, challenging the stigma and lack of information that surrounds mental illness and learning disabilities. [6077 Oct 99]

Address: Mental Health Foundation, 20/21, Cornwall Terrace, London, NW1 4QL.

Tel: 020 7535 7400. *Fax:* 020 7535 7474. *E-mail*: mhf@mentalhealth.org.uk *Website*: http://www.mentalhealth.org.uk Jul 2000

Publications catalogue
The Mental Health Foundation publishes a wide range of material on mental health. For a free copy of their catalogue please call the MHF on 020 7535 7400. 6028

Mental Health Czar

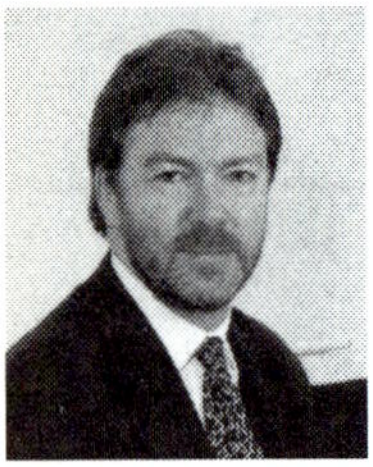

Professor Louis Appleby (pictured left) was appointed by the government in April 2000 to oversee provision of mental health services. His role is to modernise and improve mental health services in England. In particular he will be ensuring that the National Service Framework is implemented. The NSF calls for services to be more responsive to patients/service users and their families - an essential part of a modern, high quality service.

According to Professor Appleby: 'Mental health services are still in urgent need of reform. Too often, services are fractured and people fall between the cracks. I am keen to hear directly from patients, families and professionals about their experiences and the changes they would like to see.

'Mixed sex accommodation is out of place in the modern mental health services, and new guidance is going out to health authorities on this subject. We need to create a climate of privacy and dignity on the wards. It is not good enough that women and men can feel threatened in an environment that is meant to help them.

Out-of-area acute admissions, where a patient needing urgent hospital treatment must be moved to a different area because of bed shortages, are distressing to patients and families. I want to see this practice stopped as soon as possible.' Communicate your views directly to Professor Appleby.

Address: Professor Louis Appleby, National Director of Mental Health. Department of Psychiatry, Withington Hospital, West Didsbury, Manchester, M20 8LR. *Tel:* Direct Line: 0161 291 4362. *Fax:* 0161 445 9263.
E-mail: louis.appleby@man.ac.uk *Website:* www.doh.gov.uk/mentalhealthczar May 2000; 5032 Jul 2000

DDA Helpline

The Disability Discrimination Act Helpline provides information and advice about all aspects of the DDA, as well as good practice advice on the employment of disabled people. Hours are 8am to 8pm, when trained advisers are available. All calls at local rate. *Tel:* 08457 622633. 6085 Jul 2000

Further Information

Note: the following books are relevant to mental health generally, or are on topics not covered in other chapters. For books on specific topics, see in the appropriate chapters.

A History of Mental Health
A History of Mental Health and Community Care. By George Stewart. Published by Mind Information Unit. 1999. Price £0.50p. Available from Mind: 020 8221 9666.

A Shattered World
'The mental health needs of refugees and newly arrived communities'. By the CVS Consultants & Migrant & Refugee Communities Forum.

The results of a project commissioned by the Department of Health, this report describes the kinds of mental health problems that are particularly common amongst newly arrived people and what causes them, as well as looking at some of the services that have been developed to help them. With useful contact addresses.

Published by CVS, 2000. ISBN: 1-901-591-05-0. 88 pages. £7.50. Available from Mind Mail Order Service. *Tel*: 020 8221 9666. 5251

Amongst Ourselves

Amongst Ourselves - A Self-Help guide to Living with Dissassociative Identity Disorder. By Tracy Alderman Ph.D., & Karen Marshall LCSW. The first and only self-help guide written expressly for individuals with DID and MPD. Gives readers practical steps to take to cope with the condition and emerge with greater self-awareness and the skills to live a rich and rewarding life. Published by New Harbinger Press, 1998. ISBN: 1-57224-122-5. 240 pages. £10.99. Available from Mind Mail Order Service. *Tel*: 020 8221 9666. 5251

Assertive Community Treatment

Assertive Community Treatment - Treatment of persons with severe mental illness. Written by Leonard I Stein & Alberto B Santos. "Here, at last, is a practical book that describes the ACT approach as a vehicle for providing treatment, rehabilitation, supportive services and practical help." 5088

Published by W W Norton, 1998, ISBN: 0-393-70258-8. 274 pages. £19.95. Available from Mind Mail Order Service. *Tel*: 020 8221 9666.

From Loneliness to Love

'From Loneliness to Love - A Journey to Fulfilment'. By Phil Nuernberger. Loneliness has been found in every culture at every time. The answer, says the author of this book, is spiritual awakening. He provides a plan for overcoming these familiar yet powerful feelings of isolation, sadness and anxiety. Published by Element, 1999. ISBN: 1-86204-356-6. £7.99. Available from Mind Mail Order Service. *Tel:* 020 8221 9666. 5251

Hidden Selves

'Hidden Selves - An exploration of multiple personality'. Edited by Moria Walker & Jennifer Antony-Black. A book which deals with the controversial subject of multiple personality. Six therapists or counsellors respond to the story of a survivor of abuse who now experiences multiple selves, explaining how they would understand her presentation and how they would work with her therapeutically.

Published by Open University Press, 1999. ISBN: 0-335-20200-4. 134 pages. £17.99. Available from Mind Mail Order Service. Tel: 020 8221 9666. 5251

In Your Right Mind

By Dr Thomas Stuttaford & Dr Tonmoy Sharma. "Dr Stuttaford has spent 40 years as a GP, and is also *The Times'* resident doctor. This book, written with Dr Sharma of the Maudsley, aims to dispel the fear and ignorance that may keep people from the help they need. He is more interested in making people well than pushing any particular theory; his attitude is one of robust common sense. Fisher, journalist and musician". Published by Faber & Faber, £16.99. 5069

Mental Illness

Mental Illness - A guide to mental health in the workplace. 12-page A5 booklet published by the Department of Health, 1992.

Mental Illness

Mental Illness - What you can do about it. 16-page A5 booklet published by the Department of Health, 1995.

Midlife - A Manual

By Judith & Steven Erstrine. Witty first-hand insights on how to handle the major challenges of your midlife years. With advice on everything from 'empty nest' syndrome to renewing your sex life, to planning for retirement.

Published by Element, 1999. ISBN: 1-86204-690-5. 176 pages. £9.99. Available from Mind Mail Order Service. *Tel*: 020 8221 9666. 5069

Narrative Means to Therapeutic Ends

By Michael White & David Epston. A groundbreaking book that puts forth the idea that people experience problems when the stories of their lives, as they or as others have invented them, do not sufficiently represent their lived experience. It takes the view that people should be encouraged to become the 'authors' of their own life stories, and shows how this can be done. With real-life examples.

Published by Wiley, 1990. ISBN: 0-393-70098-4. 230 pages. £19.10. Available from Mind Mail Order Service. *Tel*: 020 8221 9666. [5069]

Phone At Nine Just To Say You're Alive

Written by Linda Hart. A diary kept by Linda Hart who was diagnosed as mentally ill. Published by the Abbott Press. £7.99.

Notes On The History Of Mental Health

By Katherine Darton. Published by Mind Information Unit. February 1999. Price £0.50p. Available from Mind Mail Order Service. *Tel*: 020 8221 9666.

Recovery: An Alien Concept

Written by Ron Coleman. Describing his own and others' experiences with a mental health system that seems to encourage dependence rather than recovery, Ron Coleman outlines his recovery plan for the disillusioned mental health service user.

Published by Handsell, 1994. 116 pages. £9.00. Available from Mind Mail Order Service. *Tel*: 020 8221 9666. [5251]

Relocating Madness

'Relocating Madness - From the mental patient to the person'. By Barham and Hayward. Available from Hastings Library, reference 362.2094.

From the Ashes of Experience

'From the Ashes of Experience -Reflections on madness, survival and growth'.

Edited by Phil Barker, Peter Campbell & Ben Davidson. Mental health professionals often focus on separate areas of a person's life rather than understanding their whole experience. This collection offers uniquely human, often spiritual perspectives from users and survivors.

Published by Whurr Publishers, 1999. ISBN: 1-85433-272-4. 144 pages. £24.50. Available from Mind Mail Order Service. *Tel*: 020 8221 9666. [5251]

Speaking Our Minds

Edited by Jim Read, & Jill Reynolds. Available from Hastings Library, reference 616.89009.

Staying Sane

'Staying Sane - How to make your mind work for you', by Dr Raj Persaud. Cuts through the myths surrounding mental health, identifying the tools you need to preserve your well-being and stay sane.

Published by Metro Books,1998. ISBN:1-900512-38-6. 490 pages. £12.99. Available from Mind Mail Order Service. *Tel*: 020 8221 9666.

Origins Of Unhappiness

By David Smail. *"David Smail is my touchstone for truth and reason. He is psychology's Voltaire"* - Dr Dorothy Rowe. In this book, first published in 1993, David Smail offers a radical argument that suggests that personal distress originates not from within, but from society, and overthrows common conceptions of 'mental illness' and 'treatment'.

Published by Constable, 1999. ISBN: 0-09-479340-9. 242 pages. £8.99. Available from Mind Mail Order Service.*Tel*: 020 8221 9666. [5251]

Towards Emotional Literacy

By Susie Orbach. This second collection of her Guardian columns deals with issues such as relationships, parenting, schooling, jealousy and fatigue, always advocating that people's emotions should be expressed and understood, not denied and repressed.

Published by Virago, 1999. ISBN; 1-86049-654-7. 270 pages. £10.99. Available from Mind Mail Order Service. *Tel*: 020 8221 9666. [5251]

Mind Organisation

Mind works for everyone in emotional distress, campaigning for rights, and promoting the development of locally-based services through more than 220 local associations.

Mind works for everyone in emotional distress, campaigning for rights, and promoting the development of locally-based services through more than 220 local associations. Mind offers a full range of publications, a bi-monthly magazine, *Open Mind*, (see 'Further Information', page 248), and a free quarterly newsletter. Below are given the addresses and other details of Local Mind groups. Other Mind Groups and National Mind.

Publications

Mind publishes a wide range of literature on mental health. The series *'Understanding Mental Health...'* gives clear, concise introductions to a wide range of mental health problems and treatments. Further details from Mind Mail Order Service. *Tel*: 020 8221 9666. [5369]

Local Mind Groups

East Sussex Alliance

East Sussex Alliance of Local Mind Associations (ESALMA), comprising groups in Lewes & Wealden, Eastbourne and Hastings, was formed to work co-operatively and provide mutual support. They respond collectively to national Mind campaigns and to local mental health strategy targets; in particular, those relating to advocacy and user involvement. *Contacts*: Margaret Moss, Peter Nicholls & Paddi Mobbs. *Address*: Mind Alliance, Eastgate House, Eastgate Street, Lewes, East Sussex, BN7 2LP.[5369]

Bexhill Shop

Contact: Lynne Collins, Manager. *Address*: The Mind Shop, 77, Devonshire Road, Bexhill, Sussex, TN40 1BD. *Tel*: 01424 222461. [5146]

Brighton

Contact: Andy Porter. *Address:* Brighton & Hove Mind, 79, Buckingham Road, Brighton, East Sussex, BN1 3RJ. *Tel*: 01273 749600. [5145 July 2000]

Eastbourne

Address: Eastbourne & District Mind, Avenida House, 3, Upper Avenue, Eastbourne, Sussex, BN21 3UY. *Tel:* 01323 726891. [July 2000]

Hastings

Hastings Mind (Hastings & Rother Association for Mental Health0. Hastings Mind was established in 1975, and has been involved in many aspects of promoting mental health since then. It has provided day centre facilities for many years and is still involved in the Hastings Day Centre. One of Mind's main priorities is to secure funding for and to effect the building of a new support centre. At the time of writing, the funding is looking very promising and it is hoped that the new building will be started by 2002. Aug 2000

Day Centre
Day to day management of the Hastings Day Centre transferred to Maca in July 2000. Please see 'Day Centres' chapter for further information, page 209.

Good Health Guide
This *Guide* was published in the summer of 2000 as a celebration of 25 years continuous promotion of mental health in Hastings & Rother. It is hoped that it will be updated regularly in the years to come.

Membership
If you would like to support the work of Hastings Mind, you could consider becoming a member. By becoming a member you will be helping us to combat discrimination and you will be putting your weight behind us to improve local services. It costs just £5 per year (£2 if unwaged). Please send your payment to Hastings Mind, St Peter's Place, 32/33, St Peter's Road, St Leonards-on-Sea, Sussex, TN37 6JQ. Please make cheques etc. payable to 'Hastings Mind'. Thank you.

Donations to Hastings Mind
Hastings Mind works hard to promote all aspects of mental health, this Guide being but one example. If you want to help us, please be assured that all donations, however small, are always very welcome indeed, but this is strictly optional. Please send any donations to 'Hastings Mind' St Peter's Place, 32/33, St Peter's Road, St Leonards, Sussex, TN37 6JQ. Thank you.

Executive Committee:
John Lutman, chairman; Margaret Moss, vice-chairman; Patrick Dawson, secretary; John Humphries, treasurer. Other members of the executive committee are Su Barnicoat, Peter Howard, Franco Di Francesco, Do Macnair, Liz Coleman, Anna Barnes.
Address: Hastings Mind, St Peter's Place, St Leonards, Sussex, TN37 6JQ. *Tel:* 01424 439599. *E-mail:* john@johnhumphries.co.uk

Lewes
Contact: Peter Nicholls, Local Co-ordinator. *Address*: Lewes District and Wealden Mind, c/o Community Mental Health Centre, Eastgate House, 6, Eastgate Street, Lewes, East Sussex, BN7 2LP. *Tel*: 01273 476934 AND 488660. Jul 2000

South East
Contact: Fiona Hill, Network Regional Manager. *Address:* South East Mind, First Floor, Kemp House, 152-160, City Road, London, EC1V 2NP.
Tel: 020 7608 0881. *Fax:* 020 7608 3750.
E-mail: southeast@mind.org.uk
Website: www.mind.org.uk Jul 2000

Other Mind Groups

Barnet
Has a useful website which attracts hundreds of 'hits' from all over the world. Mind in Barnet kindly allowed Hastings Mind to use material from its excellent *Mental Health Guide* published in 1999. *Contact:* Chief executive Mike O'Sullivan.
Address: Mind in Barnet, 2, Schoolway, North Finchley, London, N12 ORY. *Tel*: 0845 600 6543. *Fax*: 0208 343 5707.
E-mail: admin@mindinbarnet.org
Website: www.mindinbarnet.org 6060 Jul 2000

Mind, Manchester
Has an interesting website; an excellent mixture of campaigning, with QUDOS (Questioning the Unreliable Diagnosis of Schizophrenia), information about services and mental health issues, all presented in a lively and colourful way with some fascinating artwork. *Website:* www.mind-in-manchester.org.uk 5425

National Mind

Mind, National

Chief Executive: Judi Clements. Office hours: Mondays to Fridays 9.15am to 4.45pm. Mind is the National Association for Mental Health. It is a registered charity, and its patron is HRH Princess Alexandra, the Hon. Lady Ogilvy.

Address: Mind (The National Association for Mental Health), Granta House, 15-19, Broadway, London, E15 4BQ. *Tel*: 020 8519 2122. *Fax:* 020 8522 1725. *Website:* www.mind.org.uk [Jul 2000]

Mind*info*Line

Mind*info*Line is Mind's mental health telephone information service, which offers a vital lifeline to people in distress, their relatives and carers, as well as providing mental health information to members of the public, professionals, students; anybody with a problem or a question. People ring up wanting to find out about counselling, local support groups, different treatment options, their rights in hospital, how to access community care, disclosing sexual abuse, feeling suicidal.

The service trains people to listen and offers information about the different options available. *Hours*: Mondays to Fridays, 9.15am to 4.45pm.

Mind now uses a telephone translation and interpreting service with access to over 100 languages. It consists of a 3-way conferencing facility enabling information staff to communicate effectively through a trained interpreter.

Address: Mind, 15-19, Broadway, London E15 4BQ. *Tel*: 020 8522; Outside London: 08457 660163. [5279]

Medication

Ten per cent of calls to Mind are about medication. Mind has launched a special service operating on Thursday mornings between 9.15 and 11.45am taking calls about psychiatric drugs. The line is manned by a pharmacist from the UK Psychiatric Pharmacy Group, based at the Maudsley Hospital. *Tel:* 020 8215 2274. [5425]

MindLink

MindLink is about communication between mental health service users and National Mind. The primary purpose of MindLink is to be a consultative body to ensure that users of mental health services have a direct say in shaping Mind's policies and campaigns.

Although MindLink operates primarily within Mind, it is also part of the broader user movement and has contact with other user organisations as well as statutory bodies.

Anyone who defines themselves as a user of mental health services can join. In fact, membership of MindLink is restricted to users, past or present and membership is free.

Contacts list

Members are invited to join the MindLink Contacts List. The Contacts List is for members who are interested in communicating directly with other members and is sent out to all new members when they join. The Contacts List operates via a PO box system to help preserve privacy.

Information packs

There are regular mailings of MindLink Information Packs which contain information on Mind campaigns and policies, articles, user news, letters, reviews, adverts, etc. Information Packs provide an opportunity for members to become better informed, to share their knowledge, and to help empower themselves and support others.

Address: The MindLink Coordinator, Mind, Freepost (WD2336), 15-19 Broadway, London E15 4BQ. *Tel*: 020 8519 2122 (MindLink); 0345 660 163 (MindInfoLine). [5269]

Minds Matter

This is the company which manages all the Mind shops up and down the country. Chair: Ivor Hunt; Managing Director: Robert Monteath.

Address: Minds Matter (Trading Activities) Ltd, Granta House, 15-19, Broadway, London, E15 4BQ. *Tel*: 020 8534 4040. *Fax*: 020 8534 7733. *Website:* www.mind.org.uk [Jul 2000]

Further Information

A History of Mind

Mind - the National Association for Mental Health). By Katherine Darton. Published by MIND Information Unit, Feb. 1999. £1.36.

Open Mind

'Open Mind' is the journal of Mind (National Association for Mental Health), published every two months.

'For over 15 years *Openmind* magazine has provided progressive coverage of mental health, always recognizing it as a social and political issue as well as a clinical one.

Only *Openmind* has consistently looked at mental health from the perspective of both providers and users of mental health services. Only *Openmind* is editorially independent, non-profitmaking and does not accept advertising or other revenue from any pharmaceutical manufacturer - all enabling it to report without fear or favour.' [5278] Annual subscription, (six issues) for an individual is £20. Editor is Sara Dunn.

Address: Mind, 15, Broadway, London, E15 4BQ. *Tel*: 020 8221 9661. *E-mail:* openmind@mind.org.uk [5110]

Mental Health Guide

'The Mental Health Guide for the London Borough of Barnet' Published by Mind in Barnet, 1999; 92 pages. Available from Mind in Barnet, address as above.

Acknowledgements
Our grateful thanks to Franco Di Francesco of Hastings Day Centre for editorial assistance with this chapter.

Miscellaneous

The information given here consists of items which do not fall naturally into any of the existing chapters and which do not justify having a chapter to themselves.

Religion & mental health

'Courage To Bare Our Souls' was published, 1999, by the Mental Health Foundation, 20-21 Cornwall Terrace, London, NW1 4QL. *Tel:* 020 7535 7441. Price: £7.00. 5110

Missing Persons Helpline

Counselling, listening and practical support for anyone missing relatives or immediate family members. Call free on 0500 700 700. Jul 2000

Message Home

Confidential helpline to let someone know that you are safe if you have left home or run away. Call free on 0800 700 740. Jul 2000

Local Organisations

Hastings Area Community Trust

The HACT is an organisation that raises charitable funds and administers six existing Trust funds. Enquiries should only be made through the following agencies: HARC, Social Services, Seaview, Age Concern and the Citizens Advice Bureau. *Hours:* Mondays to Fridays 9.30 to 11.30am. *Contact Name:* Mrs Jean Fletcher.

Address: HACT, 49 Cambridge Gardens, Hastings, East Sussex TN34 1EN. *Tel*: 01424 718880. May 2000

Hastings Borough Council

Address: Hastings Borough Council, Town Hall, Queen's Road, Hastings, TN34 1QR. *Tel:* 01424 781066. Emergency information service, after hours, *Tel:* 01424 781999. Jul 2000

Hastings Police

Contact: Inspector Chris Wratten, Divisional Patrol Unit Mental Health Liaison Officer. *Address*: Hastings Police Station, Bohemia Road, Hastings, East Sussex, TN34 1PS. *Tel*: Non emergency *(low cost local rate)* 0845 60 70 999. Emergency dial 999. *Fax:* 01424 456017. May 2000

Sussex Police

Contact: Inspector Mike Fagan. *Address*: Police HQ, Malling House, Church Lane, Lewes, East Sussex, BN7 2DZ. *Tel*: 0845 60 70 999. *Fax:* 01273 404274. *Website:* www.sussex.police.uk Jul 2000

National Organisations

Charities Aid Foundation

Address: Charities Aid Foundation, Kings Hill, West Malling, Kent, ME19 4TA. *Tel:* 01732 590000. *Fax:* 01732 520001. *E-mail:* enquiries@caf.charitynet.org *Website:* www.cafonline.org Jul 2000

Crimestoppers

If you know the names of people committing crime, or dealing drugs call Crimestoppers on 0800 555 111. Your call is free and totally anonymous and you may receive a reward. Jul 2000

Social Security Enquiry Line

Social Security Public Enquiry Line, *Tel*: London 020 7712 2171. Jul 2000

Private Health Care

Private health care is widely available and millions of people in this country subscribe to one or other of the providers, some of whom are listed here.

Private health care is widely available and millions of people in this country subscribe to one or other of the providers, some of whom are listed here. An independent guide to private medical insurance is published by the Association of British Insurers, see below.

NHS National Plan
The NHS National Plan announced by the government in July 2000 states "For decades, there has been a stand-off between the NHS and the private sector providers of health care. This has to end. Ideological boundaries or institutional barriers should not stand in the way of better care for NHS patients." 6042 Jul 2000

Local Organisations

Hospitals & Clinics

Details of all private hospitals and clinics will be found in the 'Hospitals & Clinics' chapter, page 323. They include:

Bupa Hospital at Hastings
Eastbourne Clinic at Eastbourne
Godden Green Clinic at Sevenoaks, Kent
Sussex Private Clinic at St Leonards
Priory Ticehurst, at Ticehurst
Ticehurst House Hospital, (This is now known as 'Priory Ticehurst' Hospital).

Psychiatrists

Bott, Dr Michael
Consultant pyschiatrist. Qualifications: MB, BS, DPM, MRC Psych. Dr Bott sees patients at Wilbury Road and at Godden Green Clinic at Sevenoaks. Dr Bott is a general adult psychiatrist with a special interest in stress in employment and post-traumatic stress disorder. Fees are based on a standard rate. Details of fees and all appointments through Dr Bott's secretary at Hove.

Address: Dr Michael Bott, 28, Wilbury Road, Hove, Sussex, BN3 3JP. *Tel*: 01273 773838. *Fax*: 01273 820754. 5118 May 2000

National Organisations

Association of British Insurers

Publishes an independent guide to private medical insurance, available free, *Are you buying private medical insurance?* It addresses such questions as:

- What is private medical insurance?
- How do I buy private medical insurance?
- How do I choose the right cover?
- What am I covered for?
- What does my cover not include?
- What will affect my premiums?
- Will I need to provide details of my health?
- Will my cover be affected if I am disabled?
- How do I make a claim?
- How is private medical insurance controlled?

- What if I want to change to a new insurance company?

Address: Association of British Insurers, 51, Gresham Street, London, EC2V 7HQ. *Tel*: 020 7600 3333. *Fax:* 020 7696 8999. *Website:* www.abi.org.uk [5104 May 2000]

BUPA

BUPA is a provident association and there are no shareholders, which means that 'all profits are reinvested into the health care services provided.' BUPA states that it is Britain's largest independent health care organisation, with over three million clients, and 50 years' experience, and operating in over 170 countries worldwide. [5102, 5103]

Cover

BUPA offers a range of schemes for personal members (i.e. those who pay their own subscriptions) and they can opt for a scheme that covers psychiatry if they wish. For example, one of our main schemes, BUPACare includes cover for psychiatry for personal members. When cover for psychiatry is offered on BUPA schemes, this usually matches the cover set out in the BUPACare membership guide (see next paragraph). [5275]

Psychiatric treatment

BUPA offers psychiatric treatment after two years' membership as follows:

'We may, at our discretion, pay for psychiatric treatment received as day-case or in-patient treatment in a psychiatric network hospital after you have been a member of any BUPA scheme which includes cover for psychiatric treatment for the whole of the two years leading up to the treatment. We may pay for up to 45 days treatment costs each membership year. We have arrangements with psychiatric network hospitals which require them to obtain our written agreement before the treatment starts or at the earliest opportunity. We must receive full clinical details from your consultant or psychiatric network hospital before we can give our decision.' [5274]

Hospitals

BUPA hospitals in this area include the Sussex Nuffield Hospital at Brighton, the Esperance Private Hospital at Eastbourne, the BUPA Hospital at Hastings and the Hove Nuffield Hospital at Hove.

Please call 0800 600 500.

Address: BUPA House,15-19, Bloomsbury Way, London, WC1A 2BA. *Tel:* 020 7656 2000. *Fax:* 020 7656 2700. Website: www.bupa.co.uk [5105 May 2000]

Exeter Healthcare

Established 1973, Exeter Healthcare is a Friendly Society which means there are no shareholders. All surpluses are used to improve benefits for members. The Society is incorporated under the Friendly Societies Act 1992.

Address: Exeter Healthcare, Exeter Friendly Society Limited, Beech Hill House, Walnut Gardens, Exeter, Devon, EX4 4DG. *Tel:* 01392 477210. *Fax:* 01392 477235. [5824]

Insurance Ombudsman

If you have a complaint with your insurance company and you cannot sort it out with them, the Insurance Ombudsman or the Personal Insurance Arbitration Service may be able to help. Their decisions are binding on the insurance company, but do not affect your right to take legal action if you want to do so.

Address: The Insurance Ombudsman Bureau, South Quay Plaza, 183, Marsh Wall, London, E14 9SR. *Tel*: 0845 600 6666. *Fax:* 020 7964 1001. *Website:* www.theiob.org [Jul 2000]

Address: Personal Insurance Arbi-tration Service, 24, Angel Gate, City Road, London, EC1V 2RS. *Tel*: 020 7837 4483.

Fax: 020 7837 4815. *E-mail: info*@arbitrators.org
Website: www.arbitrators.org [5104 Jul 2000]

Norwich Union Healthcare

Address: Chilworth House, Hampshire Corporate Park, Templars Way, Eastleigh, Hampshire, SO53 3DG. *Tel*: 0800 142 142. *Website*: www.norwich.co.uk/healthcare [Jul 2000]

PPP Healthcare

Treatment of psychiatric illness
"Broadly, our medical insurance policies are designed to pay for treatment by specialists of medical conditions that respond quickly to treatment in the short-term. This includes treatment of psychiatric illness and our position on this is set out as follows:

We have an arrangement with psychiatric hospitals covering payment to them for treatment our members need. This arrangement covers members who require in-patient admission to a private psychiatric hospital in the United Kingdom.

It allows us to establish benefit entitlement and pre-authorise payment for psychiatric admissions. This ensures that members receive the treatment they need at a cost that represents value for money.

How does it work?

When a member is to be admitted, the hospital notifies us and provides basic membership information, treatment details and an estimated length of stay in hospital.

Once we have established that the hospital is included in the PPP healthcare directory of hospitals and that the admission is covered by the policy, payment for an initial period of hospitalisation is agreed with the hospital. If the member requires a longer stay in hospital than was originally agreed, the specialist gives us information explaining the need for an extension of the stay.

When payment for a stay in hospital has been agreed between us and the hospital, payment of benefit for that period is guaranteed. All you need to do is tell the hospital that you are a member of one of our plans and give them your membership details. Then once they have received confirmation from us, you need not worry about your benefit entitlement in respect of the agreed stay." [5174, 5175]

Address: PPP Healthcare, Phillips House, Crescent Road, Tunbridge Wells, Kent, TN1 2PL. *Tel*: 01892 512345. *Fax*: 01892 515143.
Website: www: ppphealthcare.co.uk [May 2000]

Standard Life Healthcare

Standard Life Healthcare is the UK's fourth larg-est private medical insurance provider and is part of the Standard Life Group, Europe's largest mutual life assurance company. The majority of their business is concentrated on providing quality private medical insurance to individuals and they pride themselves on giving an extremely high level of service. Their achievement of ISO 9002 and their membership of the Insurance Ombudsman are evidence of their dedication to the customer. They have pledged to simplify healthcare products for consumers and ensure that their product literature is written in plain English and made easy to understand - indeed they have won the Clear English Award for their policy documentation.

Standard Life Healthcare offers a range of private medical insurance plans designed to suit every budget. The following plans offer comprehensive cover for psychiatric and mental conditions: Prime-care, Primecare Plus, Primecare Gold, Choices, and Health Cash Plan.

What's included?

Cover includes in-patient treatment in respect of accommodation, nursing, drugs prescribed in a ward, diagnostic procedures including pathology and radiology, physicians' fees and specialist consultations. The policies provide up to 28 days' in-patient treatment per policy year in any hospital approved by their Claims department. In addition, Primecare, Primecare Plus, and Primecare Gold offer up to £1,200 per policy year towards out-patient treatment. This can include specialist consultations, ECT, and diagnostic procedures including pathology and radiology.

The recently launched Health Cash Plan pays out generous tax free cash sums to cover 24 health benefits. Starting from as little as £2.73 a week, this plan will pay a cash sum on admission to a psychiatric ward in a hospital or to a psychiatric hospital, up to a maximum of 21 nights.

Address: Standard Life Healthcare, Weyhouse, Farnham Road, Guildford, Surrey, GU1 4XS. *Tel:* 0800 77 99 55. *Fax:* 01483 553852. *Website:* standardlifehealthcare.co.uk 5829 Jun 2000

Residential, Nursing & Respite Care

Local Organisations

Care Homes Association

Contact: Mr Anthony Andrews. *Address:* Residential Care Homes Association, 74, London Road, St Leonards, Sussex, TN37 6AS. *Tel:* 01424 712982. *Fax:* 01424 443457. Jul 2000

ESCC Inspection Unit

The chief inspector is John Windebank. *Address:* ESCC Inspection Unit, 1, Grove Road, Eastbourne, Sussex, BN21 4TW. *Tel:* 01323 439994.

Crossroads

Short periods of respite care for carers who are looking after a physically and/or mentally disabled or elderly frail person at home. Referrals: Anyone can make a referral, and for all age groups. Primarily concerned with respite for the carer, through caring for the person with the disability.

For people with a mental health problem, and depending on the type of disability or illness, professional advice may be sought as to whether the scheme is appropriate before acceptance.

Address: Hastings & Rother Crossroads Care Attendant Scheme Limited, 135, Hughenden Road, Hastings, East Sussex, TN34 3TF. *Tel*: 01424 444964. *Fax*: 01424 435972. May 2000

Local Care Homes

The following list was based mainly on information kindly provided by East Sussex County Council's registered care homes' inspection unit. The list also includes some nursing homes. 5375

Acacia House

Owner: Welcare Ltd; manager: Mrs C Maitland; 23 places for older people with a dementia type illness. *Address:* Acacia House, Charles Road, St Leonards, Sussex, TN38 0JU. *Tel:* 01424 421081. Jul 2000

Alexandra House

Owners: Mr T & Mrs R Tagoe; manager: Mr T Tagoe; 8 places for people with learning disabilities; fees: £708.22. *Address:* Alexandra House, 43, Lower Park Road, Hastings, Sussex, TN34 2LA. *Tel:* 01424 426026. Jul 2000

Ashburnham Lodge

Owner and manager: Mr M Kay; 26 places for older people; fees: £213-300 per week. *Address:* Ashburnham Lodge, 62, London Road, St Leonards, Sussex, TN37 6AS. *Tel:* 01424 438575. Jul 2000

Bannow

Owners: Mr T and Mrs M Tracey; manager: Mrs K Tracey; 18 places for older people; fees: £260-£450 per week. *Address:* Bannow, Quarry Hill, St Leonards, Sussex, TN38 0HG. *Tel:* 01424 433021/433200. Jul 2000

Barchester Tower

Owners: Mr P and Mrs I Hughes; managers: Mrs V Frew and Mrs I Hughes; 21 places for older people with a dementia type illness; fees: £297-£320 per week. *Address:* Barchester Tower, 31, De Cham Road, St Leonards, Sussex, TN37 6JA. *Tel:* 01424 435398. Jul 2000

Barrington House

Owner/Manager: Mr I Pardii; manager: Mrs D Pardii; 26 places for adults with a learning disability; fees: £265 per week. *Address:* Barrington House, Rye Road, Hastings, Sussex, TN35 5DG. *Tel:* 01424 422228. Jul 2000

Bay View

Owner: Mr A Sehmi; manager: Mrs C Preston; 17 places for older people; fees: £209-375.75. *Address:* Bay View, 27,

Eversfield Place, St Leonards, Sussex, TN37 6BY. *Tel:* 01424 425565. Jul 20000

Bethune Court
Owner: Anchor Trust; manager: Mrs O Blything; 45 places for older people; fees: £209-£327 per week. *Address:* Bethune Court, 30, Boscobel Road, St Leonards, Sussex, TN38 0LX. *Tel:* 01424 719393. Jul 2000

Blackrock House
Owners: Mrs R and Mr T Thomas; manager: Mrs R Thomas; 14 places for people with a mental illness, past or present; fees: £297-£350 per week. *Address:* Blackrock House, 10, Stanley Road, Hastings, Sussex, TN34 1UE. *Tel:* 01424 421832. Jul 2000

Blair House
Owners and managers: Mr E and Mrs P Gibson; 29 places for people with a mental illness, past or present; fees: £296 per week. *Address:* Blair House, 24, Pevensey Road, St Leonards, Sussex, TN38 0LF. *Tel:* 01424 437608. Jul 2000

Blenheim House
Owners: Mr S King and Ms A Sawyers; manager: Ms A Sawyers; 6 places for older people.; fees £213 per week. *Address:* Blenheim House, 6, Brittany Road, St Leonards, Sussex, TN38 0RA. *Tel:* 01424 428247. Jul 20000

Braeburn House
Owner and manager: Miss E Murray; 11 places for people with a mental illness, past or present; fees £220 per week. *Address:* Braeburn House, 30, Laton Road, Hastings, Sussex, TN34 2ES. *Tel:* 01424 423226. May2000

Braeside Limited
Owner: Braeside Ltd.; manager: Miss E Murray; 17 places for older people with a dementia type illness; fees: £297-320 per week. *Address:* Braeside Ltd, 48, Pevensey Road, St Leonards, Sussex, TN38 0LS. *Tel:* 01424 422330. Jul 2000

Carman
Owners and managers: Mr M and Mrs C Pirouznia; 25 places for older people; fees: £215 per week. *Address:* Carman, 31-33, Sedlescombe Road South, St Leonards, Sussex, TN38 0TB. *Tel:* 01424 435500. Jul 2000

Castlemaine
Owner and manager: Mr H Garside; 43 places for older people with a mental health problem.; fees £300 per week (under review). *Address:* Castlemaine, 4, Avondale Road, St Leonards, Sussex, TN38 0SA. *Tel:* 01424 422226. Jul 2000

Chateau Fleur de Lys
Owner: Ferguson Care Ltd (Craegmoor Healthcare); regional manager: Mr Andrew Glee; manager: Mrs B Dendy. Chateau Fleur de Lys is committed to providing the highest quality of professional care within a homely, caring and stimulating environment. Up to 20 places for clients with learning disabilities. Fees: £400+ per week dependent on individual needs.
Address: Chateau Fleur De Lys, St Helen's Park Road, Hastings, Sussex, TN34 2JW. *Tel/Fax:* 01424 422030. May 2000

Clifton Court
Owner and manager: Mrs E Sullivan; 15 places for people with a mental illness, past or present; fees: £224-260 per week. *Address:* Clifton Court, 8-10, Clifton Road, Hastings, Sussex, TN35 5AP. *Tel:* 01424 428708. Jul 2000

Clinton House
Owner: Saxonthorpe Ltd; manager: Mrs J Knight; 48 places for older people with a mental health problem, past or present; fees: £225-285 per week. *Address:* Clinton House, 22-26, Clinton Crescent, St Leonards, TN38 0RN. *Tel:* 01424 434267. [*Note*: unable to confirm details, Aug 2000]

Crest House
Owner and manager: Mrs J Crawford; 25 places for older people; fees: from £260 per

week. *Address:* Crest House, 6-8, St Matthews Road, St Leonards, Sussex, TN38 0TN. *Tel:* 01424 436229. [Jul 2000]

Croft Unit, The

Owner: Parkcare Homes Ltd; manager: Mrs V Riedel; 12 places for people with a mental illness, past or present; fees: £350-£450 per week. *Address:* The Croft Unit, 25-29, Ashburnham Road, Hastings, Sussex, TN35 5JN. *Tel:* 01424 434921. [Jul 20000]

Cumberland Court

Owners: Mr R and Mrs S Caie; manager: Mrs S Caie; 20 places for older people. *Address:* Cumberland Court, 6, Cumberland Gardens, St Leonards, Sussex, TN38 0QL. *Tel:* 01424 432949. *E-mail:* office@cumberlandcourt.co.uk *Website:* www.cumber landcourt.co.uk [May 2000]

Cumberland House

Owners: Mrs D & Mr P Spencer, and Mrs L Gratton; 18 places for older people with a mental health problem; fees: £224-297 per week. *Address:* Cumberland House, 21, Laton Road, Hastings, Sussex, TN34 2ES. *Tel:* 01424 422458. [Jul 2000]

Derwent House

Owners: Mr R and Mrs E Cox; manager: Mrs E Cox; 24 places for older people; fees: £213-£250. *Address:* Derwent Hotel, 38, Sedlescombe Road South, St Leonards, Sussex, TN38 0TB. *Tel:* 01424 436044. [Jul 2000]

Draper House

Owners: Mr J and Mrs J Walton; manager: Mrs J Walton; 8 places for people with learning disabilities; fees: £256 per week. *Address:* Draper House, 7-8, Whitefriars Road, Hastings, Sussex, TN34 3LA. *Tel:* 01424 420083. [Jul 2000]

Edendale

Owners and managers: Mr G & Mrs A Fettiplace; 30 places for older people with a mental health problem; fees: £297. *Address:* Edendale, 5, The Green, St Leonards, TN38 0SY. *Tel:* 01424 429908. [Jul 2000]

Edmund House

Owner: The Penang Group; manager: Miss M Baughurst; 6 places for people with learning disabilities; fees: £703 per week. *Address:* Edmund House, 66, St Saviours Road, St Leonards, Sussex, TN38 0AR. *Tel:* 01424 432958. [Jul 2000]

Essenden Road

The home is run by Mencap; manager: Mrs K Hutchinson; 7 places for people with learning disabilities; fees: from £342.10 per week. *Address:* 4, Essenden Road, St Leonards, Sussex, TN38 0NW. *Tel:* 01424 432201. [Aug 2000]

Fairview

Owner: Mauhart Residential Homes Ltd; manager: Mrs S Kursey; 9 places for people with learning (but not physical) disabilities; fees: from £396. *Address:* Fairview, 2, Tilekiln Lane, Hastings, Sussex, TN35 5EN. *Tel:* 01424 420880. [Aug 2000]

Filsham House

Owner and manager: Mrs C Loureiro; 15 places for older people; fees: DSS rates. *Address:* Filsham House, 73, Filsham Road, St Leonards, Sussex, TN38 0PG. *Tel:* 01424 431123. [Jul 2000]

Firs, at Crowhurst

Specialist Residential Care Home. Specialist care for those with Alzheimers or dementia. Dedicated team, superb cooking, activities and outings. A client-centred approach, run to aim for the best possible quality of life. Contact: Jo Dethridge; fees: from £250 per week.

Address: The Firs, at Crowhurst, Old Forewood Lane, Crowhurst, Sussex TN33 9AE. *Tel*: 01424 830591. *Fax*: 01424 830130. [Aug 2000]

Forresters Respite Centre

Forresters Respite Centre is a country hotel which provides a holiday and respite for those who have experienced a mental illness and their carers from across the UK. *Tel*: 01703 843042. *Fax:* 023 8084 1250 [Jul 2000]

Gemini House
Owner: Saxonthorpe Ltd; managers: Mrs J, Mrs P and Mr S Knight; 35 places for people with a mental illness, past or present;. [Unconfirmed details]. *Address:* Gemini House, 8-10, White Rock, Hastings, Sussex, TN34 1JY. Tel: 01424 433613.

Gensing
Owners: Mr A Andrews and Mr W Smith; manager: Mr A Andrews; 19 places men with alcohol, mental health and physical disablement; fees: £225-315 per week. *Address:* Gensing, 76-78, London Road, St Leonards, Sussex, TN37 6AS. *Tel:* 01424 712982. Jul 2000

Glenmar
Owner: Grovestead Ltd; manager: Mrs J Couzens; 25 places for people with a mental illness, past or present; fees: DSS rates. *Address:* Glenmar, 2-3, Charles Road, St Leonards, Sussex, TN38 0QA. *Tel:* 01424 436864. Jul 2000

Glenmuir House
Owner/manager: Mr K Twist; 17 places for older people; fees: £220-£250. *Address:* Glenmuir House, 4, Branksome Road, St Leonards, Sussex, TN38 0UA. *Tel:* 01424 430203. Jul 2000

Grosvenor House
Owner: Greensleeves Homes Trust. Manager: Mrs J Fox; 28 places for older people; fees: £229 - £291 per week. *Address:* Grosvenor House, 11-14, Grosvenor Gardens, St Leonards, TN38 0AE. *Tel:* 01424 423831. *Fax:* 01424 443586. Jul 2000

Hazelbrae
Owners: Mr P & Mrs D E Fowler; manager: Mrs D Fowler; 15 places for older people with a dementia type illness; fees: £235-£288 per week. *Address:* Hazelbrae, 76, St Saviours Road, St Leonards, Sussex, TN38 0AR. *Tel:* 01424 425080. May 2000

Healey House
Owner: Hastings/Rother Voluntary Assoc. for the Blind; manager: Mrs B Quigley; 28 places for older people; fees: £246 per week. *Address:* Healey House, 3, Upper Maze Hill, St Leonards, Sussex, TN38 0LQ. *Tel:* 01424 436359. Jul 2000

Helenswood
Owners: Mr J Grey, Mr G Newton, Mrs Grey; manager: Mrs S Grey; 15 places for older people; fees: £213-£250 per week. *Address:* Helenswood, 195, The Ridge, Hastings, Sussex, TN34 2AE. *Tel:* 01424 445127. Jul 2000

Hurst, The
The owners are Mr A and Mrs Z Buckhoree; manager: Mr D Wells; 29 places for people with a mental illness, past or present; fees: £234-250. *Address:* The Hurst, 124, Hoadswood Road, Sussex, TN34 2BA. *Tel:* 01424 425693. Jul 2000

Invicta Community Care NHS Trust
Contact: Ms Sue Walter, service manager. 11 residential houses for adults with learning disabilities. *Address:* Invicta Community Care NHS Trust, High Glades, 9a, Upper Church Road, St Leonards, Sussex. *Tel:* 01424 753696. Jul 2000

Kenilworth
Owners: Dr P and Mrs E Das; manager: Mrs E Das; 24 places for older people; fees: £213-£270 per week. *Address:* Kenilworth, 13-14, Linton Road, Hastings, Sussex, TN34 1TW. *Tel:* 01424 420205. May 2000

Kingswood Nursing Home
Nursing care provided, with drugs trolley, etc. Matron: Mrs D Hogan. *Address:* Kingswood Nursing Home, 21-23, Chapel Park Road, St Leonards-on-Sea, East Sussex. *Tel:* 01424 716303. *Fax:* 01424 423737. Jul 2000

Kilncroft
Owner: Parkcare Homes, Ltd; manager: Mrs V Riedel; senior carer: Hilary Mathis. 15 places for older people with a dementia type illness. Kilncroft's aim is to provide quality care which constantly meets the expectations of its clients. It is the home's

intention to review and improve performance continuously in order to promote a high standard of care within a safe environment. Kilncroft aims to remain a specific residential home with discrete units catering for the elderly infirm. *Address:* Kilncroft, 25-29, Ashburnham Road, Hastings, TN35 5JN. *Tel:* 01424 434921. May 2000

La Chenerie
Owner: Ferguson Care Ltd (Craegmoor Healthcare); manager: Mrs C Pike; 26 places for people with learning disabilities. *Address:* La Chenerie, 57, Church Road, St Leonards, Sussex, TN37 6HJ. *Tel:* 01424 721548. May 2000

London Road
Owners: Mr J and Mrs J Walton; manager: Mrs J Walton; 8 places for people with learning disabilities. *Address:* 355, London Road, St Leonards, Sussex, TN37 6PA. *Tel:* 01424 422221. May 2000

Lower Park Road
Owner: Mencap; manager: Miss J Smith; 7 places for people with learning disabilities; fees: DSS rates. *Address:* 49, Lower Park Road, Hastings, Sussex, TN34 2LA. *Tel:* 01424 429101. Jul 2000

Merleon
Owners: Mr C and Mrs J Gower; manager: Mrs J Gower; 20 places for older people; fees: DSS rates. *Address:* Merleon, 5, Dane Road, St Leonards, Sussex, TN38 0QU. *Tel:* 01424 429287. Jul 2000

Milward Road
Owner: Mencap; manager: Mr A Heffernan; 7 places for people with learning disabilities; fees: £325.27 per week. *Address:* 19, Milward Road, Hastings, Sussex, TN34 3RP. *Tel:* 01424 429941. Jul 2000

Monks Orchard
Owner and manager: Mrs B Kilsby; 10 places for older people; fees: £213-£221 per week. *Address:* Monks Orchard, 9, St Matthews Gardens, St Leonards, Sussex, TN38 0TS. *Tel:* 01424 427755. Jul 2000

Moreton Centre
Owner: East Sussex County Council; manager: Mrs T Gallop; 18 places for older people; fees: £52-410. *Address:* The Moreton Centre, Boscobel Road, St Leonards, Sussex, TN38 0LX. *Tel:* 01424 427467. Jul 2000

Mount Denys
Owner: East Sussex County Council; manager: Mrs Maureen McAdam; 31 places for older people with a dementia type illness; fees: £52.05-£410.90. *Address:* Mount Denys, 187, The Ridge, Hastings, Sussex, TN34 2AE. *Tel:* 01424 421353. Jul 2000

Mount Hermon
Owner: Saxonthorpe Ltd; manager: Mrs J Knight; 28 places for people with a mental illness, past or present. [Unconfirmed details] *Address:* Mount Hermon, 34, Ashburnham Road, Hastings, Sussex, TN35 5JL. *Tel:* 01424 428840.

Mount Pleasant
Owner: Phoenix House Housing Assoc.; manager: Ms C Reddington; half-way house with 5 places for people with a drug dependence; fees: £289.78. *Address:* 85, Mount Pleasant Road, Hastings, Sussex, TN34 3SL. *Tel:* 01424 460469. Jul 2000

Mountside Residential Home
Owner: Mr & Mrs J R Morton; manager: Mrs F I Steuart-Pownall; 36 places for older people; fees: £213-£300 per week: *Address:* Mountside Residential Home, 9-11, Laton Road, Hastings, East Sussex, TN34 2ES. *Tel:* 01424 424144. Fax: 01424 434906. May 2000

Norton Lodge
Owners: Mr T and Mrs V Wells; manager: Mrs R Dumbrell; 9 places for older people with a mental health problem. *Address:* Norton Lodge, 20, West Hill Road, St Leonards, TN38 0NB. *Tel:* 01424 423531. May 2000

Oaklands
Owner: Ferguson Care Ltd (Craegmoor

Healthcare); Manager: Mr D Rickaby; Regional manager: Mr Andrew Gee; Clinical services director: Mr Alan Whittle.

Oaklands provides care for adults with learning disabilities and challenging behaviour. The age range is 18 to 65, with care offered to clientele suffering from autism, epilepsy and some challenging behaviour. The aim is to provide quality care and a safe, homely environment for residents. Oaklands is registered as a 27-bedded care home. *Address:* Oaklands, Old Roar Road, St Leonards, Sussex, TN39 7HA. *TelFax:* 01424 751161. May 2000

Old Hastings House
Owner: Magdalen & Lasher Charity; manager: Mrs P Davies; 44 places for older people; fees: £275 per week. *Address:* Old Hastings House, High Street, Hastings, Sussex, TN34 3ET. *Tel:* 01424 442836. Jul 2000

Park Beck Hotel
Owners/managers: Mr E and Mrs P Gibson; 37 places for older people; fees: £213-256 per week. *Address:* Park Beck Hotel, 21, Upper Maze Hill, St Leonards, Sussex, TN38 0LG. *Tel:* 01424 445855. Aug 2000

Penang
Owner: The Penang Group; manager: Mr T Tagoe; 8 places for people with learning disabilities; fees: £721 per week. *Address:* Penang, 35, Charles Road, St Leonards, Sussex, TN38 0QX. *Tel:* 01424 420484. Jul 2000

Phoenix House
Owners: Phoenix House Housing Association; manager: Ms C Reddington; 30 places for people with a history of substance misuse problems; fees: £289.78. *Address:* Phoenix House, Colwall Court, 1, Pages Avenue, Bexhill, Sussex, TN39 3AP. *Tel:* 01424 732171. Jul 2000

Priory Residential Home
Owners: Mr B and Mrs D Saumtally; manager: Mr B Saumtally; 17 places for people with a mental illness, past or present; fees: £230-£380 per week. *Address:* The Priory Residential Home, 26-28, Priory Avenue, Hastings, Sussex, TN34 1UG. *Tel:* 01424 436792. Jul 2000

Redmere Lodge
Owners/managers: Mr S MacKenzie; 15 places for older people with a mental health problem; fees: £213-296 per week. *Address:* Redmere Lodge, 67, Pevensey Road, St Leonards, Sussex, TN38 0LE. *Tel:* 01424 426676. Jul 2000

Salt Lea
Owners: Mr S and Mrs U Rekhaye; manager: Mrs M Stretton; 15 places for older people.; fees: £213-250 per week. *Address:* Salt Lea, 10, St Matthews Gardens, St Leonards, Sussex, TN38 0TS. *Tel:* 01424 428353. Jul 2000

St Dominics Nursing & Residential Home
Owner: St Dominics Nursing Home Ltd; manager: Miss M Dempsey; 15 places for older people; fees: £213-313 per week. *Address:* St Dominics, 71, Filsham Road, St Leonards, Sussex, TN38 0PG. *Tel:* 01424 436140. Jul 2000

St Helen's House
Owners: Mr G and Mrs G Williams; manager: Mrs G Williams; 31 places for older people; fees: DSS rates. *Address:* St Helen's House, 3, The Ridge, Hastings, Sussex, TN34 2AA. *Tel:* 01424 439239. Jul 2000

St James
Owner: Mr T Koonjul; managers: Mr T and Mrs T Koonjul; 15 places for people with a mental illness, past or present; fees: DSS rates. *Address:* St James, 26, Magdalen Road, St Leonards, Sussex, TN37 6EP. *Tel:* 01424 425141. Jul 2000

St Josephs
Owner: The Penang Group; manager: Miss M Baughurst; 6 places for people with learning disabilities; fees: £708. *Address:* St Josephs, 1, Edmund Road, Hastings,

Sussex, TN35 5JY. *Tel:* 01424 423094. Jul 2000

St Laurence
Owners: Mr T and Mrs R Tagoe; manager: Mr T Tagoe; 8 places for people with learning disabilities; fees: £750-£950. *Address:* St Laurence, 33, Tower Road West, St Leonards, Sussex, TN38 0RJ. *Tel:* 01424 438262. Jul 2000

St Leonards Mansions
Owners: Mrs T Hannaford and Mrs S Bazalgette; manager: Mrs Michaela Lanarth; 20 places for older people; fees: £210-£270 per week. *Address:* St Leonards Mansions, 19, West Hill Road, St Leonards, Sussex, TN38 0NA. *Tel:* 01424 441774. Jul 2000

St Marks
Owners: Mr D and Mrs F Kennard; manager: Mr P Hussey; 6 places for people with autism; fees: £850-£950 per week. *Address:* St Marks, 23, Collier Road, Hastings, Sussex, TN34 3JR. *Tel:* 01424 200854. Jul 2000

St Peter's Grange
Owners: Mr R and Mrs M Elam; manager: Mr R Elam; 44 places for older people; fees: £213-303 per week. *Address:* St Peter's Grange, 24, Upper Maze Hill, St Leonards, Sussex, TN38 0LA. *Tel:* 01424 423427. Jul 2000

Streatfield House
Owners: Mr T and Mrs Mahoney; manager: Mrs G Clusker; 16 places for people with learning and physical disabilities; also adjacent to the Home is the Evelyn Juden Day Care Centre; fees: £450-£550, including day care; fees for day care only: £20 per day. *Address:* Streatfield House, Cornfield Terrace, St Leonards, Sussex, TN37 6JD. *Tel:* 01424 439103. May 2000

Sydney Lodge
Owners: Mrs C Smith and Mr K Gilhespy; manager: Mrs C Smith; 14 places for older people; fees: £213-268. *Address:* Sydney Lodge, 48, Sedlescombe Road South, St Leonards, Sussex, TN38 0TJ. *Tel:* 01424 437653. Jul 2000

Tamarisk
Tamarisk is a private Residential Care Home for the mentally handicapped and people with learning disabilities, which opened its doors in 1988. Registered with East Sussex County Council, Tamarisk provides an environment of stimulation and motivation to encourage self-awareness and personal development.

Part of the home is a self-contained flat, a feature designed to encourage even greater independence. Long term residents are welcome, as are those of challenging behaviour or having special needs. Qualified staff are in attendance 24 hours a day and all the rooms have an emergency call system installed. *Contact:* Mrs P.Hughes, owner and manager.

Address: Tamarisk, 25, Priory Avenue, Hastings, Sussex, TN34 1UH. *Tel:* 01424 430917. *Fax:* 01424 200895. May 2000

Tenby House
Owner: Kelsey Housing Assn; Project manager: Judith Hobbs; 12 places for people with a mental illness, past or present. Referrals accepted from Community Care Act Assessors for in-patients of Hastings hospitals, and for anyone with a mental health difficulty in the Hastings and Rother area, with an identified need for a residential rehabilitation service. Providing active rehabilitation/supportive environment; encouraging individual choice in communal setting; encouraging development of social/domestic skills; educational/vocational/recreational interests in preparation for independent living. Tenby House is a joint project between MACA, ESHA and Kelsey Housing Association. Fees: £224 per week.

Address: Tenby House, 34, Boscobel Road, St Leonards, Sussex, TN38 0LX. *Tel:* 01424 440448. *E-mail:* th42@dial.pipex.com 5867, 6011 Jul 2000

Tusker House

Owners: Mr M Goonane, Miss D Kingsley and Mrs P Woolgar; manager: Miss D Kinsley; 76 places for older people with a mental health problem. *Address:* Tusker House, 57, Pine Avenue, Hastings, Sussex, TN34 3PP. *Tel:* 01424 421573 / 01424 715706. *Fax:* 01424 427578. May 2000

Victoria Road

The home is run by Mencap; manager: Mrs J Armour; 7 places for people with learning disabilities. Address: 4, Victoria Road, St Leonards, Sussex, TN37 6ER. Tel: 01424 444095. Jul 2000

Westwood

The home is run by Mencap (Hastings & Bexhill Society); manager: Mrs J Bourne; 9 places for people with learning disabilities. Address: Westwood, 55, St Helen's Park Road, Hastings, Sussex, TN34 2JJ. Tel: 01424 428805. Jul 2000

White Lights

Proprietors: Mr D Robinson & Mrs L Robinson; managers: Mrs L Robinson & Miss Kerry Clifton; 20 places for people with a mental illness, past or present; fees: DSS rates. Address: White Lights, 20, Chapel Park Road, St Leonards, Sussex, TN37 6HU. Tel: 01424 437995. Jul 2000

White Lodge

Owners: Mrs A McAuliffe and Miss J Baker; manager: Mrs A McAuliffe; 8 places for people with physical disabilities; fees: from £303 per week. Address: White Lodge, 30, Charles Road, St Leonards, Sussex, TN38 0QH. Tel: 01424 420776. Jul 2000

National Organisations

Holiday Care

Holiday Care provides holiday ideas for people with mental health needs. *Address:* Holiday Care, 2nd Floor, Imperial Buildings, Victoria Road, Horley, Surrey, RH6 7PZ. Tel: 01293 774535. May 2000

Further Information

Health Information Service

The HIS is a free and confidential 24-hour service. You can speak to staff during office hours, and you can listen to any of hundreds of tapes at any time, e.g: *Residential & nursing homes* (Tape 057).

Address: The College of Health, St Margaret's House, 21, Old Ford Road, London, E2 9PL. *Freephone*: 0800 66 55 44. 5367

Self-management

Advance directives

An 'advance directive' is a document - i.e. a piece of paper - with your instructions about what you would like other people to do for you should you become too 'high' or 'low' to do those things for yourself.

It has become apparent that it is probably far more valuable to look upon advance directives as one of the tools that can be used to try to help you get treated in the way you want, rather than to consider it as some sort of 'legal document'.

Treatment preferences

The directives can include: your own treatment preferences (with explanations why); your own personal signs and symptoms in case you are seen by a doctor who does not know you; other preferences you may have, e.g. how you want money matters handled.

We have heard of people who say they have felt really empowered by having an advance directive. They tell us that this comes from the knowledge that in the event of another high or low, several people will be aware of how they want to be helped.

And because they have written it themselves it is what they want - not what a well-meaning professional thinks they want. David Woods-Taylor, Southend MDF Self-help Group. [5069]

Self-management

The Manic Depression Fellowship has been running self-management programmes. By the end of 1999, seven London and five National programmes, as well as three training courses for facilitators had been run. More are scheduled for 2000. [5069]

Training Programme

If you are unsure what the programme is about or would like further information please write to Andy Pattison at the MDF. The Programme Manager is Amanda Harris, the Greater London Project Worker is Miles Rinald and the Training Programme Administrator is Andy Pattison.

Address: Manic Depression Fellowship, Castle Works, 21, St George's Road, London, SE1 6ES. *Tel:* 020 8546 9763. [5069]

Mood Diaries

'Mood diaries' enable people who are self-managing to keep a daily mood record which can assist in the recognition of triggers and warning signs. They also contain important reminders of the key principles of self-management.

The Manic Depression Fellowship plans to produce and distribute a version of a mood diary used as part of its self-management programme. They will be available for sale to all members of the MDF in early 2000. Please see the chapter 'Manic Depression' for more information on this topic, page 83. [5069]

Further Information

Advance Directives

By Jackie Golding. Price 40p + stamped, addressed envelope. Available from Mind. Tel: 020 8552 1725.

Inside Out

'A Guide to Self-Management of Manic Depression'. Published by the Manic Depression Fellowship, Castle Works, 21, St George's Road, London, SE1 6ES. *Tel:* 020 8974 6600.

User groups

We want to ensure that the services meet our needs. We are involved in the planning of future services and monitoring the quality of the present services. We have good relations with health care managers and planners. *Focus on Mental Health* [5048]

Quality Monitoring
The 'User Q' Project (see below), is developing a set of Quality Monitoring Standards which can be used as bencmarks. It is intended that if mental health service providers meet the standards set by the benchmarks, they will receive a 'stamp of quality approval' from the User Q group.

It is planned that all monitoring will be carried out by trained monitoring teams, made up of individuals who have had experience of using mental health services. The information gathered will be analysed and fed back to the health service providers together with indications of ways in which the service can be improved.

User Q hopes that with time it will work closely with the mental health services so that users, visitors and staff feel happy and safe in using it. [5218]

Local Organisations

Focus on Mental Health

Focus on Mental Health is a group of people from Hastings & Rother who meet each month to talk about a range of local mental health issues. Many of us have used the services in the past and some still do. We want to ensure that the services meet our needs. We are involved in the planning of future services and monitoring the quality of the present services. We have good relations with health care managers and planners who often join us to hear our opinions and respond to our concerns.

The group started about 1995, to give an organised response from the point of view of service users to the plans to close Queen Charlotte's Hospital.

Meetings - Meetings are held on the first Friday of the month at the Advocacy Centre, 42, Robertson Street, Hastings.

Group logo - This was designed by a member of the group and represents the chemical structure of the lithium atom.

Patients' satisfaction - A questionnaire to measure patients' satisfaction is being created, which will be given to all patients as they leave Woodlands Adult Mental Health Unit. [5402]

Staff - The administrator is Su Barnicoat.

Address: Focus on Mental Health, 42, Robertson Street, Hastings, Sussex, TN34 1HL. *Tel:* 01424 442435. [5048, 5215, 5867]

Mental Health Action Group

This group, chaired by Toni Wilkinson (chief executive of the Hastings & St Leonards Primary Care Group), meets monthly and is accountable to Focus. [5913 Jun 2000]

Eastbourne Patients' Council

Eastbourne Patients' Council meets every fortnight to discuss ways of improving the service. The Council has conducted in-patient surveys. Anyone interested in contacting them are requested to write to the following address.

Address: Eastbourne Patients' Council, c/o Reception, Department of Psychiatry, Eastbourne District General Hospital, Kings Drive, Eastbourne, East Sussex. [6039 Aug 2000]

Hastings Patients' Council

At the time of writing, there is no Patients' Council for Hastings & Rother.[5256] However, Focus on Mental Health is actively promoting the formation of one.

The aims would be to improve the quality of in-patient care. It would be open to anyone with a mental health problem who has or hasn't used the acute unit at Woodlands. Anyone interested in the progress of this scheme should contact Su Barnicoat at Focus on Mental Health, see above.[6092, Aug 2000]

User Q Project

An innovative project managed by the East Sussex Alliance of local Mind associations.The User Q project aims to increase user involvement in all aspects of monitoring and evaluating the quality of mental health services. The project is also involved in a range of other initiatives, including developing the county's mental health training strategy. *Contact:* Paddi Mobbs.

Address: User Q Project, Lewes District and Wealden Mind, c/o Eastgate House, 6, Eastgate Street, Lewes, East Sussex, BN7 2LP. *Tel:* 01273 488660. *Fax*: 01273 476934. *E-mail:* userq@mind1.freeserve.co.uk [5218 Jun 2000]

User Involvement Fund

The User Involvement Fund provides funding for users wishing to attend courses, conferences, workshops and meetings. It can help with the fees, travelling, telephone and postage expenses, incurred in joining and attending the above. Anyone who has received, or is receiving, psychiatric services may apply in writing for an application form. The User Involvement Fund Committee are all volunteers. *Contacts:* Helen Pain, secretary; Heather Virgo, chair; Greg Virgo, advisor. [Aug 2000]

Address: User Involvement Fund, 73a Resource Centre, 73a London Road, Bexhill-on-Sea, East Sussex TN39 3LB. *Tel*: 01424 213099. *Fax:* 01424 731867. [Jul]

Further Information

Changing Practice

'Changing Practice - Mental health nursing and user empowerment' by Peter Campbell and Vivien Lindow. 'Useful to all nurses who work with people who use mental health services, this book is written by leading trainers from the mental health service user movement. Service users and survivors who train nurses will also find it helpful in their work'. Published by Mind/RCN, 1997, 30 pages, £4.50, ISBN 1-874690-62-6.

Self-help Groups

'Self-help groups: getting started, keeping going'. Written by Judy Wilson and Jan Myers. *'... an excellent source for anyone thinking of setting up a group'* - National Association of Citizens' Advice Bureau. Based on the authors' 20 years of experience, and written for groups at all stages of their lives this book covers everything you will need to know about self-help groups, from structuring meetings to publicity, to joint meetings and fund raising. Published by R A Wilson, ISBN: 1-874259-00-3, 164 pages, price £7.99. Available from Mind Mail Order Service. *Tel*: 020 8221 9666. [5251]

Unequal Partners

'Unequal partners: user groups and community care'. Written by Marian Barnes, Stephen Harrison, Maggie Mort and Polly Shardlow. Based on detailed empirical work this report includes details of user groups and officials in mental health and disability. The authors examine both the strategies user groups adopt to seek their objectives, and explore conceptual issues relating to notions of consumerism and citizenship. Essential reading for all those concerned with the user movement.

Published by Policy Press, 1999, ISBN: 1-86134-056-7, 116 pages, price £13.99. Available from Mind Mail Order Service. *Tel*: 020 8221 9666.

User Involvement

'User Involvement and User Empowerment Information Pack'. By Jan Wallcraft. Published by MindLink, March 1993, updated December 1998. £1.36. Available from Mind Mail Order Service. *Tel*: 020 8221 9666.

Health Information Service

The HIS is a free and confidential 24-hour service. You can speak to staff during office hours, and you can listen to any of hundreds of tapes at any time, e.g: *Patient support groups* (Tape 328). *Address*: The College of Health, St Margaret's House, 21, Old Ford Road, London, E2 9PL. *Freephone*: 0800 66 55 44. [5367]

Acknowledgements
Our grateful thanks to Margaret Moss, Su Barnicoat and the members of Focus on Mental Health, Hastings & Rother, for their editorial assistance with this chapter.

Voluntary work

Volunteers are ordinary people who become very special ... If you *are* thinking of voluntary work, Hastings Voluntary Action and Hastings Volunteer Bureau could be good places to start ...

Local Organisations

Hastings Voluntary Action

Hastings Voluntary Action is a council for voluntary service in Hastings, which assists both individuals and organisations to find and allocate voluntary work. It also publishes the *Hastings Community News* (see 'Information' chapter) and helps people and organisations involved with voluntary work in a variety of ways.

To enquire about the services they offer, please telephone initially to make an appointment. HVA is located in the town centre very close to bus services, railway station and taxi rank. It has ground floor access to the meeting rooms and disabled toilet facilities. *Hours*: Mondays to Fridays 9.00am to 5.00pm. *Contact*: Katy Burbridge.

Address: Hastings Voluntary Action, 31a, Priory Street, Hastings, East Sussex, TN34 1EA.

Tel: 01424 444010. *Fax:* 01424 432877. *E-mail:* infoworker@hva.k-web.co.uk

Website: www.hastingsvoluntaryaction.bizland.com/ 5867

Volunteer Bureau

The Volunteer Bureau offers a friendly informal service to all sections of the community who wish to volunteer and provides ongoing support, advice and information to all volunteers. Enquiries for voluntary work are made to charitable or non-profit making organisations.

The Bureau will make the initial contact and set up interviews. Voluntary work means making a commitment to help and support people or projects in your community. Please phone for an appointment. *Hours*: Monday, Tuesday, Wednesday & Friday 9.30am to 2.00pm. *Contact*: Rose Austen.

Hastings Ad-News

Current volunteering opportunities are advertised by Hastings Volunteer Bureau in the local AdNews once a month.

Arrow FM

Current volunteering opportunities are advertised by Hastings Volunteer Bureau on Arrow FM (107.8 FM) on alternate Mondays at about 10.15 am.

Address: Volunteer Bureau, HVA, 31a, Priory Street, Hastings, East Sussex, TN34 1EA. *Tel:* 01424 444010. *Fax:* 01424 432877. *Website:* www.hastingsvoluntary-action.biz land.com May 2000

Voluntary Help Office

The Voluntary Help Office is based at the Conquest Hospital, but the department is responsible for all voluntary services provided by the Hastings & Rother NHS Trust within the hospitals, community clinics and with the community itself. The department was founded in 1974 with just 6 volunteers; today it has over 350. The services offered are extremely varied and include welcoming and escort service, ward helpers, the League of Friends cornershop at Conquest Hospital, bereavement service, flower arrangers, work in community clinics, drivers, work with children's outpatient departments, complementary therapy, and support for blind people. *Contact:* Helen Mitchell.

Address: Voluntary Help Office, Conquest Hospital, The Ridge, St Leonards, Sussex, TN37 7RD. *Tel:* 01424 755255, ext. 8496.

6035

National Organisations

Community Service Volunteers

A service offered to 16-35 year olds providing the opportunity to gain experience in the health/social care field for free, and the chance to live in another part of the country. Food, accommodation, travel and pocket money is provided.

Skills and interests are matched to one of 800 projects around the UK. All that is asked is that participants give a minimum of 4 months (3 months in the summer).

Questions and answers

What do volunteers do?

Volunteers are people who, unpaid and of their own free will, contribute their time, energies and skills to benefit other people in the community.

Who can volunteer?

Volunteering should be open to all sections of the community and Hastings Volunteer Bureau works to ensure that anyone wanting to volunteer is able to do so.

What commitment is needed?

Volunteering does not necessarily demand a large time commitment. Around 3 hours a week is the average. In fact it's a good idea not to over-commit yourself initially. However, it is very important to be reliable - people may be depending on you.

What can the work offer?

There are many benefits to be gained by volunteering. It can provide a new challenge to build confidence and a sense of achievement; a platform for developing a new career; work experience and a chance to gain references; social contact and the opportunity to make new friends; a chance for personal growth and development.

How does the Bureau work?

The Hastings Volunteer Bureau is based within Hastings Voluntary Action and has been set up to assist people who want to volunteer by putting them into contact with appropriate voluntary or charitable organisations and groups who need the services of volunteers.

What are the opportunities?

Voluntary work is available in a wide range of areas: Advice and advocacy; Caring and befriending; Committe work; Computing, office and admistration; Conservation; Driving and transport; Education and training; Fund-raising and collecting; Gardening; Health Service; Shop work.

How do I start?

If you have time to spare and you think people could rely on you for help, please telephone the Volunteer Bureau (see above). 5055

Contacts: Ms Jules Payne, External Relations officer; Mr Billy Dann, Regional Director, Hastings; Kerry McClellend, Assistant Regional Director; James Simister, Volunteer Director; Manju Kaushdel, Volunteer Director; Vicky Hill, Administrator.

Address: Community Service Volunteers, Wenlock House, 41-43, North Street, Brighton, East Sussex, BN1 1RH. *Tel:* 01273 748811. *Fax:* 01273 748855. *E-mail:* csv.brighton@ukonline.co.uk

Website: www.csv.org.uk [5867, 6015 Aug 2000]

National Centre

The National Centre for Volunteering is based in London.

Address: The National Centre for Volunteering, Regent's Wharf, 8, All Saints Street, London, N1 9RL. *Tel*: 020 7520 8900. *Fax:* 020 7520 8910.

E-mail: volunteering@thecentre.org.uk

Website: www.volunteering.org.uk [Jul 2000]

Further Information

Directory of Local Resources

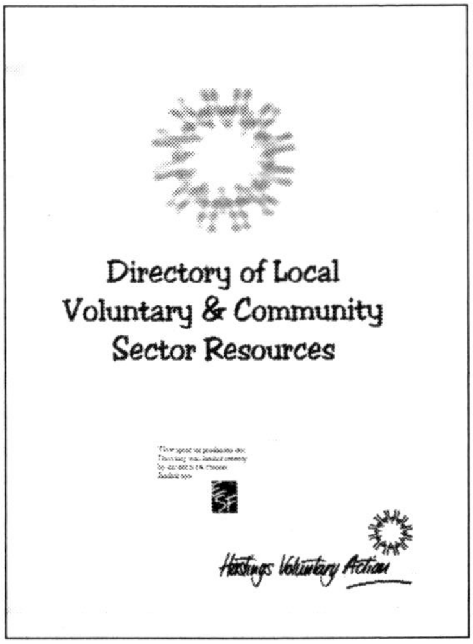

HVA publishes a 40 page, A4 sized *Directory of Local Voluntary & Community Sector Resources*, available from HVA.

Address: Hastings Voluntary Action, 31a, Priory Street, Hastings, East Sussex, TN34 1EA. *Tel:* 01424 444010. *Fax:* 01424 432877. *E-mail:* infoworker@hva.k-web.co.uk *Website:* www.hastingsvoluntary-action.bizland.com/ [5867]

See also these chapters...

Employment & training

Acknowledgements

Our grateful thanks to Rose Austen of Hastings Voluntary Action for editorial assistance with this chapter.

Your rights

Carers' rights

The Mental Health Act states that carers' views must be considered when making a mental health assessment. If you are designated the 'nearest relative' under the Mental Health Act, you will have additional rights.

Under the NHS and Community Care Act, carers have the right to have their own needs assessed at the same time as the person they are caring for is assessed.

Carers making a significant contribution to the support of a person with mental health problems have the right to expect mental health professionals to listen to them, to consider their views, and to involve them in planning services.

Initial contact with mental health professionals and the mental health system can be a frightening and demoralising experience, especially if you feel you have no control over what happens to you. It can be easy to forget that you have rights and to just accept what the professionals say, even when you feel unhappy about it.

It can be very difficult to question diagnosis, treatment or other professional advice or decisions. Knowing your rights and being able to say what you want and need will boost your confidence and help you get more out of your contact with doctors and other professionals.

Mental health professionals have a duty to listen to your views about your needs, and they should be met. If there is disagreement, you have a right to complain and ask for decisions to be reviewed (see below). [0534]

Advocacy service

Hastings & Rother has an advocacy service which can help when you do not have the confidence to speak up for yourself - please see the 'Advocacy' chapter, page 154 for more information.

Needs Assessments

You have the right to expect the health service and social services to provide care and treatment that meets your needs. The NHS and Community Care Act 1990 sets out how community care should be provided.

Under the Community Care Act 1990 your right to services depends on your needs as assessed by a professional. Social services departments have a legal duty to assess the community care needs of people with mental health problems.

They must also make sure that other services are available for people in need, including day care, supported housing, travel permits, meals on wheels and help at home. Whether or not you get a particular service usually depends on a doctor, social worker or other professional agreeing that it is necessary. [0534]

Confidentiality issues

Both the health service and social services are involved in planning your care, so information about you may need to pass between them. If you are being treated under the Care Programme Approach, your GP should be told about your treatment progress and your care plan.

Information about you will only be given to other agencies such as housing or voluntary agencies if they have a direct need to know in order to help with your care plan. In exceptional circumstances disclosure of information may be required by law, or justified in the public interest.

Patients' Charter

For details of your rights contained in this important document please see chapter 'Patients' Charter', page 338.

Your records and files

You have the legal right to see any written health records produced after November 1991 and any Social Services' files that exist about you. But you can be denied access to your records or some of them may be withheld if a senior professional thinks the content may be damaging to your physical or mental health, or if it identifies a third party.

You can ask for an explanation if you are denied access, but you may not know if information has been withheld.

You need to apply to the record holder - usually a hospital or GP - and ask for an appointment to look at your records. In-patients may be able to see their records informally and free of charge.

If you are an outpatient you may be charged a £10 fee, and, if you want copies, photocopying charges may be added on. If you disagree with anything, you can ask for the record to be corrected or to have your disagreement recorded.

You can also ask to see any medical reports prepared by your doctor for employment or insurance purposes. If there are factual inaccuracies you can ask your doctor to correct them. The doctor does not have to do this but must record your disagreement and attach it to the report.

The Advocacy Service or Mind can help if you have problems seeing your records. [0534]

Further Information

Access to Health Records

Published by the Legal Department, May 1997. Price £0.20. Available from Mind Mail Order Service. *Tel:* 020 8221 9666.

Care in the Community

Useful factsheet about your rights if you are receiving care in the community. Published August 1998 by ACHCEW. *Address:* 30, Drayton Park, London, N5 1PB. Free. [6026]

Family Doctors

'Everyone in the UK has the right to be registered with a General Practitioner'. Useful factsheet about your rights regarding treatment, access and complaints. Published April 1998 by ACHCEW. *Address:* 30, Drayton Park, London, N5 1PB. Free. [6027]

Going into Hospital

Useful leaflet about your rights on going into hospital. Available free from ACHCEW. *Address:* 30, Drayton Park, London, N5 1PB. [6025]

Health Information Service

The HIS is a free and confidential 24-hour service. You can speak to staff during office hours, and you can listen to any of hundreds of tapes at any time, e.g: *Access to GP medical records* (Tape 330); *Patient's Charter* (Tape 376).

Address: The College of Health, St Margaret's House, 21, Old Ford Road, London, E2 9PL. *Freephone:* 0800 66 55 44. [5367]

Making Choices

Finding out about your illness and consenting to treatment. Useful leaflet published by Association of Community Health Councils for England & Wales. *Address:* ACHCEW, 30, Drayton Park, London, N5 1PB. Free. [6023]

On The Record

Confidentiality and health records. Useful leaflet on confidentiality of your health records. Available free from ACHCEW. *Address:* 30, Drayton Park, London, N5 1PB. [6024]

Patients' Rights

Useful booklet published April 1999 by the Association of Community Health Councils for England & Wales. *Address:* ACHCEW, 30, Drayton Park, London, N5 1PB. Free. [6021]

See also these chapters ...

Advocacy, page 154.
Care Programme Approach, page 300.
Carers, page 159.
Community Health Councils, page 303.
Complainting, page 170.
Legal Matters, page 223.
Mental Health Act, page 330.
Patients' Charter, page 338.

alternative help

This third part of the *Guide* provides descriptions of different alternative therapies and information about local and national organisations which can provide this kind of help. For a quick overview of this section, please see the Contents on page 6.

Alternative therapies

Complementary or alternative therapies include acupuncture (see separate section), aromatherapy, herbalism, and homoeopathy. Practitioners describe their approach as 'holistic'. They see the mind and body as interlinked and pay attention to you as an individual.

Alternative therapists will spend time with you, talking and listening, which can be therapeutic in itself. Some of the relaxing therapies can be especially beneficial if you are anxious or tense.

Complementary therapies are becoming more widely available on the NHS, but normally you have to pay and it can become very expensive. Find out what is on offer by talking to your GP or the practice manager. [5224]

Alternative practitioners

Alternative practitioners will usually spend at least 45 minutes per session with you, to build up a complete picture of your symptoms in the context of your life. This time and attention can be therapeutic in itself and feels very different to a short appointment with a busy GP.

Fees can range from £10 to £35 per session and, although some practitioners will negotiate according to your income, the cost means these therapies are outside the reach of many people with mental health problems. [5224]

Alternative v. conventional

There is some disagreement within the medical profession about the value of complementary therapies, but more and more people are choosing to visit these practitioners every year.

Most people use them not as an 'alternative' but alongside, or 'complementary' to, conventional medicine, continuing to visit their doctor as well. It is important to tell your doctor about your alternative treatment in case of any drug interactions or unexplained symptoms. [5224]

Acupuncture

Please see separate chapter, page 279

Alexander Technique

Please see separate chapter, page 281

Aromatherapy

Please see separate chapter, page 283

Art

Please see separate chapter, page 284

Autogenic Therapy

Please see separate chapter, page 285

Ayurveda

"Ayurveda is the oldest medical system in the world. Derived from the two Sanskrit words 'Ayus' meaning 'Life' and 'Veda' meaning 'Knowledge', Ayurveda is usually translated as the 'Science of Life'.

Address: The Ayurvedic Company of Great Britain Ltd, 81, Wimpole Street, London, W1M 7DB. *Tel:* 0207 224 6070. *Fax:* 0207 224 6080. *E-mail:* acgb@cs.com *Website:* www.ayurvediccompanyofgreatbritain.co.uk [Aug 2000]

Bach Flower

The Remedies transform negative attitudes into positive harmonious states of mind. They help such states as anxiety, lack of confidence, panic, uncertainty, despondency, apathy and impatience.

All negative thoughts produce strife in everyday life and can create physical symptoms. The Remedies are homeopathic and can be safely taken with any other medicines without any side effects.

Practitioner: Gillian Smith. *Address:* 38, Quebec Close, Bexhill, Sussex. *Tel:* 01424 215646. [Aug 2000]

Bowen Technique

An exceedingly gentle therapy which triggers the body's own healing responses to effectively address such issues as poor vitality, migraine/head-ache, menopausal difficulties and rebalancing the body and mind.

Practitioner: Gillian Smith. *Address:* 38, Quebec Close, Bexhill, Sussex, TN39 4HX. *Tel:* 01424 215646. [Aug 2000]

Colourpuncture

Colourpuncture is claimed to be able to cure, among other things, insomnia, itching skin and migraine. It is not a form of acupuncture and no needles are used. Instead, coloured lights are focused on specific points of the skin via coloured rods of quartz glass. The system was developed about 25 years ago by a German scientist and healer, Peter Mandel.[5056]

There are about 40 practitioners in this country, one of whom is Angelika Hochadel, 'Colourpucture is a quite wonderful system', she says 'because there is always the possibility of true healing. We treat the emotional state and, if that changes, the disease changes'. *Tel:* 01732 700263, Angelika Hochadel. [5056]

However, Professor Edzard Ernst at the University of Exeter's Department of Complementary Medicine says 'I have yet to see a convincing piece of research on the subject ... I can only conclude that colourpuncture is an unproven method.' [5056]

Colour Therapy

Gabby Kinsella, Colour therapist. *Address:* The Professional Centre, High Street, Old Town, Hastings, East Sussex. *Tel:* 01424 465050. [Aug 2000]

Drama Therapy

Mary Hughes. *Tel:* 01424 430015.

Energy Field Therapy

Energy field therapists are able to detect imbalances by using their hands to scan the patient's electro-magnetic field. Whilst receiving the therapy a very deep level of relaxation is felt by the recipient. Tingling in the hands or feet, or hot and cold sensations are all a normal part of the process as the energy begins to flow and realign. [5810]

Practitioners

Carla Sher, Dip. LCM MGCP

Carla trained at the School of Psychic and Spiritual Development, the London College of Psychic Studies and at the Terton Institute in Energy Field Therapy. Carla also trained at the London College of Massage and is fully qualified in therapeutic and remedial massage as well as lymphatic drainage. She has been working with natural health therapies including yoga, keep fit and meditation since 1981 and advises on diet and hormone balancing. She is a full member of The Guild of Complementary Practitioners. *Tel:* 01580 881169. [Jul 2000]

Steve Austen, MGCP.

Steve trained with the National Federation of Spiritual Healers and has studied anatomy, physiology and pathology in depth. Steve has been practising and working with meditation, healing, yoga and relaxation techniques since 1980. He is a full member of The Guild of Complementary Practitioners. *Tel:* 01580 881169. [Jul 2000]

Herbalism

Please see separate chapter, page 286

Homoeopathy

Please see separate chapter, page 289

Hypnotherapy

Please see separate chapter, page 292

Massage

'Massage helps muscles to relax, relieves stress and tension, and helps release physical and emotional blocks. People who have massage over a period of time report changes in their attitudes towards themselves and their bodies.' [5224]

Health Information Service

The HIS is a free and confidential 24-hour service. You can speak to staff during office hours, and you can listen to any of hundreds of tapes at any time, e.g: *Massage &*

aromatherapy (Tape 481). *Address:* The College of Health, St Margaret's House, 21, Old Ford Road, London, E2 9PL. *Freephone:* 0800 66 55 44. 5367

Publications:

'Massage' - an introductory guide to the healing power of touch. By Stewart Mitchell. One by-product of emotional stress is physical tension. This book shows you how to use basic massage and self-massage techniques to help relieve this. Published by Element, 1999. ISBN: 1-86204-626-3. 128 pages. £5.99. Available from Mind Mail Order Service. *Tel:* 020 8221 9666.

Meditation

Please see separate chapter, page 293

Movement & Arts Therapy

Movement & Arts Therapy can combine several art forms, or only one. It provides a space and time to talk with a qualified therapist. The overall aim is to understand your emotional life, through images and the healing process.

It is suitable for developing a greater understanding of oneself, or for help in times of crisis - for young people and adults. The art forms used can include sandplay, clay, painting, puppets, poetry, writing, drama, dance and music.

Practitioner

Fiona Rankine, BA; PGCE; IATE. *Tel:* 01424 715961. 6087 Apr 2000

Music Therapy

Music therapist, Beryl Hope

Address: Beryl Hope, Burnt Oak Cottage, Iden, Rye, Sussex, TN31 7QA. *Tel*: 01797 280481. (See also 'Hope, Beryl, page 194). Aug 2000

Play Therapy

This therapy is specifically for children and involves, as the name suggests, playing, storytelling, drama, art and so on. Children who might otherwise find it difficult to express their feelings in words may be able to do so through this form of therapy.

Play Therapy Association

The Play Therapy Association will provide details of play therapists in this area. *Address:* Play Therapy Association, PO Box 98, Amersham, Bucks, HP6 5BL. Aug 2000

Roehampton Institute

Runs courses in play therapy leading to Diploma in Play Therapy. *Tel:* 020 8392 3000. Aug 2000

Pauline Cutler

Qualifications: M.A. Psychotherapy; Dip. Couns. Cert. Ed. Dip. Ed. Cert. Play Therapy/Child Psychotherapy; Cert. Supervisor Child Psychother-apist & Play Therapist. Play therapist and trainer. Member of Play Therapy International. *Tel*: 01892 852656. Aug 2000

Mary Dawson

Address: Family support Practitioner Team, Eversfield Hospital, West Hill Road, St Leonards-on-Sea, East Sussex, TN38 0NG. *Tel:* 01424 710105. Aug 2000

Elphinstone Family Centre

Play therapy available here.

Tall Trees, Bexhill

Play therapy available here. 5371

Poetry & Writing

Please see separate chapter, page 294

Psychotherapy

Please see 'Counselling & Therapy' chapter, page 000 for details of this approach.

Reflexology

Please see separate chapter, page 296

Reiki

Reika is a form of 'hands on' healing which you can use for yourself and others. Reiki can be used to 'restore health' and 'gain relaxations for personal growth' and as 'a

regular spiritual practice'. Once 'attuned to Reiki' you only need to place your hands on various parts of the body, either your own or another's to 'allow Reiki energy to flow through resulting in deep relaxation'. During this time, the 'body's energies are altered and re-balanced allowing healing to take place'. Reiki is taught at three levels known as First Degree, Second Degree and Third Degree Reiki. [6091, Gillian Smith]
Local practitioners are:

Marilyn Anderson
Specialist in Indian head massage, crystal healing and regression therapy. *Address:* Mrs Marilyn Anderson, 7, Old Humphrey Avenue, Old Town, Hastings, East Sussex, TN34 3BT. *Tel:* 01424 719116. [May 2000]

Gillian Smith
Gillian Smith describes herself as a 'Usui Reiki Master'. *Address:* Gillian smith, 38, Quebec Close, Bexhill, Sussex, TN39 4HX. *Tel:* 01424 215646. [6091 Aug 2000]

Relaxation
Please see 'Autogenic Therapy' chapter for more information about this form of relaxation.

'Learn to Relax' by Mike George.
'I use the book and the tape as a resource in my workshops' - Elaine Horne, Personal Development Consultant. This is a practical guide to relaxing the mind and body through easily learned exercises and techniques. It presents 25 step-by-step exercises which incorporate methods based on Eastern approaches such as mantras, mandalas and yoga. Available from Mind. *Tel:* 020 8221 9666. [5024]

Retreats
Please see separate chapter, page 297.

Shiatsu
Please see separate chapter, page 298.

Spiritual Healing
Hands on healing or spiritual healing or faith healing. The National Federation of Spiritual Healers Referral Service is on 0891 616080 (50p/min.) [Aug 2000]

Yoga
British Wheel of Yoga
British Wheel estimates that in 1997 there were 300,000 regular practitioners. For a list of qualified Yoga instructors and classes in your area, send a stamped addressed envelope to British Wheel of Yoga, 1, Hamilton Place, Boston Road, Sleaford, Lincolnshire, NG34 7ES. *Tel:* 01529 306851. *E-mail:* wheelyoga@aol.com *Website:* www.bwy.org.uk [Aug 2000]

Hastings College
Courses in Yoga are run at our local college. Contact the student advisers. *Address:* Hastings College of Arts & Technology, Archery Road, St Leonards, Sussex. *Tel:* 01424 442222. [Aug 2000]

Health Information Service
The HIS is a free and confidential 24-hour service. You can speak to staff during office hours, and you can listen to any of hundreds of tapes at any time, e.g: *Yoga* (Tape 078). *Address:* The College of Health, St Margaret's House, 21, Old Ford Road, London, E2 9PL. *Freephone:* 0800 66 55 44. [5367]

Local Clinics

Clinic of Natural Medicine
Multi-disciplinary health centre offering a wide range of complementary/alternative therapies by fifteen practitioners. Objectives are to heal the sick with natural therapeutics and encourage good preventive self-help measures also.

Address: Eastbourne Clinic of Natural Medicine, 69, Meads Road, Eastbourne,

East Sussex, BN20 7QL. *Tel/Fax:* 01323 734664. May 2000

Hale Clinic
Address: Hale Clinic, 7, Park Crescent, London, W1N 3HE. *Tel*: 020 7631 0156. *Website:* www.haleclinic.com Aug 2000

Natural Clinic
Suzanne Carmichael, ITEC, IEB. Natural Clinic, Complementary therapies & workshops in Kent & Sussex. *Tel*: 07977 256259 or 01233 822252. Aug 2000

Professional Centre
'Natural therapies, qualified practitioners.' *Address*: The Professional Centre for Holistic Health, 50, High Street, Hastings, Sussex. *Tel*: 01424 465050. May 2000

Silverhill Natural Health
The Silverhill Natural Health Centre Aromatherapy; counselling; homeopathy; Indian head massage; massage; osteopathy; reflexology. *Address:* Silverhill Natural Health Centre, 3, Battle Road, St Leonards, Sussex, TN37 7AA. *Tel:* 01424 440898. Aug 2000

Springfield Centre
The Centre provides a holistic service and training, including counselling therapy, massage, reflexology, healing and aromatherapy. Particular counselling therapy interests include eating distress, divorce recovery and stress management, alcohol abuse and couples' counselling. The hours are negotiated with the client. Contact Name: Jen Popkin MA (Education) MSc (Counselling).

Address: 4, Springfield Road, St. Leonards-on-Sea, East Sussex, TN38 0TU. *Tel:* 01424 428470. *E-mail:* jen@popkin.fsnet.com.uk Aug 2000

Dyke Road Natural Health Clinic
Specialising in homoeopathic treatment. *Address:* The Dyke Road Natural Health Clinic, 274, Dyke Road, Brighton, Sussex, BN1 5AE. *Tel:* 01273 561844 / 561845. May 2000

Wallace Clinic

The Clinic was opened in March 2000 by Dr Lera Groves. Her qualifications are: PhD, BSYA(Acu), MASC(ACD), DIHOM, DHM, mFBIH.

Address: Wallace Alternative Medical Practice, 32a, Chapel Park Road, St Leonards, Sussex, TN37 6HU. *Tel:* 01424 443435. 5403

Training Courses

Angelgate
'Angelgate' is a training school for complementary therapies. Aromatherapy, champissage, metamorphic technique, nutritional advice, reflexology, Reiki energy renewal, spinal touch treatment, therapeutic massage. *Contacts:* Gill Ayres and John Coppin, see below. 6041

Course fees

These vary enormously, from £35 for workshops to over £1,000 for a diploma course in armotherapy. 6041

Gill Ayres

Qualifications: MA, MIFA, ITEC Dip, MMA, MIFR, ALTT. Gill established the Foundation in St Leonards in East Sussex to maintain standards of training in the area. She has practised holistic therapies for many years and, with a background in communication and social policy, she has provided training to a variety of people.

Address: Gill Ayres, 6, Combermere Road, St Leonards, Sussex, TN38 0RR. *Tel/Fax:* 01424 430001. *E-mail:* lighttouch@callnetuk.com

Website: www.intenethealthlibrary.com 6041

John Coppin
John works in complementary medicine practising Spinal Touch Treatment and Body Stress Release. He established and administered a clinic in Devon before moving to Kent. He is also trained in Jungian Psychotherapy. *Contact:* John Coppin, Seekers' Trust Training Venue, West Malling, Kent. *Tel:* 01732 845133. [6041]

National Organisations

British Complementary Medicine Association
Address: British Complementary Medicine Association, Kensington House, 33, Imperial Square, Cheltenham, Glos., GL50 1QZ. *Tel:* 01242 519911. *Fax:* 01242 227765. *E-mail:* info@bcma.co.uk *Website:* www.bcma.co.uk [May 2000]

British Register of Complementary Practitioners
Address: BRCP, PO Box 194, London, SE16 7QZ.

Complete Health Care Centre
Address: Complete Health Care Centre, 160, City Road, London, EC1V 2NP. *Tel*: 020 7336 0466. *Fax:* 020 7336 8073. *E-mail:* chc@globalnet.co.uk *Website:* www.complete healthcare.co.uk [Aug 2000]

Institute for Complementary Medicine
Address: Institute for Complementary Medicine, PO Box 194, London SE16 7QZ. *Tel*: 020 7237 5165. [Aug 2000]

Apoteke 20-20
Supplier of alternative remedies. *Address*: 296, Chiswick High Road, London, W4 1PA. *Tel*: 020 8995 2293. [Aug 2000]

Body Harmonics
Supplier of alternative remedies. *Address*: 54, Flecker's Drive, Hatherley, Cheltenham, GL51 5BD. *Tel*: 01242 582168. *E-mail:* mariamercati@bodyharmonics.co.uk [Aug 2000]

Nutri Centre
Supplier of nutritional supplements by mail order. *Tel*: 020 7436 5122. [Aug 2000]

Further Information

A-Z of Complementary and Alternative Therapies
Fully revised and updated to include new and emerging therapies. Published by Mind, 2000. ISBN: 1-874690-49-9. 24 pages. £3.00. Available from Mind. *Tel:* 020 8221 9666. [5024]

Encyclopaedia of Energy Healing
Written by Andy Baggott. 'Many people believe that we are all infused with a special kind of energy or life force, which plays a vital role in determining our spiritual, emotional and physical well being.' This book provides a comprehensive look at the major popular and respected forms of healing for the body, mind and spirit.

Published by Godsfield Press, 1999, 192 pages, ISBN: 1-899434-89-5, £17.99. [5088]

From the Ashes of Experience
Reflections on Madness, Survival and Growth. Editors: Phil Barker, Peter Campbell and Ben Davidson. 'Mental health professionals often focus on separate areas of a person's life rather than understanding their whole experience. It could be argued that a more sensitive appreciation of the total reality of the 'madness experience' is the single most important development that could improve the life of people diagnosed as mentally ill. This collection offers uniquely human, often spiritual perspectives from users and survivors.'

Published by Whurr Publishers, 1999, 144 pages, ISBN: 1-85433-272-4, £24.50. Available from Mind Mail Order Service.

Tel: 020 8221 9666. [5088]

Guide to Complementary Medicine
Written by Anne Woodham, 1994. Published by the Health Education Authority.

Healing Minds
Exhaustive evidence from a research programme into complementary therapies. Published by the Mental Health Foundation, £12. [5298]

Healing Touch
Written by Marcus and Maria Webb."Our natural instinct is always to rub an injury, or touch and hold someone who is in pain. This practical, informative, full colour guide explores the many methods of touch therapy including shiatsu, reflexology, reiki, massage therapy, acupressure and aromatherapy. The book illustrates step-by-step how to use some of the techniques yourself to promote well being and health". Published by Godsfield Press, 1999, 128 pages, ISBN: 1-899434-34-8, £12.99. Available from Mind Mail Order Service. *Tel*: 020 8221 9666. [5088]

Leaflets and factsheets
Published by National Mind. Call 020 8519 2122 and ask for Mind Mail Order.

Healing Online (Website)
Founded by Brandon Klein in March 2000, Healing online is a complementary health website, holding 60,000 pages of information on drug, herb and vitamin interactions and side effects. The information on the site is being developed by the Nutri Centre and is being vetted by a team of medical advisers. *Website*: healingonline.co.uk [5266]

Abbreviations
BSYA(Acu).
DHM.
DHP (NC).
DIHOM.
MABCH.
MASC(ACD).
MCAHYP.
MFBIH.
ITEC.
MNEHP
PhD,

Acknowledgements
Our grateful thanks to Mary Dawson, Family Support Practitioner, for editorial assistance with this chapter.

Acupuncture

Known in the East for thousands of years, acupuncture is today used to treat a wide range of illnesses. 'By inserting fine needles in the channels of energy, an acupuncturist can stimulate the body's own healing response and help restore its natural balance.' There are about 2,000 registered acupuncturists practising in this country. [5086, 5087]

Acupuncture

Acupuncture is a system of healing which has been practised in China and other eastern countries for thousands of years. Often described as a means of pain relief, it is in fact used to treat people with a wide range of illnesses. Its focus is on improving the overall well-being of the patient rather than the isolated treatment of specific symptoms.

According to traditional Chinese philosophy, our health is dependent on the body's motivating energy - known as Qi - moving in a smooth and balanced way through a series of channels beneath the skin. Qi consists of equal and opposite qualities - Yin and Yang - and when these become unbalanced, illness may result.[5087]

By inserting fine needles into the channels of energy, an acupuncturist can stimulate the body's own healing response and help restore its natural balance. The flow of Qi can be disturbed by a number of factors. These include emotional states such anxiety, stress, fear, anger, grief, poor nutrition, weather conditions, hereditary factors, infections, poisons and trauma.

The principal aim of acupuncture in treating the whole person is to recover the equilibrium between the physical, emotional and spiritual aspects of the individual. [5087]

Finding an acupuncturist

Members of the British Acupuncture Council (BAcC), have completed a thorough training of at least three years in traditional acupuncture and Western medical sciences appropriate to the practise of acupuncture. They carry the letters MBAcC after their name. The BAcC maintains common standards of education, ethics, discipline and practice to ensure the health and safety of the public at all times. Members are covered by Medical Malpractice and Public/Products Liability Insurance. [5087]

How often will I need treatment?

In traditional acupuncture philosophy each person is considered as unique, and therefore the number of treatments required depends on the individual. Some change is usually felt after five treatments. Normally you are recommended to visit your acupuncturist once or twice a week at first, although some conditions may need less frequent attention. [5087]

What does it feel like?

Most people's experiences of needles is of those used in injections and blood tests. Acupuncture needles bear little resemblance to these. They are much finer and are solid rather than hollow. When the needle is inserted, the sensation is often described as a tingling or dull ache.

Needles are inserted either for a second or two, or left in place for up to 20 minutes, depending on the effect required. During treatment, patients commonly experience a heaviness in the limbs or a pleasant feeling of relaxation. [5087]

Who has acupuncture?

Many people come to acupuncture for help with specific symptoms or conditions. These might include anxiety states, arthritis, asthma, back pain, circulatory problems, depression, high blood pressure, indeterminate aches and pains, infertility, menstrual problems, migraines, rheumatism, sciatica, skin conditions or ulcers.

Acupuncture is also helpful for people trying to overcome addictions such as those related to smoking, alcohol, food or drugs. [5087]

Local Acupuncturists

The following list of practitioners working in the Hastings & Rother area was supplied by the British Acupuncture Council, May 2000. For a more detailed free list please apply directly to the BAC, address below. The British Acupuncture council cannot verify a practitioner's membership of another professional body or their qualification in a therapy other than acupuncture.

Carr-Hopkins, Bradley
Address: Clinic of Nigel Bassett, 74, Canute Road, Hastings, East Sussex. *Tel:* 01424 433991. Also at: Clinic of Nigel Bassett, 16, Ferry Road, Rye, East Sussex, TN31 7DN. *Tel:* 01797 225099. [May 2000]

Holmes, Philip D
Qualifications: BAc, MBAcC, LCSP (Assoc.)
Address: Bexhill Osteopathic Practice, 16, Ednwell Road, Bexhill-on-Sea, East Sussex, TN40 1EA. *Tel:* 01323 738784.

Also at: Ashfield House, 15A, Upper Avenue, Eastbourne, BN21 3XR. *Tel:* 01323 738784. [May 2000]

Kavanagh, Katheryne
Address: The Upper Suite, 30, High Street, Battle, East Sussex, TN33 0EN. *Tel:* 01424 775535. [May 2000]

Sofroniou, Nicholas
Address: 12, Virgins Lane, Battle, East Sussex, TN33 0JH. *Tel:* 01424 773011. [Jul 2000]

For a more detailed free list please contact the BacC at the address below. [5448]

National Organisations

British Acupuncture Council

The British Acupuncture Council was formed in 1995 to represent and govern its professionally qualified acupuncturists.

The BAcC currently has more than 1,900 members whose details are published in an annual Register of Practioner Members. A copy of the full register can be obtained by sending a payment of £3.50 to the address below.

Address: The British Acupuncture Council, 63, Jeddo Road, London, W12 9HQ. *Tel:* 020 8735 0400. *Fax:* 020 8735 0404.
E-mail: info@acupuncture.org.uk
Website: www.acupuncture.org.uk
[5086, 5087]

Further Information

A Guide to Acupuncture
By Peter Firebrace, Sandra Hill and Angela Hicks. Published by Paul Hamlyn 1989 & Constable 1994.

Acupuncture
'Acupuncture: Energy Balancing for Mind, Body & Spirit'. By Peter Mole. Published by Element Books.

Acupuncture: A Scientific Appraisal
Edited by A White and E Ernst. Published by Butterworth-Heinemann, 1999.

Principles Of Acupuncture.
By Peter Firebrace, Sandra Hill and Angela Hicks. Published by Thorsons 1997.

Abbreviations
BAcC. British Acupuncture Council.
MBAcC. Member of the British Acupuncture Council.

Acknowledgements
Our grateful thanks to Joan Maynard of the British Acupuncture Council for editorial assistance with this section.

Alexander Technique

"Alexander established not only the beginning of a far reaching science of the apparently involuntary movements we call reflexes, but a technique of connection (i.e. integration) and self control which forms a substantial addition to our very slender resources in personal education." George Bernard Shaw, playwright.

The challenges and fast-changing demands of modern life can so occupy our thoughts that we forget about that most important consideration: ourselves.

When the natural subconscious mechanisms for balance and posture are influenced by habitual misuse or injury the standard of our physical and mental functioning can be adversely affected. However, the appropriate muscular activity for posture is not something we can regain by simply trying harder. It involves 'automatic' reflex responses that, when working well, appear to support the body almost effortlessly. Jun 2000

By adopting the principles of the Alexander Technique and by learning to prevent interference with these subtle, complex mechanisms we can significantly restore their effectiveness. Breathing and speaking becomes easier; movement becomes freer, lighter and more enjoyable.

Who can benefit?

The Alexander technique can add a new dimension of awareness, well-being and creativity to most peoples' lives. Because it is concerned with the quality of movement the technique can benefit anybody with the interest to pursue it.

The Alexander technique addresses the fundamental causes on many cases of back pain, neck and shoulder tension, breathing disorders, stress-related illnesses and general fatigue where misuse and a loss of poise are contributory factors.

Sports players and the health conscious learn the Alexander technique to improve co-ordination, performance and well-being.

As a pupil you learn to appreciate the practical implications of thought and its effect on muscle activity. The teacher's hands encourage a specific quality of muscle tone. So, together with words of instruction, this helps to release inappropriate tension and allow the body to become better aligned and balanced. A few lessons can make a difference, but for continuous self-improvement a minimum of twenty lessons is recommended. Lessons usually cost between £18 and £30. Apart from a short introductory course for groups, the Alexander technique is taught individually. For comfort, ordinary loose-fitting clothes should be worn.

It is important to consult a qualified teacher. For details of teachers in your area contact the Society of Teachers of the Alexander Technique, page 282.

Local Practitioners

The list that now follows is taken from the United Kingdom list of Teachers published by the Society of Teachers of the Alexander Technique, Sept 1999. 5066 May 2000

Birnie, Deborah

Deborah covers the Brighton area. *Address:* Deborah Birnie, 55, Queens Park Road, Brighton, Sussex, BN2 2GJ. *Tel:* 01273 685873. *E-mail:* deborah@birnie-uk.com May 2000

Child, Sarah

Addresses: The Professional Centre, 50, High Street, Hastings, Sussex, TN34 3EN. *Tel:* 01424 465050;

Practice Room, 15, Bolton Road, Eastbourne, Sussex, BN21 3JT. *Tel:* 01323 734428;

Evolution Arts Centre, 2, Sillwood Terrace, Brighton, Sussex. *Tel:* 01273 729803. May 2000

Haines Sullivan, Christine

Address: Christine Haines Sullivan, Willow

House, 1, Kennet Close, Stone Cross, Pevensey, Sussex, BN24 5PN. *Tel:* 01323 461371. *E-mail:* christine.sullivan@talk21.com
Also teaches in Eastbourne. *Tel:* 01323 461371. Aug 2000

Hughes, Clare
Address: Clare Hughes, 155, Ditchling Rise, Brighton, Sussex, BN1 4QQ. *Tel:* 01273 623460. May 2000

Landau, Leah
Address: Leah Landau, Brighton, Sussex, BN1 6NH. *Tel:* 01273 386369. May 2000

Lofts, John
Address: John Lofts, Half Acre, Station Road, Northiam, Sussex, TN31 6QL. *Tel:* 01797 253216. *Fax:* 01797 253006. Jun 2000

Rolleston Smith, Mrs C
Address: Mrs C. Rolleston Smith, The Old Bakery, High Street, Wadhurst, Sussex, TN5 6AA. *Tel:* 01892 783707. Aug 2000

Sanderson, Suzie
Addresses: Suzie Sanderson, Star Gallery, Fisher Street, Lewes, Sussex, BN7 1YJ. *Tel:* 01273 605226. *E-mail:* info@alexandertechnique.org.uk *Website:* www.alexandertechnique.org.uk
Also: Sunny Glen, Balcombe Road, Crawley, RH10 3NL. Tel: 01273 605226.
Also: 7, College Place, Brighton, Sussex, BN2 1HN. Tel: 01273 605226. May 2000

Schepokat, Gudi
Address: Gudi Schepokat, Dyke Road Natural Health Clinic, 274, Dyke Road, Brighton, Sussex, BN1 5AE. *Tel:* 01273 561844.
Also: 21A, Inwood Crescent, Brighton, Sussex, BN1 5AP. *Tel:* 01273 549758. May 2000

Taraz, Margaret
Address: Margaret Taraz, 47, Dean Court Road, Brighton, Sussex, BN2 7DL. *Tel:* 01273 303382
Also: Dolphin House Clinic, 14, New Road, Brighton, Sussex, BN1 1UF. *Tel:* 01273 324790. 6007 Jul 2000

Local Organisations

Hastings College

Courses in the Alexander Technique are run at our local college. Contact the student advisers. *Address:* Hastings College of Arts & Technology, Archery Road, St Leonards, Sussex. *Tel:* 01424 442222. Jul 2000

National Organisations

Society of Teachers

The Society of Teachers of the Alexander Technique (STAT), was established in 1958 and is the internationally recognised representative body. The Society has over 1,500 members world-wide with more than 850 teaching members in the UK. They are professionally qualified, and adhere to a published code of ethics. The Society publishes a quarterly newsletter and the Alexander Journal. It holds an annual National Conference. *Tel:* 020 7284 3338. *Website:* www.stat.org.uk 5066

Further Information

Alexander Technique

STAT Books offers the world's most comprehensive selection of books and articles on of the Alexander Technique, available by mail order. Address: STAT Books, 129, Camden Mews, London, NW1 9AH. Tel: 020 7482 5369 5066 Aug 2000

Health Information Service

The HIS is a free and confidential 24-hour service. You can speak to staff during office hours, and you can listen to any of hundreds of tapes at any time, e.g: *Alexander technique* (Tape 396).

Address: The College of Health, St Margaret's House, 21, Old Ford Road, London, E2 9PL. *Freephone:* 0800 66 55 44. 5367

Aromatherapy

Aromatherapy is the systematic use of essential oils in holistic treatments to improve physical and emotional well-being. It is an especially effective treatment for stress-related problems and a variety of chronic conditions. Aug 2000

Local Aromatherapists

David Williams

Offers holistic aromatherapy for stress and stress related conditions. 'Qualified, experienced therapist.' *Tel:* 01424 715484. Aug 2000

Elizabeth Downs,

Qualification: MISPA. Is able to give advice to anyone wishing to use aromatherapy at home. *Tel:* 01424 843710. 5412

Gillian Smith

Qualifications: Dip.A. (Diploma in Aromatherapy). *Address:* 38, Quebec Close, Bexhill, Sussex. *Tel:* 01424 215646. Aug 2000

Organisations

Hastings College

Courses in Aromatherapy to diploma level are run at our local college. Contact the student advisers. *Address:* Hastings College of Arts & Technology, Archery Road, St Leonards, Sussex. *Tel:* 01424 442222. Aug 2000

Aromatherapy Council

AROMATHERAPY AOC ORGANISATIONS COUNCIL

The AOC is the UK governing body for aromatherapy. It was formed in 1991 to unify the profession through bringing together its various organisations and to establish common standards of training.

These mandatory standards were implemented in January 1994. The AOC represents the 12 professional associations, their 115 or so accredited training establishments and their 6,000 aromatherapists. AOC recognised aromatherapists are trained to the AOC standards, are fully insured to practice and abide by a Code of Conduct and Ethics. The AOC has a National Register of Aromatherapists and their contact details are available from the AOC office. It is currently seeking statutory regulation of title for aromatherapy to protect the public.

Address: Aromatherapy Organisations Council, PO Box 19834, London, SE25 6WF. *Tel:* 0208 8251 7912. *Fax:* 020 8251 7942. *Website:* www.aromatherapy-uk.org Aug 2000

Further Information

Aromatherapy and the Mind

Written by Julia Lawless. This book examines early beliefs and traditions in the light of the latest scientific research to provide a comprehensive picture of the development and role of fragrance and its power to heal the human psyche.

Published by Thorsons, 1998, 242 pages, ISBN: 0-7225-2927-9. Price: £8.99. Available from Mind Mail Order Service. *Tel:* 020 8221 9666. 5088

Health Information Service

The HIS is a free and confidential 24-hour service. You can speak to staff during office hours, and you can listen to any of hundreds of tapes at any time, e.g: *Aromatherapy & massage* (Tape 481).

Address: The College of Health, St Margaret's House, 21, Old Ford Road, London, E2 9PL. *Freephone:* 0800 66 55 44. 5367

Acknowledgements

Our grateful thanks to Elizabeth Downs, MISPA, for editorial assistance with this section.

Art

Producing any kind of art, be it painting, photography, drawing or sculpture can be therapeutic in itself. Please see also details of the discipline known as 'Art therapy', (page 176), and 'Person Centred Art Therapy', (page 179), in the 'Counselling & Therapy' chapter.

The Arts
The Arts enable us to reflect upon, understand and determine our place in the world.They allow us to challenge and change our perceptions. Art can play a positive role in maintaining good mental health.[5216.]

Mental well-being
The Arts aim to increase the level of mental well-being of participants by using a wide range of creative processes and are proving a powerful ally in fighting the debilitating effects of mental illness. They provide an alternative means of expressing needs, thoughts and aspirations.They facilitate a creative interaction between our inner and outer life, whether we are doing or seeing, artist or audience, striking the balance between the active and the passive. [5216.]

Local Organisations

Creativity & Mental Health
Margaret Moss has set up a group called 'Creativity and Mental Health' and she has put on three exhibitions of photographs, paintings and sculpture at the De La Warr Pavillion in Bexhill in 1997, 1998 and 1999. She hopes, ownership problems of the De la Warr, not withstanding, to mount a similar exhibition beginning 10th October 2000. *Contact:* Margaret Moss.

Address: Margaret Moss, Creativity and Mental Health, c/o Hastings & Rother Community Health Council, 103, Sedlescombe Road North, St Leonards, Sussex. *Tel:* 01424 433221. [5216, 6092 Aug 2000]

Autogenic Therapy

In essence, the method is about letting go of striving for results, and being the passive observer of the inner self… [5290]

What is autogenic therapy?

'Autogenic therapy (AT) is a self-help method which brings about profound relaxation and relief from the negative effects of stress. 'Autogenic' means 'generated from within'. The technique mobilises our innate systems for healing and recuperation.

AT consists of a series of simple, easily learned mental exercises which link mind and body together in association with deep relaxation. These exercises allow the mind to calm itself by switching off the body's stress responses.' [5290]

How does AT work?

'AT is more than just another relaxation technique. In essence, the method is about letting go of striving for results, and being the passive observer of the inner self. In this state, the inherent, self-regulatory mechanisms of the brain function naturally to allow re-balancing of the activities of the right and left brain hemispheres. This in turn supports the workings of the immune system, promotes healing processes, and can bring about greater emotional balance and release of creativity.' [5290]

What are the benefits of AT?

People who have learned AT commonly report: better health and emotional balance; greater coping ability; increased well-being; improved quality of sleep; reduction of anxiety levels.

In addition, AT has been clinically applied over a wide range of disorders, such as sleep disorders, panic attacks, asthma, phobias, arthritis, muscular pain and tension, migraines, fatigue, sexual dysfunction, aggression and unresolved grief. [5290]

Local Practitioners

The following people are practising autogenic therapists.

Ben Edwards

Qualifications: MNIMH, Dip Phyt, Dip AP, MBAS, ITEC, IFR, FDZ. *Address:* Ben Edwards, 3, Place Farm Cottages, Fairlight Place, Hastings, Sussex, TN35 5DT. *Tel*: 01424 812761.

Dr William Munro

Qualifications: MBCh.B; MFOM; MFCH; FRICPHH; DPH; DIH; DTM&H. *Address*: Dr William Munro (Stress Consultant), The Estana, Freezeland Lane, Bexhill, Sussex, TN39 5JD. *Tel*: 01424 219133. [Aug 2000]

Organisations

British Autogenic Society

Formed in 1984, the Society is the professional and regulatory body for autogenic practitioners in the UK. It sets the educational and qualification standards, is an information resource for practitioners and the public and liaises with its counterparts around the world. A full list of registered practitioners will be sent to you, but please send a sae.

Address: British Autogenic Society, Royal London Homoeopathic Hospital, Great Ormond Street, London, WC1N 3HR. *Tel/Fax:* 020 7713 6336. *E-mail:*autosoc@lineone.net *Website:* www.autogenic-therapy.org.uk [Jun 2000]

Acknowlegements

Our grateful thanks to Ben Edwards, Autogenic Training Teacher, for editorial assistance with this chapter and to the British Autogenic Society for providing information on this form of therapy.

Abbreviations

EAP. European Association for Psychotherapy.

ICAT. International Council for Autogenic Therapy.

MBAS. Member, British Autogenic Society.

UKCP. United Kingdom Council for Psychotherapy.

Herbalism

Herbalism in the UK is now classed as an 'alternative' discipline, but it is still the most widely practised form of medicine worldwide with over 80% of the world's population relying on herbs for health.

In this chapter the subject of medical herbalism is explored - under the heading 'National Institute', followed by details of local practitioners, then a word of warning about St John's Wort and finally, details of a mail-order supplier of herbs. [5230]

National Institute

The National Institute of Medical Herbalists is the UK's leading professional organisation of practitioners of herbal medicine (phytotherapy).

Training

Training in phytotherapy involves rigorous study of medical sciences, diagnostic skills, pharmacy, materia medica and dietetics in addition to a minimum of 500 hours supervised clinical training. A full-time course is now accredited to degree standard. All members of the Institute are governed by a comprehensive Code of Ethics and disciplinary procedure and members are covered by full professional insurance.

Treatment

Herbalists are able to treat a wide range of conditions both acute and chronic in nature. Herbalists are trained to take into account health, any medication which is being prescribed and if necessary will know when to refer an individual to a doctor or other professional.

Herbal v orthodox

Herbal medicine is not exclusive of orthodox medicine ... indeed some practitioners are working alongside doctors in a multi-disciplinary setting. It is important to clarify that herbalists *do not simply dispense remedies;* indeed many over the counter remedies may be inappropriate.

Specific treatment

Herbalists are trained to identify the underlying cause of disease and thus will treat each person (not health problem) very specifically. A course of treatment may involve specific dietary advice, helping the individual to develop healthy lifestyle skills (e.g. stress management) in addition to an individually designed prescription. Thus herbalists, in treating symptoms, aim to re-balance and strengthen the system overall.

First visit

On your first visit to a herbalist you may expect a minimum of an hour's consultation entailing the taking of a detailed case history and if required a physical examination. Following this you would commonly see the herbalist again after two weeks and then as required (this will vary).

Materials used

Herbalists use a wide range of plant based materials for internal and external use. Preparations such as tinctures, fluid extracts, syrups, capsules and creams are all produced to a very high standard.

Herbal medicine offers a safe, gentle and effective approach to health care and serves to promote health as an active state. It is suitable for all from the very young to the very old.[5230]

St John's Wort

The Committee on Safety of Medicines issued a warning in March 2000 to users of the herbal antidepressant St John's Wort. Especially at risk are people taking prescribed medicines for depression and migraine and those with epilepsy. In case of doubt consult your pharmacist or doctor. [5229]

Local Practitioners

Boys, H C

Qualifications: MNIMH. *Address:* Mr H C Boys, The Eastbourne Clinic of Natural

Medicine, 69, Meads Road, Eastbourne, Sussex, BN20 7QL. *Tel:* 01323 734664. Aug 2000

Briars Clinic, The
Address: The Briars Clinic, Gardner Street, Herstmonceux, Sussex, BN27 4LB. *Tel:* 01323 832426. Toria Horner & Carole Wallis (see separate entry for full details). May 2000

Buning-Hambly, F
Qualifications: MNIMH. *Address:* Mrs F Buning-Hambly, The Old Dairy, Durgates, Wadhurst, Sussex, TN5 6DE. *Tel:* 01892 783027. Aug 2000

Chedgey, P
Qualifications: MNIMH; Dip Phyt. *Address:* Mr P Chedgey, The Therapy Centre, 3, Hurst Road, Eastbourne, East Sussex, BN21 2PJ. *Tel:* 01323 411900. Jun 2000

Edwards, Ben
Qualifications: MNIMH; Dip Phyt. MBAS, Dip AP, ITEC, IFR, FDZ. Address: Ben Edwards, Herbal Health Clinic, 3, Place Farm Cottages, Fairlight, Hastings, Sussex, TN35 5DT. Tel: 01424 812761. Mobile: 07714 256903. E-mail: benedwards@tinyworld.co.uk

Hambly, P
Qualifications: MNIMH; Dip Phyt; Lic. Ac; MBAcC. *Address:* Mr P Hambly, The Old Dairy, Durgates, Wadhurst, TN5 6DE. *Tel:* 01892 783027. May 2000

Horner, Toria
Qualifications: B.Sc.; MNIMH. *Address:* Ms Toria Horner, The Briars Clinic, Gardner Street, Herstmonceux, Sussex, BN27 4LB. *Tel:* 01323 832426. Toria is a member of the Briars Clinic (see separate entry). May 2000

Murden, Kym
Qualifications: BA(Hons); MNIMH; MCCP. *Address:* Ms Kym Murden, The Lewes Clinic, Fuller's Passage, 196, High Street, Lewes, Sussex, BN7 2LN. *Tel:* 01273 474428. May 2000

Noakes, S
Qualifications: MNIMH. *Address:* Mr S Noakes, 70, Milward Road, Hastings, Sussex, TN34 3RR. *Tel:* 01424 443856. May 2000

Normandale, P
Qualifications: MNIMH. *Address:* Ms P Normandale, The Professional Centre, 50, The High Street, Old Town, Hastings, Sussex, TN34 3EN. *Tel:* 01424 465050. Aug 2000

Pallett, S J.
Qualifications: MNIMH. *Address:* Mrs S J Pallett, The Lighthouse, Ghyll Road, Heathfield, Sussex, TN21 0XJ. *Tel:* 01435 866369. May 2000

Stille, Samantha
Qualifications: MNIMH, Dip Phyt. *Address:* Samantha Stille,The Rock Clinic, 270, Eastern Road, BRIGHTON, Sussex, BN2 5TA. Tel: 01273 621841. (See separate entry in Counselling & Therapy chapter). May 2000

Wagner, Miss Mary C
Consultant medical herbalist incorporating nutrition. Qualifications: B.Sc. (Hons.), MNIMH, MCPP, MICHT. *Addresses:* Miss Mary C Wagner, Flat 12, Helena Court, Pevensey Road, St Leonards, Sussex, TN38 0LY. *Tel/Fax:* 01424 447064; 07703 680754 (mobile).
E-mail: mcwagner@herbalist.fsnet.co.uk Also: Equilibrium Clinic, 'Equilibrium', 16, Station Street, Lewes, East Sussex, BN7 2DB. *Tel:* 01273 470955. Fax: 01273 470975. *E-mail:* info@equilibrium-clinic.com Also: bookings@equilibrium-clinic.com May 2000

Wallis, Carole
Carole is a medical herbalist who specialises in therapeutic/sports massage as well as aromatherapy and reflexology. *Address:* The Briars Clinic, Gardner Street, Herstmonceux, Sussex, BN27 4LB. *Tel:*

01323 832426. Carole is a member of the Briars Clinic (see separate entry). May 2000

Wright, A

Qualifications: MNIMH; MCPP. Address: Ms A Wright, Pucks Hill, Heathfield Road, Burwash, East Sussex, TN19 7HN. Tel: 01435 882751. 5059 May 2000

Organisations

Hambleden Herbs

Hambleden Herbs is an organic herb farm specialist which runs a mail-order service. It was set up by Gaye Donaldson and Mike Brook and they supply herbs, spices, flowers, fruits, seeds, barks, roots, gums, mosses, algae, petals, pods, powders, sticks, teas, infusions, tinctures, flower waters, flower essences, etc. *Tel*: 01823 401205, (general enquiries); 01823 401104, (Harriet Tubbs, mail order).

Address: Mail Order Service, Hambleden Herbs, Court Farm, Milverton, Somerset, TA4 1NF.

Website:info@hambledenherbs.co.uk 5359

Higher Nature

Founded in 1994 by Brian and Celia Wright, who helped to promote the use of natural remedies in this country. They work with eight qualified nutritionists and a medical director, Dr David Smallbone. They publish a 68 page full colour catalogue of products. There is a shop for personal shoppers which is open Mondays to Fridays 9am to 5.30pm and on Saturdays to 12 noon.

Address: Higher Nature, Freepost, TN7289, Burwash Common, Sussex, TN19 7BR. *Tel*: 01435 882880. *Fax*: 01435 883720. 5338

Hastings College

Courses in Herbalism are run at our local college. Contact the student advisers. *Address:* Hastings College of Arts & Technology, Archery Road, St Leonards, Sussex. *Tel:* 01424 442222. Aug 2000

National Institute

President-Emeritus: F. Fletcher Hyde, B.Sc., FNIMH. *Address:* National Institute of Medical Herbalists, 56, Longbrook Street, Exeter, Devon, EX4 6AH. *Tel:* 01392 426022.

Website: www.btinternet.com/-nimh/ 5230

Further Information

Health Information Service

The HIS is a free and confidential 24-hour service. You can speak to staff during office hours, and you can listen to any of hundreds of tapes at any time, e.g: *Bach flower remedies & herbalism* (Tape 482).

Address: The College of Health, St Margaret's House, 21, Old Ford Road, London, E2 9PL. *Freephone:* 0800 66 55 44. 5367

Abbreviations

B.A. Bachelor of Arts.
B.Sc. Bachelor of Science.
Dip Phyt. Diploma in Phytotherapy.
FNIMH. Fellow of the National Institute of Medical Herbalists.
Lic. Ac. Licentiate of Academy.
MBAcC. Member of British Acupuncture College. (?)
MCPP. Member of the College of Practising Phytotherapists.
MNIMH. Member of the National Institute of Medical Herbalists.

Acknowledgements
Our grateful thanks to Ben Edwards, Medical Herbalist for editorial assistance with this chapter.

Homoeopathy

Homoeopaths use medicines diluted almost to extinction in the treatment of their clients' illnesses. Orthodox medicine says that it can't possibly work. But there are many practitioners and their clients who believe it certainly does.

About homoeopathy

'Homoeopathy is an effective and scientific system of healing which assists the natural ability of the body to heal itself. The principle of Homoeopathy is that of 'like curing like'. It has been known from the time of Hypocrites in ancient Greece.'[5073]

Diet, lifestyle and homoeopathy

Changes may need to be made to diet and lifestyle for the treatment to work, especially if an excess of anything is contributing to your illness. Artificial colourings, preservatives and flavourings and pesticides are all contributory factors in our diet. Seeing a GP alongside your homoeopath is also recommended. Some remedies can be used at home such as those for stings or burns and bruises. [5060]

What the homoeopath needs to know.

The right remedy for any one individual means that the homoeopath will need to know details of any complaints and how you experience them; your general energy levels and past medical history and any medicine you are already taking and the way you live are also needed.

Other treatment can affect the homoeopathic treatment and interfere with its effectiveness. If you develop a cold or serious headache or any other symptoms during treatment please discuss these as well.

How long is the treatment?

Depending upon the illness you have and your responsiveness to the treatment, it can vary considerably from person to person. A slow developing complaint that has been developing over years will not disappear overnight. Homoeopathy cures from the inside, even for skin complaints for example. Every case is treated individually and no two patients are alike.

What will happen with treatment?

After taking the remedy you may notice some changes. Some people experience feeling exceptionally well and optimistic. Sometimes the reverse is true and symptoms can become worse for a short time. This is a good sign and means that the remedy is taking effect. [5060]

What will treatment be like?

Your homoeopath will give you a remedy in the form of a tablet or occasionally as powders which should be allowed to dissolve slowly in you mouth. A liquid remedy is occasionally given with instructions. Nothing else should be put in the mouth for twenty minutes before taking the tablet, not even toothpaste or cigarettes. Coffee, peppermint and preparations containing menthol, eucalyptus and camphor should be avoided as these can interfere with the action of the homoeopathic remedy.

History of homoeopathy

'In the late 18th century a German doctor, Samuel Hahnemann (1755 - 1843) rediscovered this true approach to cure, which he called homoeopathy from the Greek 'homoios', meaning similar, and 'pathos', meaning suffering or disease.

Hahnemann tested and demonstrated the fundamental principle of nature; that if a substance can create certain symptoms in a healthy individual then it will heal another suffering from similar symptoms.

In order to restore the sick to health a homoeopathic preparation is administered, which is similar to the symptoms experienced and expressed by the patient on an intellectual, emotional and physical level; quite simply the 'totality of symptoms'.

To achieve this enhanced medicinal action and remove the problem of side-effects, a special method of preparation of the remedies was developed by Hahnemann, called 'potentisation'. The original substance from which the remedy is prepared is subjected to a series of dilutions or trituration.

Between each stage of dilution or trituration, the medicinal solution is shaken, as a process called 'succussion'. After such preparation, remedies are referred to as 'potencies' to signify the way in which the original substance has been transformed.

Living organisms are particularly sensitive to remedies prepared in this dynamic way. It is precisely for this reason that they are so effective when administered according to the 'law of similars'. 5073 May 2000

Local Practitioners

The following list has been taken from the Register of Homoeopaths published by the Society of Homoeopaths, published August 1999.

Embden, Pamela
Address: Pamela Embden, 7, Beaconsfield Villas, Brighton, BN1 6HA. *Tel:* 01273 509193. May 2000

Gonzalez, Sohani
Address: Sohani Gonzaelez, The Dyke Road Natural Health Clinic, 274, Dyke road, Brighton, Sussex, BN1 5AE. *Tel:* 01273 689 194 / 01273 561844/561845. *E-mail:* sohani
@sohani.fsnet.co.uk May 2000

Griffith, Colin
Address: Colin Griffith, 30, High Street, Tenterden, TN30 6LR. *Tel:* 01580 766575. May 2000

Hemmings, Elizabeth
Elizabeth is a member of the Society of Homoeopaths and her aim is to support practitioners and maintain ethical practice; to insure practitioners and to encourage discourse between different medical disciplines, medical doctors, etc; to provide information to the media or anyone requesting such and to support practitioners who give their service s and medicines free in such countries as Bosnia - and probably many more!

Address: Elizabeth Hemmings, Dolphin House Clinic, 14, New Road, Brighton, BN1 1UF. *Tel:* 01273 324790. May 2000

Jones, Jocelyn
Address: Jocelyn Jones, The Waytefield Clinic, 37, Preston Drove, Brighton, East Sussex, BN1 6LA. *Tel:* 01273 550727. May 2000

Josling, Susan
Address: Susan Josling, The Complementary Therapy & Healing Centre, 41, Terminus Road, Eastbourne, BN21 3QL. *Tel:* 01323 430025. *E-mail:* sjosling@aol.com Aug 2000

King, Lesley
Address: Lesley King, Silverhill Natural Health Centre, 3, Battle Road, St Leonards, TN37 7AA. *Tel:* 01424 440898 / 01424 441397. Also: 62, Paynton Road, St Leonards, TN37 7DZ. *Tel:* 01424 441397. May 2000

North, Sarah
Address: Sarah North, The Old Bakery, High Street, Wadhurst, TN5 6AA. *Tel:* 01580 212775 Aug 2000

O'Meara, William
Qualifications: RN, RS. Hom.
Address: William O'Meara, Homoeopathic Clinic, 10, Willow Drive, Seaford, East Sussex, BN25 4BZ. *Tel:* 01323 873617. May 2000

Sanders, Pema
Address: Pema Sanders, 53B, Queens Park Road, Brighton, BN2 2GJ. *Tel:* 01273 699775. Also: Dolphin House Clinic, 14, New Road, Brighton, BN1 1UF. *Tel:* 01273 324790. May 2000

Sloan, Jane
Address: Jane Sloan, Tenterden Homoeopathic Practice, 30, High Street, Tenterden, TN30 6AR. *Tel:* 01580 766727. May 2000

Taylor, Anna
Address: Anna Taylor, Therapy Rooms, St Andrews Lane, Lewes, BN7 1UW. *Tel:* 01273 486550. May 2000

Warren, Carolyn
Address: Carolyn Warren, 3, Manor Cottages, Selmeston, Nr. Polegate, Sussex, BN26 6XB. *Tel:* 01323 811977. Aug 2000

Whiting, Wanda
Address: Wanda Whiting, 5, Priory Avenue, Hastings, TN34 1UQ. *Tel:* 01424 421348. Also: 6, Springfield Road, St Leonards, TN38 OTU. *Tel:* 01424 713643. Also: Battle Wholefood, 38, High Street, Battle, TN33 0AQ. *Tel:* 01424 421348. Aug 2000

Withers, Robert
Address: Robert Withers, 113, Freshfield Road, Brighton, BN2 2BR. *Tel:* 01273 671729. Also: The Rock Clinic, 270, Eastern Road, Brighton, BN2 5TA. *Tel:* 01273 621841. 5073, 5060, 5061

Organisations

London School

London School of Classical Homoeopathy. Principal: Lesley C Gregersen, MCH, MLSH, RSHom, BRCP (Classical Homoeopathy). *Address:* Frazer House, 6, Netherhall Gardens, Hampstead, London, NW3 5RR. All enquiries and correspondence to: The School Office, 94, Green Dragon Road, Winchmore Hill, London, N21 2NJ. *Tel/ Fax:* 020 8360 8757. May 2000

Society of Homoeopaths

Address: The Society of Homoeopaths, 4a, Artizan Road, Northampton, NN1 4HU. *Tel:* 01604 621400. *Fax:* 01604 622622.
E-mail: info@homeopathy-soh.org
Website: www.info@homeopathy-soh.org
6038 Aug 2000

Further Information

Complete Homoeopathy Handbook.
By Miranda Castro, published by Macmillan.

Homoeopathy, Medicine for the New MaN.
By George Vithoulkas, Published by Thorsons.

Homoeopath, Natural Medicine for the Whole Person.
By Peter Adams, Published by Element.

Practical Homoeopathy
A Complete Guide to Home Treatment. By Beth MacEoin, published by Bloomsbury.

Homoeopathy
Homoeopathy - An introductory guide to natural medicine for the whole person. By Peter Adams. Homoeopathic remedies are increasingly popular and they can be combined with traditional medicine for effective self-treatment. An introduction for those new to the area. Published by Element, 1999. ISBN: 1-86204-663-8. 128 pages. Price £5.99. available from Mind Mail Order Service. *Tel:* 020 8221 9666. 5251

Health Information Service
The HIS is a free and confidential 24-hour service. You can speak to staff during office hours, and you can listen to any of hundreds of tapes at any time, e.g:*Homoeopathy* (Tape 162).

Address: The College of Health, St Margaret's House, 21, Old Ford Road, London, E2 9PL. *Freephone:* 0800 66 55 44. 5367

Abbreviations
MCH. Member of the London School of Classical Homoeopathy.
MLSH. Member of the London School of Homoeopathy.
RS.Hom. Register of the Society of Homeopaths.
BRCP. British Register of Complementary Practitioners.

Hypnotherapy

'Hypnosis can be a useful way of aiding relaxation, especially if you are taught how to put yourself into a deeply relaxed state. It is used for tension, addictions, anxiety and insomnia.' [5224]

Local Hypnotherapists

Brenda Riley

Help with such problems as smoking, stress, overeating, panic attacks, phobias, lack of confidence and self-esteem, insomnia, IBS or blushing, and many other stress-related problems. Caring professional approach by Registered Psychotherapist, Hypnotherapist and Stress Consultant. *Qualifications*: DHP(NC), MNRHP, UKCP. Appointments: Benenden Hospital, Cranbrook; Pinehurst Centre, St Leonards-on-Sea. *Tel*: 01424 851739. [6040 Aug 2000]

Karen Hayes

'Effective help for all problems; free initial consultation.' *Qualifications*: MCAHyp; MABCH. *Tel*: 01424 718412. [Aug 2000]

Local Organisations

Hastings College

Courses in Self-Hypnosis are run at our local college. Contact the student advisers. *Address:* Hastings College of Arts & Technology, Archery Road, St Leonards, Sussex. *Tel:* 01424 442222. [Aug 2000]

National Organisations

British Hypnotherapy Association

To find an accredited practitioner in your area, contact the professional association BHA. Founded 1958. 'The orgnisation of practitioners who have had at least four years of relevant training and who comply with professional standards of competence and ethics in hypnotherapy'.[6097.Aug 2000]

Address: British Hypnotherapy Association, 67, Upper Berkeley Street, London, W1H 7DH. *Tel:* 020 7723 4443. [ug 2000]

Further Information

Hypnosis and Hypnotherapy.

Factsheet by George Stewart. Published by MIND Information Unit, April 1998, £0.35. Available from Mind Mail Order Service. *Tel*: 020 8221 9666.

Meditation

Meditation
This involves adopting a comfortable posture, regulating your breathing and focusing on an object, for example, an idea or image, your breathing or a repeated word or phrase (mantra).

The aim is to focus completely on one thing and empty your mind of other thoughts and worries. Meditation has significant effects on the mind and the body: it slows down your heart rate, reduces your blood pressure and calms your breathing. 5224

What is meditation?
'Meditation uses a variety of mental techniques to attain a state of complete relaxation' writes Dr Sarah Brewer, 'the GP who looks for alternatives'.

She continues 'The form known as transendental meditation, or TM was developed by the Maharishi Mahesh Yogi, to be practised easily (15-20 minutes twice a day) despite our busy way of life.

TM uses a variety of Sanskrit mantras, each of which is a short word or phrase that, when repeated in the mind, helps the user still their thoughts to find a deeper level of conciousness, while remaining fully alert. It leaves you feeling refreshed mentally and physically, calmer and able to think more clearly.

It can reduce blood pressure, stress, anxiety and cholesterol levels and improves the quality of sleep as well as helping people cut back on, or stop smoking, drinking, or drug abuse.

TM is practised by many healthcare professionals, including doctors, and is taught througout Britain. A course of four consecutive sessions lasting one and half hours each is recommended'. 5276

Organisations

Transendental Meditation
Address: Transendental Meditation, Freepost, London, SW1P 4YY. Monday to Friday 10am to 5pm. *Tel*: 0990 143 733. *Fax:* 01695 727499.
E-mail: tminfo@maharishi.org.uk *Website*: www.transendental-meditation.org.uk Aug 2000

Hastings College
Courses in Meditation are run at our local college. Contact the student advisers. *Address:* Hastings College of Arts & Technology, Archery Road, St Leonards, Sussex. *Tel:* 01424 442222. Aug 2000

Further Information

Learn to meditate
By David Fontana. Meditation can be of great benefit to general mental health. This beautifully illustrated book presents over twenty practical meditations in the form of affirmations, exercises and visualisations, which draw upon the world's great meditative traditions especially Zen and Tibetan Buddhism. Published by Duncan Baird, 2000. ISBN: 1-900131-91-9. 160 pages. £10.95. Available from Mind. *Tel:* 020 8221 9666. 5024

Meditation
'An introductory guide to relaxation for mind and body. By David Fontana. With photographs and exercises to try, this book is an ideal introduction to meditation as a way of relieving stress and anxiety. Published by Element, 1999. ISBN: 1-86204-627-1. 128 pages. £5.99. Available from Mind. *Tel*: 020 8221 9666. 5251

Poetry & Writing

Survivors' Poetry 'provides survivors with opportunities to actively participate in writing or performance training workshops, poetry performances and publishing projects throughout the UK.' [5323]

Poetry evenings
The Manic Depression Fellowship runs 'Bipolar Poetry Evenings', see 'Manic Depression Fellowship, below.

Local Organisations

Shorelink Community Writers
Creative writing for adults who lack confidence in their ability; have communication difficulties including language barriers; have mental/emotional health problems; need support or encouragement to enable them to write for any reason.

Open to anyone who feels they would benefit from coming to the workshops, regardless of writing/reading ability. Support is offered and sessions include time to read out own work and have constructive criticism and feedback from the group, as well as some writing exercises. There are also projects such as performance poetry/plays. *Contact:* Mrs Ashley Jordan. *Hours:* Every Tuesday morning from 10am to 12 noon at the Children's Library Resource Centre, Robertson Street, Hastings (not during school holidays). There are no sessions at local schools.

Address: Shorelink Community Writers, 25, Cumberland Road, Sidley, Bexhill, East Sussex, TN39 5BU. *Tel:* 01424 730647. *E-mail:* ashley@jordana.screaming.net [5867 Jun 2000]

Survivors' Poetry
Bexhill Survivors' Poetry is linked to Survivors' Poetry in London and currently meets in members' homes. The Bexhill Group hopes to do things which include: having readings of poetry, inviting guest speakers, publishing an anthology, inviting members from other groups, running a poetry competition, publishing a newsletter, running a workshop, discussing & encouraging writers in the group, attracting sponsors and purchasing or otherwise acquiring a computer.

If interested please contact Cliff Bevan on 01424 225153. [5246 Jun 2000]

National Organisations

Manic Depression Fellowship
For details of 'Bipolar Poetry Evenings', contact Luke Chatterton of the Manic Depression Fellowship on 020 7793 2600. 5069 [Jul 2000]

Survivors' Poetry
Survivors' Poetry is a national literature and performance organisation dedicated to promoting poetry by survivors of mental distress through workshops, performances, readings and publications to audiences all over the UK. It was founded in 1991 by four poets with first-hand experience of the mental health system.

Community Outreach
Their community outreach work provides survivors with opportunities to actively participate in writing or performance training workshops, poetry performances and publishing projects throughout the UK. The organisation supports the formation of a nationwide network of survivors' writing groups and works in partnership with local and national arts, mental health, community and disability organisations.

Workshops
Regular workshops are held in London at the Diorama Arts Centre, NW1, and many one-off projects in London and throughout

the UK are organised.

Performances

Regular performances are held twice a month at two separate venues in central London. These give space for new and established survivor poets to read or perform their work in relaxed surroundings.

Writers' group

If you are involved in a writing or poetry group you may find that there are benefits in your group becoming an affiliated member of the Survivors' Poetry national network of writing groups. They offer workshop facilitator training and other training opportunities for members of your group.

There are opportunities to visit or take part in literary festivals and the chance to share skills and information with other writers and writing groups throughout the UK. Contact the organisation for further details. May 2000

Address: Survivors' Poetry, Diorama Arts Centre, 34, Osnaburgh Street, London, NW1 3ND. *Tel*: 020 7916 5317. *Fax*: 020 7916 0830. *E-mail*: survivor@survivorspoetry.org.uk 5323

Further Information

Beyond Bedlam

Poems written out of Mental Distress. Edited by Ken Smith & Matthew Sweeney. 'Witty, brittle, serene, remote, tortured' Published by Anvil Press in co-operation with Survivors' Poetry, 1997. ISBN 0 85646 296 9. 160 pages. Paperback. Price £7.95. Available from Survivors' Press. *Tel*: 020 916 5317.

Beyond Bedlam

A commemorative anthology of poetry. 'This anthology, written and illustrated by users and staff for the 750th anniversary of Bethlem Royal Hospital, dramatically reflects many of the issues that prevail in the contemporary mental health debate.'

Published by Bethlem and Maudsley NHS Trust, 1997. 60 pages. Price £3.50. Available from Mind Mail Order Service. *Tel*: 020 8221 9666. 5106

Fresher Than Green, Brighter Than Orange

An Anthology of poetry by Irish women living in London in 1999. Edited by Eamer O'Keeffe & Lisa Boardman. Published by Survivors' Poetry Press, 1999. ISBN 0 9535455 0 4. 42 pages. Paperback. Price £2.95. Available from Survivors' Press. *Tel*: 020 916 5317.

From Dark To Light

An illustrated anthology of poetry. Edited by Frank Bangay, Joe Bidder & Hilary Porter. 'This is a beautifully produced anthology, full of fascinating insights, images and illustrations' - Geoff Lowe, Psychopoetica.

Published by Survivors' Press, 1992. ISBN 1 874595 00 3. 128 pages. Paperback. Price £5.95. Available from survivors' Press. *Tel*: 020 916 5317.

Under The Asylum Tree

An illustrated anthology of poetry. Edited by Jenny Ford, Colin Hambrook & Hilary Porter. This beautifully produced anthology was short-listed for the 'Mind Book of the Year Award'. Published by Survivors' Press, 1995. ISBN 1 874595 01 1. 208 pages. Paperback. Price £7.95. Available from Survivors' Press. *Tel*: 020 916 5317.

Mind Readings

Mind Readings: writers' journeys through mental states. Edited by Sara Dunn, Blake Morrison and Michele Roberts, published by Minerva, £7.99.

Writing Well

Creative writing and mental health. By Deborah Philips and others. Published 1998. ISBN: 1-853-0265-0. Price £15.95. 5069

Acknowledgements
Our grateful thanks to Roy Holland of Survivors' Poetry for editorial assistance with this chapter.

Reflexology

The hard-wearing soles that transport you about your daily business can often be neglected and uncared for, but reflexologists claim that the feet are a map to the whole physical body. By massaging the feet using a special method, reflexologists say that they can improve mental and physical health.

Chinese medicine

The ideas behind reflexology are not dissimilar to traditional Chinese medicine beliefs about energy lines or meridians. In reflexology these energy lines are seen to run through the body linking up remote body parts and terminating in the feet. Disease is seen to arise when these energy lines become blocked or energy manifests in a certain area.

Standards

Reflexologists massage areas on the feet and say that this stimulates the flow of energy and improves health. There are a number of registering bodies that promote themselves as professional organizations for reflexology. As a result practitioners can train and register under varying academic and practical standards, so choosing a reputable practitioner is very important.

Mental health

There has been very little research into reflexology and mental health.In fact, there has been very little good quality research undertaken to substantiate any of the claims of reflexologists. That said, mental health service users who have tried reflexology often report benefits such as relaxation and release of tension.

A typical session starts with a sequence of relaxation techniques, so perhaps it is not surprising that people find this type of foot massage to be relaxing and pleasurable. Nonetheless, more rigorous research in this area is warranted. [5110]

Local Organisations

Hastings College

Courses in reflexology to diploma level are run at our local college. Contact the student advisers. *Address:* Hastings College of Arts & Technology, Archery Road, St Leonards, Sussex. *Tel:* 01424 442222. [Aug 2000]

Further Information

Health Information Service

The HIS is a free and confidential 24-hour service. You can speak to staff during office hours, and you can listen to any of hundreds of tapes at any time, e.g: *Reflexology* (Tape 444).

Address: The College of Health, St Margaret's House, 21, Old Ford Road, London, E2 9PL. *Freephone:* 0800 66 55 44. [5367]

Retreats

Why not get away from it all? Find peace of mind in the tranquility of a retreat ... Some of this country's top retreats are listed here.

Why not get away from it all? Find peace of mind in the tranquility of a retreat. Here is a list of some of the country's retreats.

Abbey, The
Inter-Faith retreat offering space and support. *Address:* The Abbey, Sutton Courtenay, Oxon, OX14 4AF. *Tel:* 01235 847401. [Jun 2000]

Barn, The
A Buddhist retreat enabling people to work on the land. *Address:* The Barn, Lower Sharpham Barton, Ashprington, Totnes, Devon. *Tel:* 01803 732661. [Jun 2000]

Eagle's Wing
Contemporary Shamanism retreat. *Address:* Eagle's Wing Centre for Contemporary Shamanism, 58, Westbere Road, London, NW2. *Tel:* 020 7435 8174. [Jun 2000]

Kagyu Samye Ling
Tibetan monastery retreat in Eskdalemuir. *Address:* Kagyu Samye Ling Tibetan Centre, Eskdalemuir, Langholm, Dumfriesshire. *Tel:* 01387 373232. [Jun 2000]

Launde Abbey
Built by Thomas Cromwell in 1540. Anglo-Ecumenical retreat. *Address:* Launde Abbey, East Norton, Leicestershire, LE7 9XB. *Tel:* 01572 717254. [Jun 2000]

Marygate House
Historical inter-denominational place still visited by pilgrims. *Address:* Marygate House, Holy Island, Berwick-upon-Tweed, Northumberland,TD15 2SD. *Tel:* 01289 389246. [Jun 2000]

Monkton Wyld Court
Holistic Education for mind, body & spirit. *Address:* Monkton Wyld Court, Charmouth, Dorset. *Tel:* 01297 560342. [Jun 2000]

Sancta Maria Abbey
Roman Catholic retreat. *Address:* Nunraw Guest House, Garvald, Haddington, East Lothian, EH41 4LW. *Contact tel:* 01620 830228. [Jun 2000]

Shambhala Healing Centre
Retreat on the ancient holy site of Glastonbury Tor. *Tel:* 01458 831797. [Jun 2000]

Tekels Park Guest House
Retreat set in a wildlife sanctuary. *Address:* Tekels Park Guest House, Tekels Park, Camberley, Surrey, GU15 2LF. *Tel:* 01276 23159. [Jun 2000]

Organisations

National Retreat Assocation

Address: The National Retreat Association, Liddon House, 24, South Audley Street, London, W1Y 5DL. *Tel:* 020 7493 3534. [5885]

Further Information

The Good Retreat Guide
The Good Retreat Guide or Away From It All: A Guide To Retreat Houses And Centres For Spiritual Renewal. [5885]

Shiatsu

Shiatsu is a traditional Japanese healing art, which is an increasingly popular form of complementary medicine. Shiatsu treatment can help a wide range of conditions, from specific injuries to more general symptoms of poor health. It is also very relaxing and enjoyable.[5478]

Local Practitioners

Annie Cryar
(Teacher), St Leonards-on-Sea, East Sussex, *Tel*: 01424 441743. [Aug 2000]

Rosamunde Parke Jordan
(Teacher), Hastings, East Sussex, TN34 *Tel*: 01424 460355 ext. 20. [Aug 2000]

Sarah Tomisson
(Practitioner), Hastings, East Sussex TN35. *Tel*: 01424 433991; Battle, East Sussex TN33. *Tel*: 01424 870857. [5186]

Organisations

Shiatsu Society

The Shiatsu Society is the national network for everyone interested in Shiatsu. They link all the major schools and approaches to Shiatsu, and run a quarterly newsletter with articles relating to Shiatsu and oriental medicine and philosophy in general.

The society also maintains a register of qualified practitioners, designated by the letters MRSS (Member on the Register of the Shiatsu Society). Members of the public may obtain names of MRSS practitioners in their area by contacting the Shiatsu Society.

Address: The Shiatsu Society, Eastlands Court, St. Peters Road, Rugby, CV21 3QP. *Tel:* 01788 555051. *Fax:* 01788 555052. *E-mail:* admin@shiatsu.org
*Website:*www.shiatsu.org [5478]

nhs & social services

This fourth part of the *Guide* gives information about the NHS, hospitals and clinics (both NHS and private) and social services. For a quick overview of this section, please see the Contents on page 6

Care Programme Approach

Probably few mental health services users have ever heard of the 'Care Programme Approach'. It is the ideal standard upon which actual delivery of mental health care is based. Unfortunately, we do not live in a perfect world ...

What is the CPA?

The Care Programme Approach (CPA) is used nationally by the specialist mental health services. It is a way to identify your needs with you, then agree and arrange a care plan.

What will happen?

1.You will be involved in an assessment of your health and social care needs.
2. After consultation you will be allocated somebody (known as your care co-ordinator) who will co-ordinate and monitor your care.
3. A care plan will be negotiated with you to meet your specific needs. You, and with your agreement your carer, will have a copy of your agreed care plan.
4. At least every six months your care co-ordinator, yourself and anyone else concerned in your care will take a fresh look at your current needs. This is called a review.

What information will be kept?

1. Your personal details, e.g. name, address, date of birth, general information about your assessment, care plans, review dates, records of review meetings and care plan summaries. You will have access to this information. Your information is confidential to yourself, your care co-ordinator and other professionals involved in your care.
3. No other person will have access to this information without your permission, apart from exceptional circumstances.
4. If you wish to access your Health and Social Services records your care co-ordinator will help you with this process.

Your rights under the CPA

You have a right to:
1. Refuse/withdraw from some or all parts of the CPA process at any time.
2. A care co-ordinator and to know how to contact them.
3. Full involvement in care planning and a copy of agreed care plan.
4. An advocate, friend or carer to support you throughout the process, participating in all meetings and reviews.
5. Ask for a review at any time.
6. Access all your CPA care plans and review forms.
7. Know who has access to your personal information.
8. Request another opinion on any aspect of your care.
9. Complain if dissatisfied with any aspect of your care. [5220]

New guidelines

In 1999, the Government issued new guidelines for what is called the Care Programme Approach, a framework for effective mental health care. This forms part of the Government's National Framework Document for mental health services. These new guidelines aim to simplify the CPA procedure by first reducing the amount of paperwork needed to record a patient's progress during a CPA programme.

Needs Assessment

At the centre of this is the *Needs Assessment Document,* a yellow booklet that covers all of that individual's mental health history. There are plans to computerise this document in the future. For now, however, it is kept solely by the patient's care co-ordinator, who will be the most involved professional. The *Needs Assessment Document* also incorporates a care plan, which may be written in collaboration with Community Link Nurses when a patient is discharged from hospital, though this may be ammended by the care co-ordinator as the care programme progresses.

Levels

There are to be two levels of Care Programme Approach; *standard* and *enhanced.* Standard means that just one professional health worker is involved, whilst enhanced requires the involvement of several mental health professionals, depending on the extent of the individual's needs.

Categories

Similarly, there will be just four categories of diagnosis locally. As a general guide, the first category will cover patients who have been compulsorily hospitalised. The second category will be those who have been voluntarily hospitalised. The third category will be mental health outpatients who have not been hospitalised and the fourth category will be individuals who have no formal mental health diagnosis. [5094 5221]

Further Informaion

Community Care - 2

'Community Care - 2. The Care Programme Approach' by Gail Hewitt. Published by Mind Information Unit. January 200. Available from Mind Mail Order Service. Price £1.36. *Tel*: 020 8221 9666.

Acknowledgements

Our grateful thanks to Christine Lockwood (Community Link Nurses, Woodlands) and Steve Loynes (CPA Systems Co-ordinator, St Anne's) for editorial assistance with this chapter.

Case Management

Community Care Plan

Social Services have a statutory duty to publish this plan, updated every year. It is now closely aligned with Joint Investment Plans (JIPs) for different services, which are part of the Health Improvement Programme (HImP). [5993 Jun 2000]

In 1999, East Sussex Social Services Department and the East Sussex, Brighton and Hove Health Authority jointly published this plan. To quote from the foreword:

"This plan reviews achievements and developments in community care over the past year, and updates objectives and targets for the next three years.

This is bound to be a period of considerable change, with the creation of Primary Care Groups, and the development of Joint Investment Plans and the Health Improvement Programme.

All these developments can be summed up in the word 'partnership'. The essence of partnership is effective communication and co-operation which involves not just statutory services and voluntary organisations, but also service users and their carers."

For a free copy of the 120 page document please apply to David Archibald, Director of Social Services, PO Box 5, County Hall, St Anne's Crescent, Lewes, East Sussex, BN7 1SW. *Tel:* 01273 481141. [1570 May 2000]

Local Organisations

Case Management

This service is specifically aimed at adults living in the community who are suffering from severe and enduring mental health problems. Case Managers work with other agencies and staff to create individual care programmes. Enquiries should be made through the patient's GP to the Sector Team Co-ordinator at the address below. This service is being replaced by 'assertive outreach'. [5993 Jun 2000]

Address: Case Management, Westwood House, 7, Holmesdale Gardens, Hastings, East Sussex, TN34 1LY. *Tel:* 01424 714366. *Fax:* 01424 439537. [0528 Jul 2000]

Further Information

Community Care - 1

Community Care - 1. The NHS and Community Care Act. Gail Hewitt. Published by Mind Information Unit, January 2000. Price £1.36. Available from Mind Mail Order Service. *Tel*: 020 8221 9666.

Community Care - 3

Community Care - 3. Addressing the needs of Carers. Gail Hewitt. Published by Mind Information Unit, January 200. Price £1.36. Available from Mind Mail Order Service. *Tel*: 020 8221 9666.

Community Care - 4

Community Care - 4. Commissioning. Gail Hewitt. Published by Mind Information Unit, January 200. Price £1.36. Available from Mind Mail Order Service. *Tel*: 020 8221 9666.

Community Care - 5

Community Care - 5. Services. Gail Hewitt. Published by Mind Information Unit, January 200. Price £1.36. Available from Mind Mail Order Service. *Tel*: 020 8221 9666.

See also these chapters ...

Care Programme Approach, page 300.
National Service Framework, page 334.
Primary Care Groups, page 339.
Social Services, page 347.

Community Health Councils

CHCs are the NHS Watchdogs and have consultation, information and visiting rights. Our local CHC is based at Silverhill, St Leonards-on-Sea

Community Health Councils
CHCs were set up in 1974 as local independent bodies to represent the public's interest in the health service. Commonly known as the NHS Watchdog, or CHCs, the volunteer members work with local people to help all sections of the community make their views heard by health service managers. They also identify services which are needed but not provided, and use lots of different ways to find out what people think of the NHS in their district.

CHCs have statutory rights (through an Act of Parliament) to be consulted on major changes in the health service, to information and to visit NHS premises to monitor how services are provided.

CHCs also provide information and advice to the public and assist people who have a complaint. CHC staff provide this part of the CHC's service. 5897, 6022

Local Organisations

Eastbourne CHC

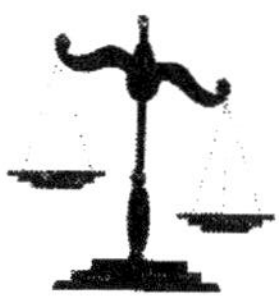

Information, representation, evaluation, consultation. Chief Officer: John Faulds, MA. *Address*: Eastbourne, Seaford & Wealden Community Health Council, Senlac House, 53-59, Seaside, Eastbourne, East Sussex, BN22 7NE. *Tel/Minicom*: 01323 737925. *Fax*: 01323 410142. May 2000

Hastings & Rother CHC

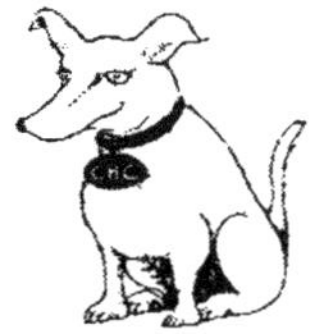

This is our local CHC. The area covered is from Camber along the coast to Cooden and to Ticehurst in the north and takes in the whole districts of Hastings Borough Council and Rother District Council. There are 20 volunteer members, between 5 and 10 co-opted members and 3 full-time staff.

Advice and Information Service
Staff are able to provide you with information about local health services, such as finding a GP or NHS dentist, or whether a health service you need is available locally. You can ask for advice about the local health services, and staff will support you if you feel you need to make a complaint about any of the local health services you receive, such as your local doctor, nurse, hospital staff, dentist, pharmacist or optician. Advice and information is free and confidential.

Representing the public's interest
Volunteer members of the CHC meet at the CHC's office in Silverhill. They are nominated as CHC members by local authorities, voluntary organisations and the regional office of the NHS Executive. Members set themselves objectives each year to undertake pieces of work around issues which local people have said are

important issues for them.

The provision and quality of mental health services has been a key CHC priority for a number of years and members are constantly in touch with people who use mental health services in Hastings and Rother to find out what they think works well and what does not. These views will be put to those who provide care and may also prompt the CHC to undertake a specific piece of work such as a series of visits to hospital wards and out-patient clients, a patient satisfaction survey or an event or public meeting to raise awareness of what is going on.

CHC priorities

Identify gaps in Mental Health Servces for children and adolescents; find out from patients and carers how hospital and community services are meeting the needs of people with Alzheimer's Disease.

Lobby for a Youth Assessment Unit at the Conquest Hospital for the elderly mentally ill; keep under review the future operational changes proposed for adult mental health services and consult on any changes which affect patients. Continue to support Focus on Mental Health user group. [5921]

Staff

Patricia Marston, chief officer; Christopher Raeburn, deputy chief officer; Sharon Dewis, office manager.

Opening hours

Mondays 2pm to 4pm; Tuesdays to Fridays 10am to 4pm. It is advisable to book an appointment if you have a problem to discuss, as staff are not always immediately available.

CHC Council

The Council meets, in public, four times a year and the public is welcome to attend. There are opportunities to raise questions and air views at these meetings. Contact the CHC office for more information. Larry Fisher, CHC chairman; Margaret Moss and Tony Moore, vice-chairmen. [5897]

Address: Hastings and Rother Community Health Council, 103, Sedlescombe Road North, St Leonards-on-Sea, East Sussex, TN37 7EJ. *Tel:* 01424 433221. *Fax:* 01424 433595.

National Organisations

ACHCEW

The Association of Community Health Councils for England and Wales (ACHCEW). Set up in 1977 to provide a forum for member CHCs, to provide information and advice to CHCs and to represent CHCs at national level. It has direct links with the Department of Health and other branches of government.

CHCs are not obliged to be members of ACHCEW, but most are. Its main function is to provide information to member CHCs and organise a wide range of training events designed for CHC members. Chair: Joyce Struthers. Director: Donna Covey. [5897]

Address: Association of Community Health Councils for England & Wales, Earlsmead House, 30, Drayton Park, London, N5 1PB. *Tel:* 020 7609 8405. *Fax:* 020 7700 1152. *E-mail:* mailbox@achcew.org.uk *Website:* www.achcew.org.uk [May 2000]

Further Information

Health Information Service

The HIS is a free and confidential 24-hour service. You can speak to staff during office hours, and you can listen to any of hundreds of tapes at any time, e.g: *Community Health Councils* (Tape 187)

Address: The College of Health, St Margaret's House, 21, Old Ford Road, London, E2 9PL. *Freephone:* 0800 66 55 44. [5367]

Community Mental Health Teams

CMHTs represent a real breakthrough in the provision of mental health care. By the autumn of 2000, the services previously offered by two completely independent bodies, (Social Services and the NHS Trust) will be merged to form joint teams, the CMHTs. It seems that we must get used to two new expressions, 'CMHT' and 'CMHN'.

CMHTs

CMHTs are community mental health teams. Each team is multi-disciplinary and consists of a team manager and one or more of the following: psychiatrists, psychologists, social workers including approved social workers (ASWs), community mental health nurses (CMHNs), occupational therapists, community support workers. Accommodation officers form a separate team.

Each team operates from a single address with a single point of referral and a joint assessment process and forms. They will ultimately use a single records system and joint budget, with full integration of all functions previously carried out separately by social services and the NHS Trust staff. [5336]

Amalgamation

CMHTs are an amalgamation of Social Services and NHS Trust staff. They started to come into being in the summer of 2000.

There are four CMHTs for this area: Bexhill, Hastings, Rural Rother and St Leonards. All four CMHTs report to the 'locality manager', see below. Anyone can refer you to these teams. [5336, 5343, 5408, 5993]

CMHNs

What are CMHNs?

CMHNs are community mental health nurses. All CMHNs are now based at separate CMHTs. In Hastings, CMHNs visit patients in their own homes and hold clinics at GPs' surgeries.

People living in Hastings and St Leonards, who want to see a CMHN, should first discuss this with their GP or a consultant psychiatrist.

What do CMHNs do?

CMHNs are nurses with mental health training and work in CMHTs (community mental health teams) alongside psychiatrists and social workers. CMHNs usually give home visits, give medication, and provide emotional support.

They can also teach stress management techniques and specialise in alcohol or drug problems or even eating disorders. A CMHN may also co-ordinate your care as part of the Care Programme Approach (see Care Programme Approach). You will need to see a GP, a psychiatrist, or someone from the Community Crisis Intervention Service. They can they refer you to the CMHN. [5224]

CPNs

CPNs are community psychiatric nurses, now re-named as CMHNs; see above.

Integrated Teams

Phil Gander of Social Services said, in November 1999, that integrated community health teams will be jointly managed by Health and Social Services and will eventually be working to exactly the same policies, and are working towards pooled budgets, although not all budgets will be combined. He believes the contribution from social work and approved social workers training could 'bring in the care principle from a non-medical perspective.' Social Services, HART, PCGs, and the Health Authority all share this view. [5074, 5993]

Mental health & the elderly
For information about services for people over 65, please contact Christine Thomas, Service Manager, at Ridgeway, 125, St Helen's Down, Hastings, Sussex, TN34 2AR. *Tel:* 01424 443893; *fax:* 01424 434931. [Aug 2000]

Local CMHTs

Duty Team
Manager: Madeleine Iddison. [6013 Jul 2000]

Hastings CMHT
Manager: Madeleine Iddison. *Address:* Hastings CMHT, Westwood Centre, 7, Holmesdale Gardens, Hastings, East Sussex, TN34 1LY. *Tel:* 01424 714366. *Fax:* 01424 439537. [6013 Jul 2000]

Eastbourne CMHT
Address: Eastbourne CMHT, 2-4, Birling Street, Eastbourne, Sussex, BN21 1RL. *Tel:* 01323 532110. *Fax:* 01323 532118. [5928 Jun 2000]

St Leonards CMHT
Manager: Stephen Jones. *Address:* St Leonards CMHT, Westwood Centre, 7, Holmesdale Gardens, Hastings, East Sussex, TN34 1LY. *Tel:* 01424 714366. *Fax:* 01424 439537. [6013 Jul 2000]

Accommodation Team
Manager: Stephen Jones. *Address:* 8, London Road, Bexhill-on-Sea, East Sussex, TN39 3JU. *Tel:* 01424 730512. *Fax:* 01424 732249. [6013 Jul 2000]

Bexhill CMHT
"We provide a cohesive service that makes a positive difference to the life of our users."

Consultant psychiatrist: Dr Gillian Smith; Psychologist: Ms Marchiene Van Der Veen; Senior community mental health nurse: Mr Jean-Pierre Parmainteny.

Located on the first floor of the Bexhill Health Centre, the Bexhill CMHT provides a service for adults (16 - 65) who suffer from mental health difficulties. Facilities include: out-patient clinic, psychology, counselling and psychotherapy, day services and occupational therapy. Manager: Kalpana Darliker.

Address: Bexhill CMHT, Bexhill Health Centre, Bexhill Hospital, Holliers Hill, Bexhill-on-Sea, East Sussex, TN40 2DZ. *Tel:* 01424 735608. *Fax:* 01424 735609. [6013 May 2000]

Rural Rother CMHT
This CMHT covers all the rural areas outside Hastings, St Leonards and Bexhill, extending as far as Ticehurst in the north, Wadhurst and Rye in the east.

The team consists of a consultant psychiatrist, Dr Michael Birkett; a clinical psychologist, Terry Kohler; an occupational therapist, Nicky Mehdi, two community mental health nurses, Paul Templeman and Rose Legg; a support worker, Lynne Mockett; a case manager, Jerry Edouard; two social workers and a rural Mind project worker, Su Barnicoat; Manager: Kalpana Darliker.

Address: Rural Rother CMHT, Eversfield Hospital, West Hill Road, St Leonards, Sussex. *Tel:* 01424 710111. [5668, 6013]

Locality manager
The locality manager is Morag Murray. The CMHT managers report to the locality manager:

The locality manager reports in turn to both Phil Gander, Head of Mental Health Services for the Social Services Department, and to Sarah Holmes-Smith, Director of Mental Health of the NHS Trust. [6013]

Abbreviations

CMHN. Community Mental Health Nurse.

CMHT. Community Mental Health Team.

Acknowledgements

Our grateful thanks to Madeleine Iddison for editorial assistance with this chapter.

Doctors

Your GP will normally be your first port of call if you are seeking help with a mental health problem, either for yourself or for a friend or relative [5224]

Your GP will normally be the first port of call if you are seeking help with a mental health problem, either for yourself or for a friend or relative. Your GP can refer you on to your local community mental health team or in an emergency to the Community Crisis Intervention Service.

Mental health

Most GPs both deal with mental health problems and prescribe medication themselves. Some GPs have practice nurses or counsellors on site - you may be offered sessions with a nurse on stress management, for example. If you need more specialist help your GP may refer you for an outpatient appointment with a psychiatrist, or arrange for you to be visited at home by a member of the community mental health team. [5224]

Emergencies

In an emergency, or out of hours, a GP may contact the Community Crisis Intervention Service on your behalf. You do have a choice of GP, so ask around for recommendations, study the practice leaflets and phone up several practices before you register. Ask to speak to the practice manager, who may be able to answer your queries and tell you about the GPs' interests and training. You could ask to meet any prospective GP for a pre-registration chat (but not many GPs will give you their time in this way). [5224]

Out-of-hours service

When the surgery is closed, all GPs operate an emergency service, e.g. Seadoc, see below. This is only for medical problems that cannot wait until the next surgery to be treated.

Here's what to do if you need advice outside normal surgery hours:

- Have a pen and paper handy because you might get a recorded message giving another telephone number to call.
- Make sure you can give a contact telephone number, so that the doctor or nurse can call you back if they need to.
- Make a list of your symptoms and any questions you have before you call.
- If you are calling on behalf of someone else, get as many details from them as possible.
- Remember to mention any other conditions which you or the patient may suffer from (e.g. asthma, diabetes or allergies).
- Do phone if your condition (or the patient's) improves. It may be that medical treatment is no longer needed. [5095]

Seadoc

Seadoc is the local out of hours services. Many GPs belong to 'Seadoc', a co-operative of local GPs working on a rota system. Calls to GPs' surgeries are automatically transferred to 'Seadoc'. You may be asked to attend the 'Seadoc' base surgery located in Little Ridge Avenue. [5928 Jun 2000]

Community liaison workers

As a pilot project for one year, Wellington Square Surgery has a community liaison worker. She takes referrals from the doctors at the surgery with the specific aim of supporting patients to contact appropriate community and voluntary resources. She also aims to remove some of the obstacles to accessing help experienced by mental health service users. She does not provide counselling or therapy services. 5833 Jun 2000

Doctors - by name

The following list gives details of the GPs working in the Hastings and Rother area. They are arranged in alphabetical order of surname. Doctors' surgeries are listed separately in this chapter under the heading 'GPs Surgeries'.

Al-Ansary, Dr Y....................Buckhurst Rd
Al-Saleem, Dr M A W...........South Saxon
Ashby, Dr S M...........................Albert Rd
Ashby, Dr S M.........................Turkey Rd
Blackburn, Dr A M T..................Belmont
Blackburn, Dr A M T. ....Ticehurst
Blundell, Dr R J ....Northridge
Bryden, Dr P. .... Lower Glen
Cameron, Dr D J.................Silver Springs
Cameron-Wood, Dr R A.........Carisbrooke
Carroll, Dr J. ....Northiam
Chinery, Dr C G. ....Roebuck
Chinery, Dr C G........................Guestling
Chishick, Dr H B J ....Postern Gate
Chisholm-Batten, Dr R E .....Harold Road
Clarke, Dr R C ....Martins Oak
Collis, Dr A ....Wadhurst
Collis, Dr A...............................Ticehurst
Cooper, Dr T F M ....Wellington Sq
Das, Dr P. ....Priory Road
Dewhurst, Dr P D ....Little Common
Dewing, Dr C ....Wish Valley
Dhalla, Dr P N. ....Harold Road
Digby, Dr R...........................Wish Valley
Dinwiddie, Dr J F ....Northiam
Dinwiddie, Dr J F ....Brede
Dunfield-Prayero, Dr A...............Roebuck
Dutchman, Dr D A......................Roebuck
Eaton, Dr J C R.....................Albert Road
Eaton, Dr J C R ....Turkey Road
Elias, Dr R G ....Sea Road
Elliot-Pyle, Dr E M ....Oldwood
Emmanuel, Dr J H ....Albert Road
Emmanuel, Dr J H ....Turkey Road
Ferguson, Dr N J ....Postern Gate
Francis, Dr K M ....Shankill
Freeman, Dr M P ....Churchwood
Furley-Smith, Dr E A.............Carisbrooke
Gonzalez, J.....................Bexhill Old Town
Griffin, Dr A L ....Postern Gate
Griffith, Dr D ....Martins Oak
Hadley, Dr L A.............Bexhill Old Town
Hargreaves, Dr C...................Sedlescombe
Hargreaves, Dr C........................ Westfield
Hawley, Dr W L...........Bexhill Old Town
Head, Dr A C.......................Harold Road
Heber, Dr M J ....Churchwood
Henry, Dr J G ....Shankhill
Herbert, Dr P M L............Warrior Square
Higginson, Dr B M.......Wellington Square
Horsley, Dr I T.....................Harold Road
Howie, Dr F J T.........................Shankhill
Hughes, Dr H E ....Wellington Square
James, Dr P M ....Northiam
Janes, Dr D P...................Beaconsfield Rd
Jardine-Brown, Dr T ....Sedlescombe
Jardine-Brown, Dr T ....Westfield
Jeelani, Dr M ....Cinque Ports
Jeelani, Dr R..........................Cinque Ports
Jones, Dr D ....Churchwood
Kaliniecki, Dr J P. ......Sedlescombe House
Kemm, Dr I ....Ninfield
Kinch, Dr H W A ....Albert Road
Kinch, Dr H W A ....Turkey Road
Kinloch, Dr D ....Essenden Road
Kremer, Dr D J......................Albert Road
Kremer, Dr D J ....Turkey Road
Kyu, Dr R ....Roebuck
Lawton, Dr D J ....Albert Rd & Turkey Rd
Lee, Dr J V................St Michael's Hospice
Maxwell, Dr T G..............Little Common
McCarthy, Dr N E.................Carisbrooke
Mehta, Dr P A........................Battle Road
Mogan, Dr J E ....Martins Oak
Moynagh, Dr D...................Silver Springs
Newell, Dr D N ....Albert Road

Newell, Dr D N ....Turkey Road
Nicholson, Dr H P..................Stone Street
Offord, Dr C ....Belmont
Offord, Dr C...............................Ticehurst
Packham, Dr B A..........................Fairfield
Paget, Dr S E...............................Roebuck
Parker, Dr L............Guestling & Roebuck
Player, Dr P ....Northridge
Plumpton, Dr H P ....Albert Road
Plumpton, Dr H P ....Turkey Road
Pronger, Dr E ....Silver Springs
Radia, Dr K..................Beaconsfield Road
Rajbee, Dr T Y ....Little Ridge Ave
Rice-Oxley, Dr C P................Martins Oak
Rivett, Dr J G ....Martins Oak
Roche, Dr D ....Belmont
Roche, Dr D ....Ticehurst
Rowan, Dr J ....Roebuck
Sapper, Dr M E......................South Saxon
Schneider, Dr R K ....Silver Springs
Schofield, Dr R.......................... Sea Road
Seal, Dr P L ....Wellington Square
Searson, Dr J ....Warrior Square
Sengupta, Dr G ....Essenden Road
Sharma, Dr R ....Sea Road
Shepherd, Dr M A W ....Warrior Square
Singh, Dr G ....Collington
Singh, Dr G ....Ninfield
Sitwell, Dr I A H ....Little Common
Southward, Dr S P.......................Sea Road
Sparkes, Dr R.............Sedlescombe House
Stern, Dr S R.........................Sedlescombe
Stern, Dr S R.............................Westfield
Taggart, Dr G E.....................Postern Gate
Tate, Dr P M ....Carisbrooke
Thomson, Dr A G.........Bexhill Old Town
Thomson, Dr S R.............Little Common
Van der Plas, Dr F ....Wish Valley
Walter, Dr N R.......................Albert Road
Walter, Dr N R.....................Turkey Road
Warden, Dr D J ....Collington
Wilcox, Dr G G E................Harold Road
Wong, Dr M ....Lower Glen
Wong, Dr M K Y ....Lower Glen
Wood, Dr A ....North Ridge
Woodgate, Dr J E..........................Fairfield
Young, Dr A J.......................Silver Springs

[May 2000]

GPs Surgeries - by town

If you are not sure which surgeries are in your area, the following list shows the surgeries arranged by town.

Battle.........................Martins Oak Surgery
Bexhill ....Albert Road Surgery
Bexhill ....Bexhill Old Town
Bexhill ....Buckhurst Road Surgery
Bexhill ....Collington Surgery
Bexhill..................Little Common Surgery
Bexhill.............................Sea Road Surgery
Bexhill.......................Turkey Road Surgery
Brede ....Brede Surgery
Burwash...........................Fairfield Surgery
Guestling........................Guestling Surgery
Hastings/St Leon ....Battle Road
Hastings/St Leon ....Beaconsfield
Hastings/St Leon ....Carisbrooke
Hastings/St Leon ....Churchwood
Hastings/St Leon....................Essenden Rd
Hastings/St Leon.......................Harold Rd
Hastings/St Leon ....Little Ridge
Hastings/St Leon Lower Glen Family Pract
Hastings/St Leon........................Priory Rd
Hastings/St Leon ....Roebuck
Hastings/St Leon.........Sedlescombe House
Hastings/St Leon ....Shankill
Hastings/St Leon..................Silver Springs
Hastings/St Leon ....South Saxon Hse
Hastings/St Leon ....Stone Street
Hastings/St Leon ....Warrior Squ
Hastings/St Leon...........Wellington Square
Hawkhurst.............................North Ridge
Hawkhurst ....Wish Valley
Ninfield...........................Ninfield Surgery
Northiam ....Northiam Surgery
Robertsbridge ....Oldwood Surgery
Rye ....Cinque Ports
Rye.......................................Postern Gate
Sedlescombe ....Sedlescombe
Ticehurst ....Ticehurst Surgery
Wadhurst ....Belmont Surgery
Westfield ....Westfield Surgery

GPs Surgeries - by name

Here is listed the GPs' surgeries and medical practices in the Hastings and Rother region. For convenience they are arranged by the name of the surgery. If you aren't sure which surgeries are in your area, please refer to the table above which shows which surgeries are in each area.

Albert Road, Bexhill

Dr S M Ashby

Dr J C R Eaton

Dr J H Emmanuel

Dr H Kinch

Dr D Kremer

Dr D J Lawton

Dr D N Newell

Dr H Plumpton

Dr N R Walter

Practice manager: Mrs Haslett. *Address*: 24, Albert Road, Bexhill, Sussex, TN40 1DG. *Tel*: 01424 730456. *Fax*: 01424 734430. May 2000

Battle Road, St Leonards

Dr P A Mehta

Practice manager: Mrs Mowat. *Address*: 355, Battle Road, St. Leonards, Sussex, TN37 7BE. *Tel*: 01424 851706. *Fax*: 01424 853210. May 2000

Beaconsfield Road, Hastings

Dr K Radia

Dr D Janes

Practice manager: Mrs C Bowditch. *Times*: Mondays to Fridays 8.30 to 6.30; Saturdays 8.30 to 12.30. *Address*: The Surgery, 21, Beaconsfield Road, Hastings, Sussex, TN34 3TW. *Tel*: 01424 422389. *Fax*: 01424 531500. Mar 2000

Belmont, Wadhurst

Dr A J Collis

Dr A M T Blackburn

Dr C M Offord

Dr D Roche

Practice manager: Mrs Pilbeam. *Address*: Belmont Surgery, St James' Square, Wadhurst, Sussex, TN5 6BJ. *Tel*: 01892 782121. *Fax:* 01892 783989. Jul 2000

Bexhill Old Town

Dr W L Hawley

Dr L A A Hadley

Dr A Thomson

Dr J Gonzalez

Practice manager: Tricia Busbridge. *Address*: Bexhill Old Town Surgery, 13, De la Warr Road, Bexhill, Sussex, TN40 2HG. *Tel*: 01424 219323. *Fax*: 733940. May 2000

Brede Surgery

Dr J F Dinwiddie

Practice manager: Linda Cox. *Times*: Mondays & Tuesdays 8.30 to 1.00; Wednesdays 2.00 to 6.30; Thursdays & Fridays 8.30 to 1.00. There is wheelchair access. *Address*: The Surgery, Reedswood Road, Broad Oak, Brede, Sussex, TN31 6DH. *Tel*: 01424 882394. *Fax:* 01424 882827. Jul 2000

Buckhurst Road, Bexhill

Dr Y Al-Ansary

Address: 7, Buckhurst Road, Bexhill, Sussex, TN40 1QF. *Tel*: 01424 214757. *Fax*: 01424 733811. May 2000

Carisbrooke House, St Leon.

Dr N McCarthy

Qualifications: MB., ChB., (Liverpool 1977), DRCOG, DOccMed. FHSA list Minor Surgery. Maternity. Child Health

Surveillance. Trainer in General Practice. Local GP tutor. Diploma in Occ. Health.

Dr Elizabeth Furley-Smith
Qualifications: MB., BS. BSc, (London 1983), DRCOG, FHSA list Minor Surgery. Maternity. Child Health Surveillance. Family Planning Certificate.

Dr Patricia M Tate
Qualifications: MB., BS. BSc Hons. (London, 1970). DRCOG. FHSA list Minor surgery. Maternity. Child Health Surveillance. Family Planning Certificate.

Dr Robert A Cameron-Wood
Qualifications: MB., BS., (London, 1990), DRCOG, MRCGP. FHSA list Minor Surgery, Maternity, Child Health Surveillance.

Health visitor: Mrs Lizzie Buckley. Practice Manager: Mrs D Reddie. *Times*: Mondays 8.30am to 12 noon and 2.30 to 6.30pm; Tuesdays to Fridays 8.30am to 12 noon and 2.00 to 6.00pm. Closed 12 noon to 2pm. Open Saturday mornings for emergencies only 9 to 10am by appointment. Closed Sundays.

Appointments: please telephone 01424 432925 between 9am and 12 noon or between 2 and 5pm, or simply call at the surgery. Emergencies: please telephone 01424 422864 or 423190, any time. Emergency calls outside surgery hours are automatically transferred to 'Seadoc', a co-operative of local GPs working on a rota system.

Well Person Check: All patients aged from 5 to 75 are eligible for a 'Well Person Check'. There is good access for the disabled at the surgery and all clinical rooms are on a single level and a disabled toilet is provided.

Address: Carisbrooke House, Stockleigh Road, St. Leonards, Sussex, TN38 0JP. *Tel*: 01424 423190 or 422864. *Admin:* 01424 432280. *Fax*: 01424 460473. Health visitor: 01424 01424 448120. May 2000

Churchwood Medical Practice

Dr Emlyn Jones
Qualifications: MB BS MRCGP DRCOG

Dr Michael Heber
Qualifications: MB BS MRCGP DRCOG

Dr Mark Freeman
Qualifications: MA BM BCh MRCGP DCH

Practice manager: Mrs Christine Smith. *Address*: Churchwood Community Surgery, Tilebarn Road, St Leonards, Sussex, TN38 9QU. *Tel*: 01424 853888. *Fax*: 01424 850190. May 2000

Cinque Ports House, Rye

Dr M S W Jeelani

Dr R A Jeelani

Practice manager: Karen Osborne. Practice nurse: Janet Sinclair. *Times*: Mondays to Fridays 8.30 to 5.30; Saturdays 9.00 to 10.00am. There is wheelchair access. *Address*: Cinque Ports House, Cinque Ports Street, Rye, Sussex, TN31 7AN. *Tel*: 01797 223230. *Fax*: 01797 227234. Mar 2000

Collington Surgery, Bexhill

Dr G Singh

Dr D Warden

Practice manager: Mrs Jill Jarrett. *Address*: Collington Surgery, 23, Terminus Road, Bexhill, Sussex TN39 3LR. *Tel*: 01424 217465. *Fax*: 01424 216675. 5297

Cornwallis Gardens

Details of this surgery withheld at the request of the practitioner. May 2000

Essenden Rd, St Leonards

Dr G Sengupta

Dr D Kinloch

Practice manager: Annette Tayan. *Times*: Mondays 8.30am to 6.30pm; Tuesdays 8.30am to 5.30pm; Wednesdays 8.30am to 6.30pm; Thursdays 8.30am to 12 noon, closed pm; Fridays 8.30am to 6.30pm; Saturdays 9.00 to10.00am emergencies only. Closed for lunch from noon to 2pm. There is wheelchair access.

Address: 49, Essenden Road, St Leonards, Sussex, TN38 ONN. *Tel*: 01424 720866. *Fax*: 01424 445580. May 2000

Fairfield Surgery, Burwash

Dr J Woodgate

Dr B Packham

Practice manager: Stephen Fowler. *Address:* Fairfield Surgery, High Street, Burwash, Etchingham, Sussex, TN19 7EU. *Tel*: 01435 882306. *Fax*: 01435 882064. Mar 2000

Guestling Surgery

Dr Chris Chinery

Dr Linda Parker

Surgery: Purpose built, with a large car park. This is a dispensing practice. Practice nurse, Mrs Chinery.*Times*: Mondays 8.30 to 11.00am; Tuesdays 9 to11.00am; Wednesdays 4.00 to 6.00 p.m.; Fridays 8.30 to 11.00am by appointment. *Address*: Guestling Surgery, Chapel Lane, Guestling, Sussex, TN35 4HN. *TelFax*: 01424 814332. May 2000

Harold Road, Hastings

Dr R E Chisholm-Batten

Dr A C Head

Dr G G E Wilcox

Dr I Horsley

Dr P Dhalla

Practice managers: Mrs Williams; Mrs S Fairbrother. *Address*: Harold Road Surgery, 164, Harold Road, Hastings, Sussex, TN35 5NH. *Tel*: 01424 720878. *Fax*: 01424 719525. 5315

Little Common, Bexhill

Dr P D Dewhurst

Dr T Maxwell

Dr I Sitwell

Dr S Thomson

Practice Manager: Judy Coates. *Times*: Mondays to Fridays 8.30am to 12.30pm & 2.00 to 6.30pm. *Address*: 82, Cooden Sea Road, Little Common, Bexhill, Sussex, TN39 4SP. *Tel*: 01424 845477. *Fax*: 01424 848225. May 2000

Little Ridge, St Leonards

Dr T Rajbee

Practice manager: Mrs Rajbee. *Address*: The Surgery, 38, Little Ridge Avenue, St Leonards, Sussex, TN37 7LS. *Tel*: 01424 755355. *Fax*: 01424 755560. May 2000

Lower Glen Family Practice

Dr Peter Bryden

Qualifications: B.Sc MB BS MRCGP DGM

Dr Monica Wong

Qualifications: MB BS, DRCOG, DFFP.

Quality Manager: Mrs Sharon Hitchman. *Times*: Mondays to Thursdays 8.00am to 6.30pm; Fridays 8.30am to 6.30; Saturdays 8.30am to12 noon emergencies only - telephone first. There is wheelchair access.

Address: Lower Glen Family Practice, 174, Lower Glen Road, St Leonards, Sussex, TN37 7AR. *Tel*: 01424 721616 (general enquiries, visits and emergencies); 01424 852270 (appointments only). *Fax*: 01424 854812.

E-mail: lglen@bryden.clara.net

Website: home.clara.net/bryden/lglen May 2000

Martins Oak, Battle

Dr C P Rice-Oxley

Dr J Mogan

Dr J Rivett

Dr R C A Clarke

Practice manager: Anne Edmead. *Address*: Martins Oak Surgery, 36, High Street,

Battle, Sussex, TN33 OEA. *Tel*: 01424 772263. *Fax*: 01424 775569. Mar 2000

Ninfield Surgery

Dr I Kemm

Dr G Singh

Practice Manager: Julia Scotcher. *Address*: The Surgery, High Street, Ninfield, Battle, Sussex TN33 9JP. *Tel*: 01424 892569. *Fax*: 01424 893233. May 2000

Northiam Surgery

Dr J Carroll

Dr J F Dinwiddie

Dr P M James

Practice Manager: Linda Cox. *Times*: Mondays to Thursdays 8.30am to 6.45pm; Fridays 8.30am to 5.00pm; Saturdays 9.00 to 11.30am. There is wheelchair access. *Address*: The Surgery, Main Street, Northiam, Rye, Sussex, TN31 6ND. *Tel*: 01797 252140. *Fax*: 01797 252077. May 2000

North Ridge, Hawkhurst

Dr C J R Lewis

Dr P V Player

Dr Ann Wood

Dr R J Blundell

Practice manager: Miss L Adamson. *Address*: North Ridge, Rye Road, Hawkhurst, Kent, TN18 4EX. *Tel*: 01580 753935. May 2000

Oldwood, Robertsbridge

Dr E Elliot-Pyle

Practice manager: P. Golding. *Address:* Oldwood Surgery, Station Road, Robertsbridge, Sussex, TN32 5DG. *Tel:* 01580 880790. May 2000

Postern Gate, Rye

Dr H B J Chishick

Dr N J Ferguson

Dr A Griffin

Dr G E Taggart

Practice manager: Mrs Shirley Harris. *Address:* Postern Gate, Cinque Ports Street, Rye, Sussex, TN31 7AP. *Tel:* 01797 223333 / 224924. *Fax*: 01797 226858. May 2000

Priory Road, Hastings

Dr P Das

Qualifications: MB.B.S (Cal. 1960), FRCS (Edin. 1969). Male.

Practice manager: Mrs Godden. Practice nurse: Sr. Heather Henry. Clinics available: Asthma; Chiropody; Diabetes; Family Planning; Hypertension/Chd; Minor surgery; Smokers Clinic. The surgery provides disabled access.

Consultation times: Mondays: 8.30 to 10.30 am and 4.15 to 6.15pm. Tuesdays: as Mondays. Wednesdays: 8.30 to 10am, closed in afternoon. Thursdays and Fridays: as Mondays. Saturdays: emergencies only rota system. Sundays: closed.

Emergencies: between the hours of 7pm and 7am, the emergency cover is by 'Hastings & Bexhill Doctors on Call'. *Address*: The Surgery, 83, Priory Road, Hastings, Sussex, TN34 3JJ. *Tel*: 01424 430800. *Fax*: 01424 465555. Mar 2000

Roebuck House, Hastings

Dr Chris Chinery

Qualifications: LRCP, MRCS, MBBS, DRCOG. Dr Chinery works from Roebuck Surgery and Guestling Surgery. *Tel:* 01424 452802 (Roebuck); 01424 814332 (Guestling). 0532

Dr John Rowan

Qualifications: MBChB, DRCOG, MRCGP. Qualified in Leeds University Medical College in 1976. *Tel:* 01424 452801 (Roebuck Surgery).

Dr David Dutchman

Qualified at St George's Hospital in 1978. Qualifications: MBBS, MRCGP, DCH, DRCOG. *Tel:* 01424 452803 (Roebuck Surgery).

Dr Sally Paget
Qualifications: MBBS, MRCP (UK), MRCGP. Qualified at Guy's Hospital in 1981. *Tel:* 01424 452804 (Roebuck Surgery). May 2000

Dr Andrew Dunfield-Prayero
Qualified at Manchester in 1989. Qualifications: BSc, MBChB, MRCGP, DCH, DRCOG, DFFP. *Tel:* 01424 452800 (Roebuck Surgery).

Dr Linda Parker
Qualifications: MB, B.Chir.,MA (Cantab.), DCH, DRCOG, MRCGP, DFFP. *Tel:* 01424 452802 (Roebuck Surgery). May 2000

Dr Rosita Kyu
Qualifications: MBBS, DA. *Tel:* 01424 452804. May 2000

Roebuck Surgery has five practices, with 7 GPs, all working within one building, each doctor having his own staff. This enables a personal service to be given to all patients.

The staff for each doctor are available Mondays to Fridays from 8.30 am to 1.00 pm and 2.00 to 5.00 pm. Saturdays: emergency surgery 8.30am to 12.30pm. Emergency service: Mondays to Fridays 5.00 to 7.00 pm covered by duty doctor. Emergencies out of surgery hours are covered by Seadoc. The surgery is purpose built with lift access to all floors. Practice manager: Mrs G Brooks.
Address: Roebuck House, High Street, Old Town, Hastings, Sussex, TN34 3EY. *Tel*: 01424 420378; *Fax*: 01424 452821; *Emergencies*: 01424 420378. Mar 2000

Sea Road, Bexhill

Dr R G Elias

Dr R Sharma

Dr S Southward

Practice manager: Kay Davey. *Address*: 39, Sea Road, Bexhill, Sussex. *Tel*: 01424 211616. *Fax*: 01424 733950. May 2000

Sedlescombe Ho, St Leonards

Dr J P J Kaliniecki

Dr R Sparkes

Practice manager: Mrs A Brewer. *Address*: Sedlescombe House, 8, Sedlescombe Road South, St Leonards, Sussex, TN38 OTA. *Tel*: 01424 720574. *Fax*: 01424 440199. Jul 2000

Sedlescombe Surgery

Dr T Jardine-Brown

Dr Steven Stern

Dr C Hargreaves

Practice manager: Mrs Judy Collins. *Address*: The Surgery, Brede Lane, Sedlescombe, Sussex. *Tel*: 01424 870225. *Fax*: 01424 870912. May 2000

Shankill Surgery, Hastings

Dr K M J Francis

Dr G Henry

Dr F Howie

Practice manager: Sarah Farrant. *Address*: Shankhill Surgery, 21, Fairlight Road, Hastings, Sussex, TN35 5ED. *Tel*: 01424 421046. *Fax*: 01424 425177. Jul 2000

Silver Springs, St Leonards

Dr D J Cameron

Dr A Young

Dr R K Schneider

Dr E Pronger

Practice manager: Malcolm Wright. *Times*: Mondays to Fridays 8.30am to 6.30pm; Saturdays 8.30 to10.30am emergencies only. The Practice uses Seadoc. There is wheelchair access. *Address*: Silver Springs Medical Practice, Beaufort Road, St Leonards, Sussex, TN37 6PP. *Tel*: 01424 422300. *Fax*: 436400. *E-mail*: doctors@silverspringssurgery.freeserve.co.uk Jul 2000

South Saxon House, St Leonards

Dr M A Al-Saleem

Dr M Sapper

Practice manager: Mrs Avril Chambers. *Address*: South Saxon House, 150a, Bexhill Road, St Leonards, Sussex, TN38 8BL. *Tel*: 01424 441361. *Fax*: 01424 461799. Jul 2000

St Michael's Hospice

Dr J V Lee

Address: St Michael's Hospice, 25, Upper Maze Hill, St Leonards, Sussex. *Tel*: 01424 445177. *Fax*: 01424 721255. Jul 2000

Stone Street, Hastings

Dr H Nicholson

Practice manager: Marion Nicholson. *Address*: The Surgery, 4, Stone Street, Hastings, Sussex, TN34 1QD. *Tel*: 01424 427015. *Fax*: 01424 427633. May 2000

Ticehurst Surgery

Dr D Roche

Dr C M Offord

Dr A J Collis

Dr A M T Blackburn

Address: Wisteria Cottage, High Street, Ticehurst, Sussex. *Tel*: 01580 200317. Jul 2000

Turkey Road, Bexhill

Dr S M Ashby

Dr J C R Eaton

Dr J H Emmanuel

Dr D Kremer

Dr D J Lawton

Dr D N Newell

Dr H Plumpton

Dr H Kinch

Dr N R Walter

Practice manager: Mrs Haslett. *Address*: 44, Turkey Road, Bexhill, Sussex. *Tel*: 01424 210555. *Fax*: 01424 225615. Jul 2000

Warrior Square, St Leonards

Dr P Herbert

Dr J Searson

Dr M A W Shepherd

Practice manager: Mrs Val Best. *Times:* Mondays to Fridays 8.30am to 12.30pm & 2.30 to 6.00pm. Special services: Counselling; Hypertension Clinic; Family Planning Clinic; Well Woman/Smear Clinic; Diabetes & Asthma Clinics. There is wheelchair access - just one step to manoeuvre. *Address:* Warrior Square Surgery, 1-3 Warrior Square, St Leonards, Sussex, TN37 6BA. *Tel:* 01424 430123. *Fax:* 01424 433706. Jul 2000

Wellington Square, Hastings

Dr T F M Cooper

Dr P. Seal

Dr B Higginson

Dr H E Hughes

Practice manager: Malcolm Wright. Community liaison worker: Rose Fordham. *Address*: Wellington Square Medical Centre, 45 Wellington Square, Hastings, Sussex TN34 1PN. *Tel*: 01424 722366 (Dr Seal); 01424 722866 (Dr Higginson); 01424 722166 (Dr Hughes); 01424 722066 (Dr Cooper). *Faxes*: 01424 718385. May 2000

Westfield Surgery

Dr T Jardine-Brown

Dr Caroline D Hargreaves

Dr Steven Stern

Practice manager: Mrs J Collins. *Address*: The Surgery, Main Road, Westfield, Sussex, TN35 4QE. *Tel*: 01424 751609. *Fax*: 01424 755984. Jul 2000

Wish Valley, Hawkhurst

Dr C R Dewing

Dr F van der Plas

Dr K Vale

Practice manager: Christine Paddock. *Address*: Wish Valley Surgery, Talbot Road, Hawkhurst, Kent TN18 4NB. *Tel*: 01580 753211. May 2000

Local Organisations

Health Visiting

Health Visiting & School Nursing Service. This is the central contact point for Health Visitors, who are based in GP surgeries and clinics. Health Visitors can offer health advice and counselling, including women's health counselling, advice on parenting and post natal depression.

Hours: Mondays to Fridays 9.00am to 5.00pm. Enquiries can be made about Health Visitors either direct, or at surgeries and clinics.

Address: Health Visiting and School Nursing Service, Arthur Blackman Clinic, Battle Road, St Leonards-on-Sea, East Sussex, TN37 7AN. *Tel*: 01424 851225 / 852656. *Fax:* 01424 852745. May 2

Further Information

Netdoctor

This internet service has GMTV's Dr Hilary Jones heading the "ask a doctor service", which enables users to pose their questions and receive answers from a panel of doctors on the site's interactive zone. It includes a psychotherapist for questions on sex and relationships, and an obstetrician.

The site also provides information on diseases and medical conditions, accompanied by full details of symptoms, causes and treatment options and a 'chat room' where visitors can express opinions and discuss medical matters.

Website: www.netdoctor.co.uk 5195

Surgery door

An internet service created by Intouch with Health Limited, which provides touch-screen information kiosks to the NHS. Media doctor Mark Porter is in charge of the editorial content. The site's 'on-line multi-store for health' has a pharmacy and health bookshop. It sells mother and baby products, get-well gifts, cards and healthy foods. *Website:* www.surgerydoor.co.uk 5195

Embarrassing problems

This website, launched by Health Press, was created by Dr Margaret Steam, an Oxford doctor, with advice on over seventy conditions. When many people cannot bring themselves to ask their doctor about sensitive complaints, this website offers a discreet solution. *Tel:* 01235 523233. *Website:*www.embarassingprob lems.co.uk

Planet Medica

"Takes a magazine-style approach, with articles looking at the baby blues, period pains and stress management. Those who cannot tell how ill or unfit they are can visit the Assessment Centre for a quick-and-dirty analysis of their well-being, though the list of ailments is so comprehensive that if you can't find something wrong with you, there must be something wrong with you."

Website: www.planetmedica.co.uk 5213

Which doctor

Website which locates a doctor whose qualifications and specialisms meet your specific requirements. It is not a referral service; a discussion with your own doctor is always required before referral.

Website: www.which-doctor.co.uk

Health Information Service

The HIS is a free and confidential 24-hour service. You can speak to staff during office hours, and you can listen to any of hundreds of tapes at any time, e.g: *Changing your GP* (Tape 029); *Talking to your doctor* (Tape 053). This service is due to be replaced in October 2000 by NHS Direct, see below.

Address: The College of Health, St Margaret's House, 21, Old Ford Road, London, E2 9PL. *Freephone*: 0800 66 55 44. 5367

NHS Direct

NHS Direct will be available locally from October 2000 and is a 24 hour nurse-led, confidential helpline providing advice and information on what to do if you are feeling ill; health concerns for you or your family; local health services; self-help and support organisations. *Tel:* 0845 4647.
Website: www.nhsdirect.nhs.uk 5928 Jun 2000

Abbreviations.

BCh
B.Chir
BS
BSc Bachelor of Science
ChB Bachelor of Surgery; from Latin 'Chirurgiae Baccalaurens'.
DCH
DFFP
DOccMed
DRCOG
DTM&H
FHSA
FRCS
GP General Practitioner (family doctor).
LRCP
MB Bachelor of Medicine.
MBBS
MBChB
MCh Master of Surgery; from Latin, Magister Chirurgiae.
MD Doctor of Medicine; from Latin, Medicinae Doctor.
MRCGP
MRCP(UK)
MRGS

Acknowledgements
Our grateful thanks to Dr Chris Chinery and staff of Roebuck Surgery for providing editorial assistance with this chapter.

ECT

Everyone remembers the disturbing scenes involving ECT from *One Flew Over The Cuckoo's Nest.* But what are the facts about this controversial treatment?

What is ECT?
ECT (electroconvulsive therapy) is sometimes given to people with severe depression who have not responded to drugs.

It has always been a controversial treatment which some people find helpful but others find extremely distressing and ineffective. ECT involves an electrical current being passed through a person's brain while under a general anaesthetic.

Immediate effects of ECT can include confusion, headache and dizziness. Memory loss is also common but usually temporary.
0534

Dose titration
Electroconvulsive Therapy (ECT) involves the patient being anaesthetised and injected with muscle paralysing drugs to control the violent convulsions that would otherwise occur. Since breathing is inhibted this also requires respiratory support.

Electrodes are placed on the temples and an electric current of a measured strength is applied for a measured time. The purpose of this is to cause a fit to occur. The minimum dose of electricity that will just cause the fit is called the threshold dose. This dose can vary over a range of 1 to 40 between one patient and the next.

The only way to measure a patient's threshold dose is to test for it by giving a series of increasing shocks until a fit occurs. This process is known as dose titration. 6068
Aug 2000

Government survey
A Government ECT survey provides the first reliable statistics in England for ten years. In the first three months of 1999 there were 16,482 administrations of ECT, involving 2,835 people.

This represents a reduction in treatments from 105,466 in 1990-1 to an estimated 65,930 in 1998-9. Over two-thirds of the people having ECT were women, although there was little gender difference among the under 25s.

Forty-one per cent were aged 65 and over (848 women, 328 men). The lower number of men in the population at this age accounts for some of this difference, but in the middle age-groups the rate for women is almost twice that for men.

Ninety-six per cent of those whose ethnic origin was reported were white (higher than their 93 per cent representation in the general population) but for eight per cent the ethnic origin was not known or not given.

Twenty-five per cent of people receiving ECT were formal patients under the Mental Health Act. Of these, 59 per cent did not consent to treatment, rising to 71 per cent of those treated as emergencies are added in.

Analysed by NHS regional office areas, London has the lowest rate of use of ECT (3.7 per 100,000 population), the North West the highest (7.1). Four per cent of treatments were given in private facilities.

[Electro Convulsive Therapy: Survey

Covering the Period from January 1999 to March 1999, England. Bulletin 1999/22, Department of Health. Available from DoH, PO Box 777, London SE1 6XH. [5110]

ECT - some facts

Although there has been a reduction in use, 10,000 people a year are still prescribed ECT in this country. [1571]

Wales has the second highest rate of ECT use in Europe. A survey in Wales found that 90% of people who had ECT were improved or much improved following treatment. [1571]

It has been argued that the risk of serious unwanted effects is small compared with the 15% lifetime risk of suicide in people who are depressed. [1571]

It is recognised that careful monitoring of local use of ECT is needed. [5993]

Organisations

ECT Anonymous

This organisation campaigns vigorously *against* the use of ECT and publishes numerous leaflets and newsletters to support its case. Phone or write for further information. *Contact:* Pat Butterfield. Office hours are 10am to 3pm Tuesdays and Wednesdays and 10am to 2pm Thursdays.

Address: ECT Anonymous, 14, Western Avenue, Riddlesden, Keighley, West Yorkshire, BD20 5DJ. *Tel:* 01535 661493. *Fax:* 01535 602736.
E-mail: ect.anon@ndirect.co.uk 6033, Jan 2000; July 2000

Self-help Groups

For enquiries about ECT self-help groups please contact Una Parker. *Address:* Una Parker, 8, Wenthill Close, Ackworth, Pontefract, WF7 7LP. *Tel:* 01977 704659. 6086 Aug 2000

Further Information

ECT Anonymous

This organisation publishes a number of information sheets on ECT, see above.

ECT

'Making Sense of Treatments & Drugs - ECT'. A 32-page booklet published by Mind, 1995. Contents include: What is ECT used for? What ECT involves. How effective is ECT? Adverse effects. ECT and consent. Available from Mind. *Tel:* 020 8221 9666.

See also these chapters ...

Mental Health Act for details of ECT use.

Health Authorities & NHS Trusts

National Health Service

The NHS is probably the largest organisation in Europe, employing a million people and receiving billions of pounds from the Government each year.

The Department of Health is the government department responsible for the National Health Service. The NHS is divided into a number of regions, one of which is the NHS South East Region.

This body in turn is subdivided into various Health Authorities, one of which is the East Sussex, Brighton and Hove Health Authority (ESBHHA), see below. And within the ESBHHA are six primary care groups and six NHS Trusts, see below. which are responsible for most of the hospital and community NHS services for local people.

Alan Milburn is the Secretary of State for Health. Appointed 11th October 1999.

Health Improvement Programme

During the summer of 1999, many people across the county discussed what action was needed to confront the causes of ill health, including poverty, deprivation and social exclusion.

Conferences were held in Hastings and in Rother, where people from the statutory, voluntary and private sectors discussed what they felt were the local priorities for improving health and agreed areas for joint action that could improve the health of local people.

The Plan charts a course for the health and social services for East Sussex, Brighton and Hove. It sets out some of the actions which have been agreed to improve health, reduce health inequalities and modernise services. National priorities include improvements to mental health and modernisation of the NHS.

Local priorities include improved partnership working to improve health and well-being. The action to be agreed includes areas of mental health, substance misuse and families under stress.

The HImP was published in 2000. To obtain a copy of the current HImP please contact Zoe Nicholson. *Address*: East Sussex, Brighton and Hove Health Authority, 36-38, Friars Walk, Lewes, Sussex, BN7 2PB. *Tel*: 01273 485300. Jun 2000

Joint Investment Plan

JIPs came about through the government's White Paper 'Better Services for vulnerable people' and will eventually take the place of Community Care Plans. They are basically templates for what the commissioners (Health & Social Services) plan to spend their money on. 5362, 5404

ESBHHA

EAST SUSSEX, BRIGHTON AND HOVE
Health Authority

The East Sussex, Brighton and Hove Health Authority, (ESBHHA) and primary groups are responsible for improving the health of the local population, and ensuring that appropriate, high quality health care services are in place which respond to the health needs of local people. Members of ESBHHA are:

Chairman. . . . . John Lewis
Chief exec. . . . . Alan Bedford
Public health . . . . Dr Graham Bickler
Mental health . . . . David Fordham
Performance . . . . Steve Phoenix
Finance . . . . Ronald Marshall

Development . . . . Kate Money
Health improvement. . . . . Zoe Nicholson

Address: East Sussex, Brighton and Hove Health Authority, 36-38, Friars Walk, Lewes, Sussex, BN7 2PB. *Tel:* 01273 485300. *Fax:* 01273 485400, minicom: 01273 403590. *E-mail:* nhs@esbhhealth.cix.co.uk
Website: www.esbhhealth.ndirect.co.uk
5090 May 2000

Emergency Services
Free leaflets are available on the local NHS emergency health services from East Sussex, Brighton and Hove Health Authority Communications Department. *Tel*: 01273 403550 during office opening hours. *Website*: www.healthesussex.co.uk Jul 2000

Mental Health Promotion

Mental Health Promotion aims to enhance mental well-being and positive attitudes to mental health. It is not simply about promoting individual mental ill-health, but is also about addressing the structures and processes that influence mental health. The Health Authority's Health Promotion Department has two Mental Health Promotion Advisers who work with other agencies in the community to achieve mental health improvement. They work across Hastings and Rother, as well as the rest of East Sussex, Brighton and Hove.

Martina Pickin
Mental Health Team Co-ordinator. *Address:* Brighton Health Promotion Office, Ivory Place, Morley Street, Brighton, Sussex. *Tel:* 01273 703100. *E-mail:* hpbrighton@mistral.co.uk Jun 2000

Barbara Hardcastle
Health Promotion Advisor (Mental Health). *Address:* Eastbourne & Wealden Health Promotion Office, Centenary House, The Avenue, Eastbourne, East Sussex, BN21 3XY. Tel: 01323 430003. Fax: 01323 644687. E-mail: hpeastbourne@mistral.co.uk May 2000

Hastings office
Address: Hastings & Rother Health Promotion Office, 3rd Floor, Hanover House, Marine Court, St Leonards-on-Sea, Sussex, TN38 0DX. *Tel:* 01424 441933. *Fax:* 01424 433776. *E-mail:* hphastings@mistral.co.uk Jul 2000

NHS Trusts

The six NHS Trusts within the East Sussex, Brighton & Hove Health Authority are:

Brighton

Address: Brighton Health Care NHS Trust, The Royal Sussex County Hospital, Eastern Road, Brighton, BN2 5BE. *Tel*: 01273 696955. *Fax*: 01273 626653. Jul 2000

Eastbourne & County

Address: Eastbourne & County Healthcare NHS Trust, Bowhill, The Drive, Hellingly, Sussex, BN27 4EP. *Tel:* 01323 440022. *Fax:* 01323 842868. Jul 2000

Eastbourne Hospitals

Address: Eastbourne Hospitals NHS Trust, Eastbourne District General Hospital, Kings Drive, Eastbourne, Sussex, BN21 2UD. *Tel*: 01323 417400. *Fax*: 01323 414966. Jul 2000

Hastings & Rother

Mental Health Directorate
The Mental Health Directorate acts as the main contact point for all enquiries concerning mental health services provided by the Hastings & Rother NHS Trust. *Hours:* 8.30am to 5.00pm. Jul 2000

Anna Barnes
Project manager, Mental Health.

Margaret Brett
She was appointed by the Secretary of State for Health as chairman of the Hastings & Rother NHS Trust. She is a qualified nurse

and a senior lecturer at South Bank University. [5321]

Michael Birkett
Clinical Director, Mental Health Services. [Jul 2000]

Sarah Holmes-Smith
Director of Mental Health Services. All mental health staff including nurses are ultimately managed by Sarah Holmes-Smith. [5913 Aug 2000]

Address: Mental Health Directorate, Hastings & Rother NHS Trust, St Anne's House, 729, The Ridge, St Leonards-on-Sea, East Sussex, TN37 7PT. *Tel:* 01424 754889. *Fax:* 01424 754263. [5913 Jun 2000]

Sussex Ambulance

Address: Sussex Ambulance Service NHS Trust, 40-42, Friars Walk, Lewes, Sussex, BN7 2XW. *Tel*: 01273 489444. *Fax*: 01273 489445.

South Downs

Address: South Downs Health NHS Trust, Brighton General Hospital, Elm Grove, Brighton, Sussex, BN2 3EW. *Tel*: 01273 696011. *Fax*: 01273 693812. [Jul 2000]

National Organisations

NHS Confederation

Registered charity formed 1997 when NAHAT (National Association of Health Authorities & Trusts) and the NHS Trust Federation merged. Chief executive: Stephen Thornton. "We are uniquely placed to be the voice of NHS management, as the only membership body for all NHS organisations. Our members include over 95% of NHS trusts, health authorities, health boards and health and social services boards."

Address: NHS Confederation, 26, Chapter Street, London, SW1P 4ND. *Tel*: 020 7233 7388. *E-mail:* suzanne.hughes@confed.co.uk Website: www.nhsconfed.net [5405]

NHS Direct

NHS Direct will be available locally from October 2000 and is a 24-hour nurse-led, confidential helpline providing advice and information on what to do if you are feeling ill; health concerns for you or your family; local health services; self-help and support organisations. *Tel:* 0845 4647.
Website: www.nhsdirect.nhs.uk [5928]

Acknowlegements
Our grateful thanks to Anna Barnes, Mental Health Project Worker, and Madeline Mayhew, ESBHHA, for editorial assistance with this chapter.

Hospitals & Clinics

Here are listed in alphabetical order, the hospitals, clinics and day hospitals mainly in the Hastings and Rother region, but including some from outside the area. Both private and NHS units are included. For GPs' surgeries please see the 'Doctors' chapter, page 307.

Amberstone

Eastbourne & County Health Care NHS Trust. Mental health rehabilitation unit for working age adults. *Contact:* Gareth Miller, Charge Nurse.

Address: Amberstone, Carters Corner, Hailsham, East Sussex, BN27 4HU. *Tel:* 01323 444104. *Fax:* 01323 844676. Jul 2000

Arthur Blackman Clinic

Hours: Mondays to Fridays 8.30am to 5.00pm. Plus some evening services.

Address: Battle Road, St. Leonards-on-Sea, East Sussex, TN37 7AN. *Tel:* 01424 851225 and 852656. *Fax:* 01424 852745. Jul 2000

Bexhill Health Centre

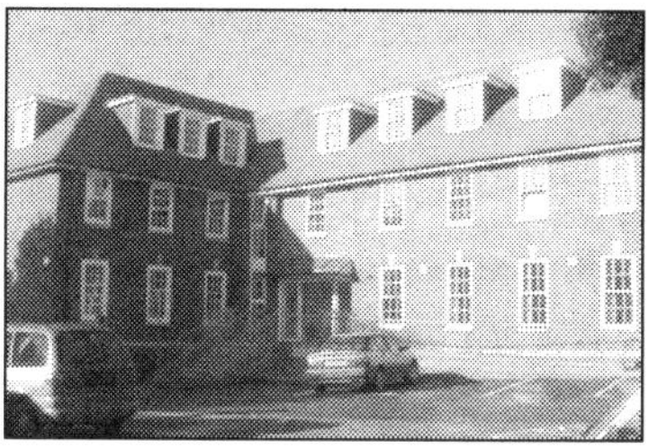

Opened in March 2000, this £1m building was in fact a nurses' home, built in the 1930s, which had lain vacant for some years. The first floor provides a base for the Bexhill Community Mental Health team and a venue for Mental Health out-patient services including input from occupational therapists, community mental health nurses, psychiatrist, and psychologist.

Address: Bexhill Health Centre, Holliers Hill, Bexhill, Sussex, TN40 2DZ. *Tel:* 01424 735608; *Fax:* 01424 735609 (for Bexhill Mental Health Services); 01424 735606 (for Bexhill Clinic Reception). 6032 Mar 2000; Jul 2000

Bexhill Hospital

Facilities include Day Surgery Unit, Out patient Department, Physiotherapy, Radiology, Renal Unit and Irvine Unit with 49 beds and a Day Hospital service.

Address: Bexhill Hospital or Irvine Unit, Holliers Hill, Bexhill, Sussex, TN40 2DZ. *Tel:* 01424 730077. *Fax:* 01424 213250. May 2000

League of Friends

The League of Friends provided £300,000 towards the cost of the Bexhill Health Centre. *Address:* Mr N Bennett, The League of Friends of the Bexhill Hospital, 14, Hartfield Road, Cooden, Sussex. *Tel:* 01424 843268. 5321

BUPA Hospital, Hastings

Consultant Psychiatrist: Dr C. Ramachander; Clinical Psychologist: Dr M. Bowles; Sexual Dysfunction therapist: Mrs D. Palmer; General Manager: Linda Dineen; Business Development Manager: Judith Bonner. Private hospital out-patient clinics to named consultants or counsellors.

Address: BUPA Hospital Hastings, The Ridge, St Leonards-on-Sea, East Sussex, TN37 7RE. *Hours:* Mondays to Fridays 8.00am to 8.00pm. *Tel:* 01424 757400. *Fax:* 01424 757424. *E-mail:* hastingshosp@bupa.com *Website:* www.bupa.com 5200 May 2000

Conquest Hospital

The Conquest Hospital opened for business in July 1992 and provides specialist facilities for out-patient consultations, departments to help in the diagnosis and treatment of illnesses, theatres and an Accident & Emergency department. The BUPA wing was added by the end of 1997. Chief executive: Mr Geoffrey Haynes.

Mental health

The mental health 'wing' of the Conquest Hospital is Woodlands, please see separate entry, page 327.

Address: Conquest Hospital, The Ridge, St Leonards, Sussex, TN37 7RD. *Tel:* 01424 755255. Accident and emergency 24-hour helpline: 01424 758106. 6035 Jul 2000

Conquest Hospital League of Friends

The aim of the League of Friends is to raise funds for equipment and services for the benefit of patients and staff in the Hospital. *Contacts:* Mr Ken Clarke, chairman; Mrs Jean Harman, membership secretary.

Address: League of Friends, Conquest Hospital, The Ridge, St Leonards on Sea, TN37 7RD. *Tel:* 01424 772471. Jun 2000

Eastbourne Clinic

Private psychiatric clinic offering in-patient, day-patient and out-patient care for all psychological disorders. Accredited by the major health insurance companies, services offered include all single rooms, most with en-suite facilities; separate mother and baby unit; friendly day hospital. *Contact:* Julia Wood, Clinic Manager.

Address: The Eastbourne Clinic, 21, Grange Road, Eastbourne, East Sussex, BN21 4HE. *Tel:* 01323 430831. 5497
Fax: 01323 320832. Jul 2000

Eastbourne District Gen Hospital

Address: Eastbourne District General Hospital, Kings Drive, Eastbourne., East Sussex. *Tel:* 01323 417400.
May 2000

Eversfield Hospital

All calls to Conquest Hospital. *Tel:* 01424 755255. Note: We are advised that the League of Friends is in the process of being wound up. 5353

Godden Green Clinic

Godden Green Clinic is a private psychiatric clinic set high in the Kentish Weald providing a high quality environment and excellent clinical care for all manner of psychological and emotional problems. They believe that an eclectic approach to emotional problems is the best form of care when individuals are in a vulnerable state and they make a conscious effort to evolve a tailor-made treatment plan for each individual.

Services

The Clinic offers out-patient, day-patient and in-patient care in addition to a day hospital with a range of services and a programme of groups. Treatment is available for the following psychological and emotional problems: depression, stress/anxiety management, obsessive-compulsive disorders, alcohol and substance abuse, post traumatic stress disorder, psychological assessment, phobias, elderly assessment, eating disorders, psychosomatic disorders and counselling.

24 hours emergency and admissions. *Contacts:* Vicky McNally, Hospital Director; Rick Lord, Director of Nursing. Part of Cygnet Health Care, plc. Staff includes Dr Bott, psychiatrist.

Address: Godden Green Clinic, Godden Green, Sevenoaks, Kent, TN15 0JR. *Tel:* 01732 763491. *Fax:* 01732 763160. *E-mail:* vickymcnal
ly@cygnethealth.co.uk 5510; 5198

Maidstone Hospital

Address: Maidstone Hospital, General wing, (all depts.) Hermitage Lane, Maidstone, Kent, ME16 9QQ. *Tel:* 01622 729000. *Fax:* 01622 224114 (gen. admin.) Jul 2000

Memorial Care Centre, Rye

Chairman: John Stevenson; Administrator:

Tony Pickett; Fund-raising Administrator: Ann Hostler. *Address:* Peasmarsh Road, Rye, East Sussex, TN31 7UD. *Tel:* 01797 223810. [May 2000]

New Wealden Clinic

Address: New Wealden Clinic, 1, Clayfield Mews, Newcomen Road, Tunbridge Wells, Kent, TN4 9PA. *Tel/Fax:* 01892 545443. [Jul 2000]

Ore Clinic

A wide range of services is available at the clinic as an alternative to those delivered within GP surgeries or local hospital. Hours: Mondays to Fridays 8.30am to 5.00pm. Plus some evening services. Ore clinic is closed for refurbishment until approximately September/October 2000. *Contact:* Babs Martin, Clinic Manager.

Address: Ore Clinic, 407, Old London Road, Hastings, TN35 5BH. *Tel:* 01424 420801. [May 2000]

Pembury Hospital

Address: Maidstone & Tunbridge Wells NHS Trust, Pembury Hospital, Tonbridge Road, Pembury, Kent, TN2 4QJ. *Tel:* 01892 823535. *Fax:* 01892 824267 (gen. admin.) [Jul 2000]

Priory Ticehurst Hospital

Private hospital specialising in adult, adolescent mental health-care, including self-harm and brain injury trauma.

Hospital director: David Anderson; acute services manager: Michael Byrne; trauma services manager: Jayne Gibb; adolescent services manager: Tina Irwin; bed bureau manager: Beau Cackett. *Contacts:* Jane Bacon, Marketing manager; Beau Cackett, bed bureau manager.

Address: The Priory Ticehurst Hospital, Ticehurst, Nr Wadhurst, Sussex, TN5 7HU. *Tel:* 01580 200391. *Fax:* 01580 201006. *E-mail:* bcackett@whc.co.uk *Website:* www.prioryhealthcare.co.uk [May 2000]

Queen Charlotte's Hospital

Opened 1986, closed 16th December 1999, when all staff and patients moved to Woodlands, at the Conquest Hospital.

All calls to Woodlands, *tel:* 01424 755255.

St Anne's Centre

Day Hospital. *Address:* St Anne's Centre, The Ridge, St Leonards-on-Sea, East Sussex. *Tel:* 01424 755255. *Fax:* 01424 757061. [Jul 2000]

St Michael's Hospice

Their motto is 'Sharing the caring', providing specialist palliative care to the people of Hastings and Rother. *Address:* St Michael's Hospice, 25, Upper Maze Hill, St Leonards, East Sussex, TN38 0LB. *Tel:* 01424 445177. *Fax:* 01424 721255. Registered Charity No. 288462. [Jul 2000]

Sussex Private Clinic

Private clinic offering in-patient, out-patient and day care for people who have physical and psychological problems. Services include hydrotherapy, physiotherapy and physio gym for physical rehabilitation; all single rooms, most with en-suite bathrooms/shower rooms; additional disabled facilities; separate mother and baby unit. *Contact:* Nichola Cox, Clinic Director. Owned by Eastbourne Clinic.[5497]

Address: The Sussex Private Clinic, 1, Hollington Park Road, St Leonards, Sussex, TN38 0SY. *Tel:* 01424 439439. *Fax:* 01424 718806. [Jul 2000]

Westwood Centre

A mental health centre. *Contacts:* Linda Bishop, Case Management; Maria Jones, Lead Nurse.

Address: Westwood Centre, 7, Holmesdale Gardens, Hastings, Sussex, TN34 1LY. *Tel:* 01424 714366. *Fax:* 01424 439537. [Jul 2000]

Westwood Centre Day Services

We work either individually or in groups, as part of the Day Service, with people experiencing functional difficulties due to mental health problems. Our group programme consists of a variety of practical domestic, creative and work skills groups, anxiety management, support groups and psychosocial groups on a sessional basis. Referrals are accepted via the Mental Health Teams. *Contacts:* Debbie Rimmer and Teresa Frank.

Address: Westwood Centre, 7, Holmesdale Gardens, Hastings, East Sussex. *Tel:* 01424 714366 (ext. 132). [5992]

Westwood Day Hospital

Westwood Day Hospital welcomed its first client on December 16th 1998. The hospital is described as an "intensive multi-disciplinary assessment and treatment centre, offering an alternative to in-patient admission for up to 15 individuals experiencing acute mental health problems."

Its reason for existence is "to prevent and reduce hospital admissions." The staff includes Hugh Maxwell, (charge nurse) and Debbie Rimmer (head occupational therapist). Facilities include a well-equipped woodwork room and a similar sized art room, with good facilities. There is a group work lounge with books and magazines and there is a separate smoking room. Relaxation classes are held every day. Simple meals are provided.

Address: Westwood Day Hospital, Westwood Centre, 7, Homesdale Gardens, Hastings, Sussex, TN34 1LY. *Tel:* 01424 714366. [5992]

My experience of the day hospital

"To begin with I was not keen to go to the day hospital. It was the word 'hospital' that put me off. However, I found it a very useful, supportive and stimulating environment. The staff were helpful, friendly and sympathetic.

The approach is gentle and 'low key'. The exercises help to develop confidence and encourage a positive attitude. It was also good to be part of a group. Sometimes it is helpful to gain support from others who have experienced similar problems.

One does not feel alone and can learn things from other people. It did not feel like a hospital because it was relaxed. If we went outside there was a noticeboard to say where we had gone.

I also liked the 'key worker' nurse system - that was very helpful. I have found the day hospital a very positive support system; it was a good experience." [5058]

'Jacky'

Woodlands

If you are so ill that you have to stay in hospital, Woodlands, our £3.5m brand new, adult mental health unit, offers somewhere bright, pleasant and safe, with private rooms, modern facilities and dedicated professional help to get you well again.

About Woodlands

Woodlands is a mental health unit offering in-patient services for the people in the Hastings & Rother area. [5206]

It opened its doors to patients and staff when Queen Charlotte's Hospital closed in December 1999. The unit contains 33 patient rooms all with en-suite facilities, communal and recreational areas, therapy rooms and office accommodation. There is a courtyard with a water feature, The unit was officially opened on March 24th, 2000, by television celebrity Jo Brand, who used to be a psychiatric nurse. [5212]

Facilities at Woodlands

There is a choice of menu and special diets can be catered for. There is a public pay telephone available for patients' use; a postbox, daily newspapers and books are available. A computer is available for patient use during weekdays. Local shops are within walking distance. Smoking is only allowed in the main quadrangle and in certain rooms. A chaplain visits regularly and your own pastor is welcome if you wish. [5206, 6013 Jul 2000]

Going home

"When you go home, we will try to ensure you get the help and support you need. We will contact your GP, you will have an appointment with a doctor who has been caring for you whilst in hospital, and also a community worker. Prior to discharge we will discuss other necessary arrangements with you and your relatives. On discharge

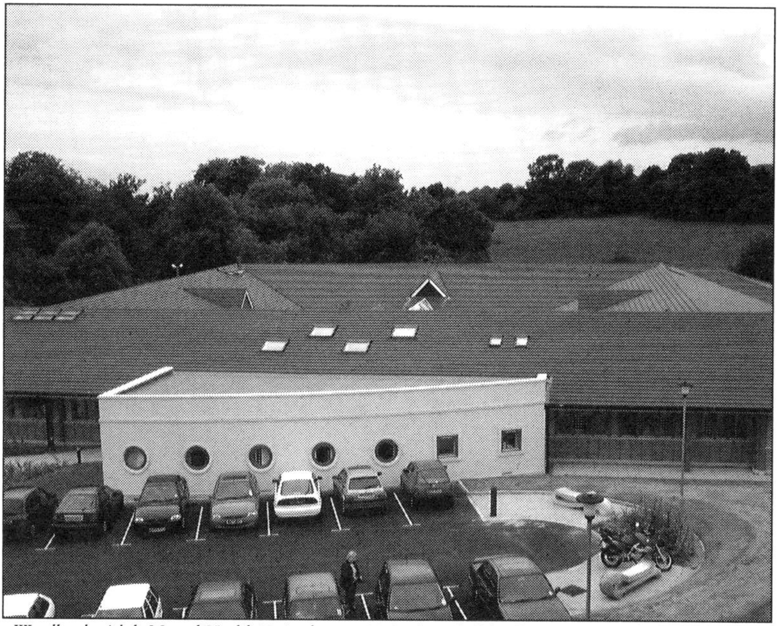

Woodlands, Adult Mental Health Unit, the new £3.5m 'wing' of the Conquest Hospital which opened its doors in Dec. 1999

you will receive a care plan informing you of the support you will receive." [5206]

Community Link Nurses

Community Link Nurses provide a service to resettle mental health patients who are newly discharged from hospital or after treatment at home from the Crisis Response Service to help them to live independently. This service is offered for a six week period from the time they leave hospital. *Hours:* Seven days a week 8.30am to 5pm. *Contacts*: Christine Lockwood, team leader.

Address: Community Link Nurses, Woodlands, Conquest Hospital, The Ridge, Hastings, East Sussex, TN37 7RD. *Tel*: 01424 755255. Ext. 2606. [May 2000]

Community meetings

Gemma Townsend leads community meetings at Woodlands which are held on a weekly basis.

At the community meetings in-patients raise matters which are of concern to themselves. The comments are fed back to the management who can effect the appropriate action. Minutes of the meetings are also circulated to the Focus on Mental Health group (see under 'User Groups' page 263).

Community meetings are held on 6 week turnaround by the Drug Dependency Unit and the Community Alcohol Team. [5402, 5795]

Groups

Various patients' groups are running or planned, including a gardening group, an introduction group for new admissions, a leavers' group, an aerobics' group, a newspaper discussion group and a therapy group. Also planned are relaxation sessions. [6013 Jul 2000]

King's College, London

The NHS Trust has joined forces with King's College, London, on a national quality initiative. This is a two-year project concentrating on the quality of care in inpatient units. The link with King's College - who will carry out research into what works well and publish the results - will help to set high quality standards for this new Hastings service. See also National Practice Development Network, this page. [5048]

Legal advice

Free legal advice is provided to patients by the local firm of solicitors, Herringtons. At present this 'clinic' is run weekly on Thursday afternoons. [6013 Jul 2000]

Mental Health Act Commission

From time to time the hospital is visited by members of the Mental Health Act Commission, an independent group set up to make sure that the mental health laws are being run properly. They will be happy to meet you when they visit, but if you want to contact them directly, please see their entry on page 333. [5206]

National Practice Development Network

This body has been set up by the Centre for Mental Health Services and the Florence Nightingale Division of Nursing Studies, King's College, London. It is an initiative to support National Health Trusts throughout the country which want to make a difference and improve acute in-patient care for mental health service users.

Service users now have higher demands about quality of mental health care and about being treated as partners in making decisions about their treatment and care.

For further information contact Penny West or Elizabeth Kurtz. *Address:* Centre for Mental Health Service Development, Friars House, 157-168, Blackfriars Road, London, SE1 8EZ. *Tel:* 020 7633 0241. *Fax:* 020 7928 4101. [6050]

Patient centred care

"At Woodlands we provide patient centred care which is individual, comprehensive and continuous for people aged between 16 and 65 years who are experiencing an episode of acute mental ill health and cannot be treated in their own home environment.

Care is delivered in a safe, secure and therapeutic environment. We believe that everyone admitted to Woodlands is entitled to high quality service, and treated with respect, dignity and as equal human beings. We also believe in the on-going development of best practice." 5206

Staff at Woodlands

When you are at Woodlands a team of trained staff will look after you and be responsible for your treatment. The team includes doctors, nurses, occupational therapists, psychologists and social workers. 5206 May 2000

Visitors

Visitors are always welcome, but are requested to check with the ward prior to arrival to avoid interruption to the patient's therapeutic programmes wherever possible. A safe place is provided for children who visit. Patients wanting their children to visit are asked to notify the nursing staff. 5206 May 2000

Address: Woodlands Mental Health Unit, Conquest Hospital, The Ridge, Hastings, Sussex, TN37 7RD. *Tel*: 01424 755255. *Patients' telephone*: 01424 755255, ext. 2522. *Fax:* 01424 445755. 5071

Acknowledgements
Our grateful thanks to Jacqui Wilson, senior clinical nurse, and colleagues at Woodlands, for editorial assistance with this chapter.

Mental Health Act

Most people in a psychiatric ward will be voluntary or 'informal' patients who can leave when they want and whose consent is needed before treatment can be given. 'Formal' patients are detained under a 'section' of the Mental Health Act 1983 and some may be given treatment without their consent.

Compulsory detention

Compulsory detention, or 'sectioning' cannot take place unless the criteria in the Act are met and there is no suitable alternative. Only a team of mental health professionals can detain you for longer than 72 hours, and only after a careful assessment, with compulsory detention as the last resort. Anyone detained in hospital is entitled to full information about their rights.

Code of Practice

The Mental Health Act 1983 is the law which states how people can be admitted to and detained in hospital. It is very complex and open to different interpretations. National Mind produces a series of rights guides to help users, relatives and professionals understand the Mental Health Act. The Mental Health Act Code of Practice is a government document containing good practice guidance on how the Mental Health Act should be used; it was updated in April 1999 and emphasises the importance of user's rights and the Care Pogramme Approach. This document is available from Mind Mail Order Service. *Tel*: 020 8221 9666.

Your right to information

All mental health professionals should keep you fully informed of what is happening, explaining things in a way you can understand. Ask if there is anything you want to know or are unsure about.

If you are admitted to hospital under a section of the Mental Health Act, this should be explained to you at the time. On arrival in hospital, staff have a duty to tell you about the section you are being held under, and about your right to appeal to the hospital managers and to the Mental Health Review Tribunal (see below).

They should also tell you about your rights regarding discharge and consent to treatment and give you information about the Mental Health Act Commission, (see below).

You should be given this information *in writing*. The hospital gives the same information to your nearest relative, including notice of when you will be discharged from hospital. Your approved social worker has a duty to inform your nearest relative that you have been admitted to hospital.

Your right to refuse treatment

Most people who are admitted to hospital are voluntary patients - free to leave or to refuse treatment when they wish. If you are detained under the Mental Health Act you may be lawfully held in hospital against your will, but if you are held under sections 4,5, 135 or 136 you can refuse to have any treatment.

Informal patients can sometimes find that when they attempt to leave hospital they are held under section 5, and then become formal patients. This can only happen after an assessment by two doctors and an approved social worker.

If you are held under section 3, you have more say in your treatment after three months. However, you can be given treatment against your will if it is deemed necessary to save your life, or if you are a serious threat to others.

ECT

You can refuse electro-convulsive therapy (ECT), under any section unless an independent psychiatrist, appointed by the Mental Health Act Commission, interviews you and decides it is necessary.

Mental Health Assessments

A formal mental health assessment considers whether or not a person should be admitted to hospital under the Mental Health Act. Three people are needed: a doctor, (usually a GP) an approved doctor with mental health experience, (usually a psychiatrist) and an approved social worker who has special training in mental health assessment.

Friends, relatives or carers may ask for a mental health assessment. If the 'nearest relative' asks for one, the approved social worker must consider it and give reasons in writing if hospital admission does not result. The approved social worker arranges the assessment and will also make the practical arrangements for taking the person into hospital if need be.

They will usually have a number of discussions with family members and professionals to consider all the circumstances before arranging an assessment. You can ask your GP to arrange an assessment.

Sections

Section 2 (up to 28 days)
Section 2 is used when detention in hospital is in the interests of the patient's health or safety, or to protect others. The approved social worker or the nearest relative may make the application, founded on two doctors' recommendations. Treatment may be given, and, as with section 3, in some circumstances consent may not be needed

Section 3 (up to 6 months)
This is most likely to be used when the hospital knows the person and the treatment needed is clear. An application is made by an approved social worker or the nearest relative, supported by two doctors.

Consent is not needed, but an application can only be made if the nearest relative does not object. You have more say in your treatment after three months under this section. At the end of six months, the section can be renewed.

Section 4 (up to 72 hours)
This section is used where admission is urgently needed and an assessment under section 2 would take too long to arrange. An application is made by an approved social worker or nearest relative, with one doctor's recommendation. There is no power to treat the person against their wishes.

Section 5(2) (up to 72 hours)
The hospital doctor in charge of treatment may recommend the use of this section to prevent a voluntary patient leaving hospital. There is no power to treat the person against their wishes, and a proper mental health assessment should be arranged as soon as possible.

Section 5(4) (up to 6 hours)
If a doctor is not available, a psychiatric nurse may authorise detention for up to six hours under this section.

Section 136 (police powers)
A person who is in a public place and who

appears to be mentally disordered and in need of immediate care and control can be taken to a hospital or police station under this section for up to 72 hours. There is no power to treat the person against their wishes and an approved social worker and a doctor must do an assessment as soon as possible.

Section 135 (court warrant)
An approved social worker can apply to a magistrate for a warrant authorising the police, accompanied by an approved social worker and a doctor, to gain entry to a person's home and if necessary remove them to a place of safety for up to 72 hours.

There must be grounds for believing the person is suffering from a mental disorder and is being neglected or ill-treated or is unable to care for themselves. A full assessment must take place afterwards.

Section 62 (urgent treatment)
Urgent treatment may be given without consent to any hospital patient if any of the following applies:
- Treatment is needed to save the person's life.
- Treatment is needed to prevent serious deteriortation - drugs or ECT can be given.
- Treatment is needed to alleviate serious suffering or prevent violent or dangerous behaviour - drug treatment may be given.

Treatment may only be given for as long as it takes to bring the emergency to an end.

Section 7 (guardianship)
A mental health assessment may result in an application for guardianship as opposed to hospital admission. This involves placing the person under the care of either the local authority or someone approved by them. The person may be required to live in a particular place, attend for treatment, and allow access to any doctor or approved social worker. But there is no power to give treatment without consent.

Guardianship lasts for six months initially. An application for guardianship can be made by either the nearest relative or an approved social worker.

Section 25 (supervision registers)
Since April 1994, all health authorities must keep a register of people thought to be at serious risk of suicide, at risk of severe self-neglect or who may be violent to others. The registers do not create any new powers.

Follow-up under the Care Programme Approach is arranged for people who are registered. You must be informed if your name is on the register, except where to inform you would cause serious harm to your physical or mental health. The local trust will usually keep the register.

Section 26 (nearest relative)
The Mental Health Act 1983 gives a number of rights and responsibilities to what is called the 'nearest relative'. The Act specifies who the nearest relative is by a set of rules.

This means that he or she is not necessarily the most closely involved or most suitable. If the nominated person prefers not to act as the nearest relative, he or she can nominate any other suitable person to take on the role. If necessary, speak to an approved social worker about this.

Compulsory treatment

The Government's Green Paper, *Reform of the Mental Health Act 1983* was published in November 1999. It includes provisions for Compulsory Treatment Orders (CTOs), for those who posed a 'substantial risk of serious harm' to themselves or others.

Consistently, all membership mental health voluntary sector organisations, including the MDF, have opposed the introduction of further compulsion. MDF's consultation survey, carried out in 1998, showed that 90% of those with a diagnosis of manic depression who responded, opposed CTOs.

When asked what effects members

thought CTOs might have on their own willingness to seek help in a crisis, over 70% indicated that the existence of such compulsory powers to treat in the community would deter them from seeking help.

The MDF will continue to oppose CTOs. "Further compulsion will not improve access to treatment, nor will it improve the under-resourced and inadequate levels of services currently available - acute and community based. By making these new proposals overwhelmingly a public safety issue, this government is avoiding the real issue - the need to improve the quality of services and treatments available in mental health." 5069

National Organisations

Mental Health Act Commission

The MHAC was set up to look after the rights and concerns of patients who are detained under the Mental Health Act 1983. It visits hospitals and meets with detained patients, and keeps the operation of the Act under review. The Commission can help to ensure that complaints receive full and proper investigation. It also administers the Second Opinion service required under the Act.

Address: Mental Health Act Commission, Maid Marion House, 56, Hounds Gate, Nottingham, NG1 6BG. *Tel*: 0115 943 7100. *Fax*: 0115 943 7101. May 2000

Mental Health Review Tribunal

The Mental Health Review Tribunal acts on behalf of people who are detained in psychiatric hospitals under the Mental Health Act 1983, and who want to appeal against this detention.

Address: Mental Health Review Tribunal, Crown Offices, Block 3, Kingston Bypass Road, Surbiton, Surrey, KT6 5QN. *Tel*: 020 8268 4520. *Fax*: 020 8268 4532. May 2000

Further Information

Mental Health Act 1983

"This revised edition provides guidance to registered medical practioners, managers and staff in hospitals and mental nursing homes, and approved social workers on how they should proceed when undertaking duties under the Mental Health Act 1983." The *Mental Health Act 1983 Code of Practice* is published by Stationery Office Books, 1999. ISBN 0-11-322111-8. 170 pages, £7.50. Available from Mind Mail Order Service. *Tel*: 020 8221 9666. 5088

Mind The Law

'Mind the Law: Mind's evidence to the Government's Mental Health Act review team'. By Margaret Pedler. The full text of Mind's policy recommendations sent to the Mental Health Act Review Team consulting on possible changes to the Mental Health Act. This book provides a clear report of the views of mental health service users and workers throughout Mind's networks. Published by Mind, 1999. ISBN: 1-874690-79-0. 60 pages. £7.50. Available from Mind Mail Order Service. *Tel*: 020 8221 9666. 5251

Mind the Law

'Mind The Law: Mind and the Mental Health Act Series. 1. Advocacy'. Issues arising out of the proposed reform of the Mental Health Act. Published by Mind, 2000. ISBN: 1-874690-91-X. 18 pages. £1.36. Available from Mind Mail Order Service. *Tel*: 020 8221 9666. 5251

Reform of the Mental Health Act 1983

Published by the Stationery Office, £10.50. Also available online. Ref. 0101448023. 5069

National Service Framework

First National Standards

National standards to drive up quality and cut wide variations in services were set out in Sept 1999 in the first National Service Framework for Mental Health, launched by Health Secretary, Frank Dobson. [5099]

The framework sets national standards based on clinical evidence, and sets out best practise for promoting mental health and treating mental illness. It promises national and regional support for health and social services and establishes the progress which should be made within certain timescales.

National Service Frameworks fulfil the Government's commitment to tackle significant causes of ill health and disability.

Frank Dobson said: "In the past, people with mental health problems have been let down by unacceptable variations in health care. I want services that offer the highest quality to everyone, regardless of their gender, age, race or where they live". The framework for mental health requires health and social services to:

* Promote mental health for all and combat discrimination against people with mental health problems.
* Identify the needs of patients with mental health problems and ensure they are offered effective treatments.
* Ensure that all mental health service users on the Care Programme Approach (CPA) receive care which prevents or anticipates crises and reduces risk.
* Provide a hospital bed or suitable alternative bed for those who need it in an environment close to home that protects them and the public.
* Make sure carers who look after someone on the CPA have their own caring, physical and mental health needs assessed on an annual basis.
* Reduce the level of suicide.

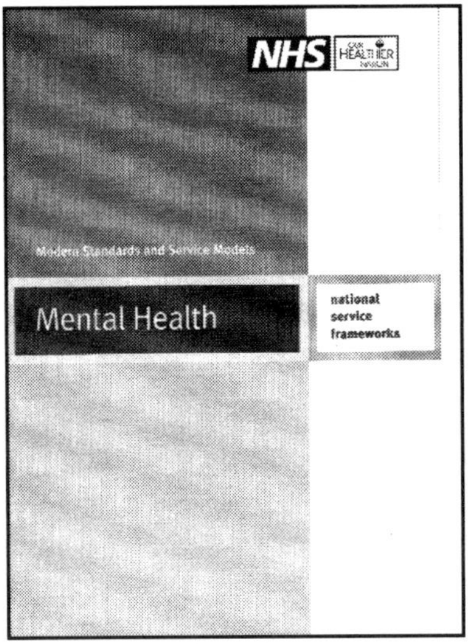

The National Service Framework For Mental Health. This bulky 150-page document was published by the Dept of Health in Sept 1999. The NSF 'will help drive up quality and remove the wide and unacceptable variations in provision'.

Mental health problems

Mental health problems are both common and diverse. As many as one in six adults suffer from mental health problems at any one time. This ranges from depression to rare but severe mental illness such as schizophrenia.

Mental health care

Mentally ill people depend on effective mental health care for their own well-being, independence and safety. Despite the public's fears, most seriously mentally ill people are not dangerous and indeed are more likely to harm or kill themselves than anyone else.

Suicide

Each year in England alone, around 4,000 people take their own lives. With proper care, intervention and support, many of these lives might be saved, and for thousands of others we can help to reduce the trauma.

One way or another, everywhere in the country, mental health services will be challenged by the National Framework's new standards. We are now being explicit about our expectations - successes will win praise, serious failures will bring intervention. I believe these new standards give us an opportunity we cannot afford to miss.

Care Programme Approach

The Care Programme Approach is an important aspect of mental health care and in support of the framework, it has been reviewed separately. The new arrangements will strengthen care co-ordination, achieve a consistent approach nationally, reduce bureaucracy and achieve greater focus on the needs of those being cared for. Under the new arrangements, health and local authorities will be expected to work together to co-ordinate delivery of care, through explicit, individually tailored plans, to minimise loss of contact with services and maximise the effect of therapeutic intervention."

The Seven Standards

The seven standards are:

Standard One

Health and social services should: promote mental health for all, working with individuals and communities; combat discrimination against individuals and groups with mental health problems, and promote their social inclusion.

Standard Two

Any service user who contacts their primary health care team with a common mental health problem should: have their mental health needs identified and assessed; be offered effective treatments, including referral to specialist services for further assessment; treatment and care if they require it.

Standard Three

Any individual with a common mental health problem should: be able to make contact round the clock with the local services necessary to meet their needs and receive adequate care; be able to use NHS Direct as it develops for first level advice and referral on to specialist helplines or to local services.

Standard Four

All mental health service users on the Care Programme Approach (CPA), should receive care which optimises engagement, anticipates or prevents a crisis, and reduces risk; have a copy of a written care plan which includes the action to be taken in a crisis by service users, their carers, and their care co-ordinator; be able to access services 24 hours a day, 365 days a year.

Standard Five

Each service user who is assessed as requiring a period of care away from their home should have: timely access to an appropriate hospital bed or alternative bed or place, which is in the least restrictive environment consistent with the need to protect them and the public, and as close to home as possible; a copy of a written after-care plan agreed on discharge which sets out the care and rehabilitation to be provided, identifies the care co-ordinator, and specifies the action to be taken in a crisis.

Standard Six

All individuals who provide regular and substantial care for a person on CPA should: have an assessment of their caring, physical and mental needs, repeated on at least an annual basis; have their own written care plan which is given to them and implemented in discussion with them.

Standard Seven

Local health and social care communities should prevent suicides by implementing the other six standards and: ensure that staff are competent to assess the risk of suicide among individuals at greatest risk; support local prison staff in preventing suicides among prisoners; and develop local systems for suicide audit to learn lessons and take any necessary action.

Monitoring standards

The National Service Framework is based on wide ranging evidence brought together by the independent External Reference Group, chaired by Professor Graham Thornicroft from the Institute of Psychiatry, Kings College, London. The group brought together health and social care professionals, service users and carers, health and social service managers, partner agencies and others.

The Commission for Health Improvements, the Social Service Inspectorate, and the Audit Commission will rigorously monitor local progress on meeting these standards. Performance indicators: local health and social care communities will also agree local milestones with the NHS Executive regional offices and social care regions.

Further Information

Natioanl Service Framework

Copies of the National Service Framework for mental health are available from the Department of Health Media Centre. *Tel:* 020 7210 5221. July 2000

Implementation

For information about the implementation of the National Service Framework under Hastings & Rother, please contact Anna Barnes. *Tel*: 01424 755255, ext. 6392. Jul 2000

Occupational Therapy

Occupational Therapists

Occupational Therapists (OTs) are trained to help people with physical or mental health problems cope with daily living. They work in hospitals, GP surgeries and a wide variety of community settings.

They offer help to enable people to develop the skills they need to manage difficulties such as anxiety or lack of confidence. OTs also run ongoing supportive groups for people with long-term mental health problems living in the community.

If you are a patient in hospital, or attending one of the day services, occupational therapy is one of the services you may be offered. Your GP is also able to refer you by contacting the occupational therapists within the Community Mental Health Teams, see page 305. [5224]

Local services

Occupational therapists currently offer services at Bexhill Day Service, within the Community Mental Health Teams, Westwood Day Hospital, Westwood Day Service, and Woodlands. They can work with people individually and in groups depending on their needs.

The treatment is mostly of a practical nature directed at building skills to enable individuals to function in the areas of self-care, domestic tasks, work and leisure. Hours: are Mondays to Fridays 9am to 5pm. [5634]

Local Organsiations

Westwood Centre

Day Services, Community & Day Hospital For all enquiries please contact Debbie Rimmer. *Address:* Westwood Centre, 7, Holmesdale Gardens, Hastings, Sussex, TN34 1LY. *Tel:* 01424 714366, extension 129. [Jul 2000]

Woodlands

The contact for inpatient services is Teresa Franks. *Address:* Woodlands, Conquest Hospital, 729, The Ridge, St Leonards, Sussex, TN37 7PT. *Tel:* 01424 755255 extension 2527. [Jul 2000]

Acknowledgements
Our grateful thanks to Debbie Rimmer for editorial assistance with this chapter.

Patients' Charter

The Patients' Charter
Under the Patients' Charter you have the right to have any treatment, its risks and options fully explained to you. Most of us want to have a say in what happens to us and we may have strong preferences for one form of treatment rather than another.

Mental Health Services
The Patients' Charter details rights for mental health services:
- You have the right to receive detailed information about mental health services in your area. This includes information on the type of care available and the standards of service you can expect. You should be given time to consider your options before you make a choice.

- You have the right to have any proposed treatment explained, including any risks involved in that treatment and any alternatives before you decide whether to agree to it.

- If your GP thinks you need to see a consultant, you have the right to be referred to one acceptable to you. You also have the right to be referred for a second opinion if you and your GP agree this is a good idea.

- If you have a complaint, you have the right to have it investigated and to receive a full and prompt reply.

- If you are detained in hospital under the Mental Health Act, you have a right to ask for a complaint to be investigated by the Mental Health Act Commission. 0534

Patients' Charter 2001

The government's NHS National Plan, announced in July 2000, makes specific proposals for the Patients' Charter. There will be more information about GPs' surgeries; for example: the number of people on the doctors' lists, how the surgery compares with national targets for waiting and appointment delays. Patients will be able to see the letters written about them by their consultants. The new Patients' Charter is due to be published in 2001. 6042 Jul 2000

Further Information

The Patient's Charter & You

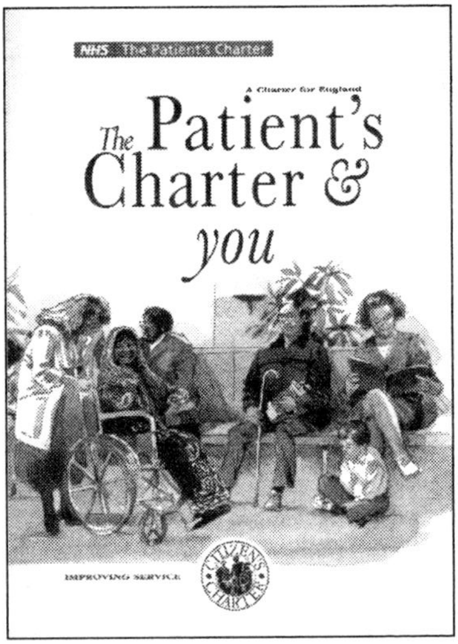

This 32-page document, published by the Department of Health, is available in many foreign languages, including Bengali, Gujarati, Hindi Chinese, Greek, Turkish and Polish. It is also available as an audio cassette and in braille and large print versions. To order your free copy, simply telephone the Department of Health on freephone 0800 555777. 6030 Jun 99; Jul 2000

Primary Care Groups

What are Primary Care Groups?

NHS primary care groups combine the expertise of GPs and practice teams, community nurses, social services, the health authority and representatives of their local community. The priorities of PCGs are to: improve the health of, and reduce health inequalities in their area; develop primary care and community services; advise on, or commission directly, a range of hospital services which meet patients' needs. [5928]

Expertise

Introduced in the White Paper *"A New NHS"*, PCGs are local groups of GP practices that bring together the expertise of GPs and practice teams, community nurses, social services and lay representatives of local people (as well as a Health Authority representative).

Responsibility

Initially set up as sub-committees of the Health Authority, PCGs take responsibility for commissioning the majority of hospital and community health services for a local population. They will be accountable to the Health Authority but will have freedom (within the guidelines of the local Health Improvement Plan) to decide how to deploy their resources, depending on the level of their operation. [5090]

Primary Care Teams

Primary Care Teams are the people who typically work from a GP surgery to provide a range of services for local patients (includes GPs, practice nurses and other specialists often including health visitors and community nurses). [5090]

Primary Care Trusts

Some PCGs may wish to become free-standing Primary Care Trusts (with some eventually combining commissioning responsibilities with providing community health services). [5090]

Hastings & Rother Primary Care Group is hoping to become a Primary Care Trust from April 2001. This new body would be "a free-standing NHS organisation, monitored by East Sussex Brighton and Hove Health Authority for commissioning care, and for the provision of local community services currently provided by Hastings & Rother NHS Trust." [6016]

Primary Care Groups

The six PCGs in this area are listed below in alphabetical order.

Bexhill & Rother

The population of Bexhill & Rother is 81,000 and is served by 45 GPs in 13 practices. Chair: Dr Peter Dewhurst; Chief Executive: Rick Stern; Commissioning: Simon Lawrence.

Address: Bexhill & Rother Primary Care Group, 53b, High Street, Battle, East Sussex, TN33 0EN. *Tel:* 01424 777025. *Fax:* 01424 777026.

E-mail: slawrence@esbhhealth.cix.co.uk [1570 May 2000]

Brighton and Hove

Chair: Dr Xavier Nalletamby; Chief Executive: Gary Needle. *Address:* Brighton and Hove Primary Care Group, Brighton Town Hall, Bartholomews, Brighton, BN1 1JA. *Tel:* 01273 295490. *Fax:* 01273 295461. [Jul 2000]

Eastbourne Downs

The population of Eastbourne downs is 167,000 and is served by 89 GPs in 24 practices. Chair: Dr Mark Barnes; Chief Executive: Angela Knight.

Address: Eastbourne Downs Primary Care Group, 3rd Floor, Greencoat House, 32, St Leonards Road, Eastbourne, East Sussex, BN21 3UT. *Tel:* 01323 417714. *Fax:* 01323 416161. [1570 May 2000]

Hastings & St Leonards

The population of Hastings & St Leonards is 90,000 and is served by 47 GPs in 25 practices.

Chair: Dr Gregory Wilcox; Chief Executive & Chair of the Mental Health Action Group: Toni Wilkinson.

Address: Hastings & St Leonards Primary Care Group, 3rd Floor, St Michael's Hospice, 25, Upper Maze Hill, St Leonards-on-Sea, East Sussex, TN38 0LB. *Tel:* 01424 204143. *Fax*: 01424 204145. *E-mail:* hastingspcg@esbhhealth.cix.co.uk 1570 May 2000

High Weald

The population of High Weald is 90,000 and is served by 48 GPs in 15 practices.

Chair: Dr Deveda Redman; Chief Executive: Peter Brooke.

Address: High Weald Primary Care Group, Ground Floor, Rother House, The Office Village, River Way, Uckfield, East Sussex, TN22 1SL. *Tel*: 01825 768688. *Fax:* 01825 768689. 1570 May 2000

Ouse Valley

The population of Ouse Valley is 64,000 and is served by 38 GPs in 10 practices.

Chair: Dr Rob Ferns; Chief Executive: Denise Rendell.

Address: Ouse Valley Primary Care Group, Springman House, 8, North Street, Lewes, East Sussex, BN7 2PB. *Tel:* 01273 485310. *Fax*: 01273 485304. 1570 May 2000

Further Information

A Primary Care Trust

'A Primary Care Trust in Hastings & St Leonards' published by the NHS July 2000. 6016

Acknowledgements

Our grateful thanks to Toni Wilkinson, Hastings & St Leonards Primary Care Group, for editorial assistance with this chapter.

Psychiatry

Psychiatrists

The psychiatrists working locally in the NHS are listed below in alphabetical order. For private psychiatrists see 'Private Health Care' chapter. And for details of the community mental health teams, please see the 'Community Mental Health Teams' chapter. The psychiatrists listed here are the *consultant* psychiatrists and are helped by a number of assistant psychiatrists of different grades.

A *liaison* psychiatrist such as Dr Declan Fitzpatrick at the Conquest, deals with mental health issues that arise from a patient having a physical difficulty.

Staff grade psychiatrists do not wish to become consultants but are fully qualified psychiatrists. [6092 Aug 2000]

Psychiatric team

Psychiatrists are medical doctors with specialist experience and qualifications in mental illness and emotional disorders and, like other doctors, work closely with nurses. In psychiatry there are hospital psychiatric nurses and community mental health nurses (CMHNs) who visit homes and various centres outside hospital.

Psychological & social aspects

However, there is more to psychiatry than that. There are different kinds of mental illnesses. These are not only medical problems; they have important psychological and social aspects. Psychiatry is concerned with all aspects of mental health and these often call for expert knowledge and skills of three other groups of professional people - clinical psychologists, occupational therapists, and social workers.

Overall view

The five professions make up the the psychiatric team, working in partnership by collecting facts, bringing the information together to obtain an overall view of the problems of each individual patient, and co-ordinating plans of treatment. So each patient stands to benefit from the presence of the multi-professional team. [5232]

Psychiatrists

The following are psychiatrists working in the local NHS.

Birkett, Dr Michael

Consultant psychiatrist for Rural Rother Community Mental Health Team and Clinical Director of the Mental Health Services for Hastings & Rother NHS Trust. *Address*: Dr Michael Birkett, Admin. Unit, Eversfield Hospital, West Hill Road, St Leonards-on-Sea, East Sussex, TN38 0NG. *Tel:* 01424 710106. [5048 Jun 2000]

Fitzpatrick, Dr Declan

Liaison psychiatrist, Conquest Hospital. *Address*: Dr Declan Fitzpatrick, Woodlands, Conquest Hospital, The Ridge, St Leonards, Sussex. *Tel*: 01424 755255. [5048 Jul 2000]

Malik, Dr Shakil J

Consultant psychiatrist for Hastings. Dr Malik is a general adult psychiatrist with special interest in community psychiatry. *Address*: Dr Shakil Malik, Woodlands, Conquest Hospital, The Ridge, St Leonards, Sussex. *Tel*: 01424 755255 / 01424 716366. [5048 May 2000]

Naz, Dr A Q

Dr Naz is a Staff Grade Psychiatrist working under Dr S J Malik. He has a special interest in community psychiatry. *Tel:* 01424 755255 / 01424 716366. [May 2000]

Raj-manickam, Dr Thiru

Joined the NHS Trust in November 1999, as consultant psychiatrist for St Leonards. She had previously been working in the north-west and is interested in researching women's post-natal mental health among doctors and other health care professionals. *Address*: Dr Thiru Raj-manickam,

Woodlands, Conquest Hospital, The Ridge, St Leonards, Sussex. *Tel*: 01424 755255. 5048 May 2000

Shyam, Dr
Works at Westwood House under Dr Rajmanickam.

Smith, Dr Gillian
Dr Smith has worked locally for the last ten years and is now consultant psychiatrist for adult services in Bexhill. She is especially interested in mental health services outside hospital settings. 5048 May 2000

Organisations

Psychiatry Research Trust

Registered Charity No. 284286. *Contact*: Mrs S. Refault. *Address:* Psychiatry Research Trust, De Crespigny Park, London, SE5 8AF. *Tel*: (Direct Line) 020 7703 6217. *Fax:* 020 7703 5796. *Switchboard:* 020 7703 5411. May 2000

Further Information

Psychiatry
Website. 'Psychiatry' is a big US database linked to other useful medical databases. *Website:* www. psychiatry.medscape.com

Couch Questions
'Couch Questions: a guide to psychiatrists'. This is an excellent video giving an oversight of psychiatry and tackling all sorts of issues such as what mental illness is and explanations of the different types of illnesses. Further details from MDF. *Tel*: 020 7793 2600. 5298

See also these chapters ...

Children & Young People (Psychiatry Services), page 40.
Community Mental Health Teams, page 306.
Elderly Mental Health (Psychiatry Services), page 59.
Learning Disabilities, (Community Learning Disability Service), page 77.
Legal Matters (Forensic Psychiatry Services), page224.
Psychology, page 343.

Abbreviations
MB.
BS.
DPM. Diploma in Psychological Medicine.
MRC.Psych. Member of the Royal College of Psychiatrists.

Acknowledgements
Our grateful thanks to Dr Michael Birkett for editorial assistance with this chapter.

Psychology

What are psychologists?
Clinical psychologists work with people with problems ranging from anxiety and phobias to severe mental illness. They are not doctors, and do not prescribe medication, but usually offer psychological treatments such as behaviour therapy, cognitive therapy or psychotherapy.

Behaviour therapy
Behaviour therapy aims to help people change problem behaviour. For example, relaxation techniques will be used to manage fears, phobias or obsessive behaviour.

Cognitive therapy
Cognitive therapy helps people identify destructive thought patterns and change them to more constructive ones.

Psychotherapy
Psychotherapy is focused more on underlying issues and childhood experiences. Often a combination of approaches (integrative therapy) will be utilised.

Access
You may gain access to psychologists via the Community Mental Health Teams, please see page 305. 6019

Local Organsiations

Dept of Clinical Psychology
This local NHS department is based in Holmesdale Gardens. Comprehensive clinical psychology service for adults covering assessment, individual and group psychotherapy, counselling, consultation, training and research. You need to be referred through your GP or other mental health professionals.

Head of Department: Mr Johann Korf, clinical consultant psychologist. *Other staff:* Dr Angela Busittil, chartered clinical psychologist; Dr Ruth Rushton, clinical psychologist; Mr Peter Connor, clinical psychologist; Dr Michael Bowles, chartered clinical psychologist; Mary Locke, consultant clinical psychologist and head of adult psychological services.

Address: Department of Clinical Psychology, NHS Trust, Braybrooke House, 9, Holmesdale Gardens, Hastings, TN34 1LY. *Tel*: 01424 435066; fax: 01424 428964. Apr 2000

Rye & Bexhill
Mr Terry Kohler, chartered clinical psychologist is based in Rye. Marchienne van der Veen, chartered clinical psychologist based in Bexhill. 0534 Jun 2000

Further Information

Health Information Service
The HIS is a free and confidential 24-hour service. You can speak to staff during office hours, and you can listen to any of hundreds of tapes at any time, e.g: *Psychological problems: services available* (Tape 251).

Address: The College of Health, St Margaret's House, 21, Old Ford Road, London, E2 9PL. *Freephone*: 0800 66 55 44. 5367

Rehabilitation

Local Organisations

Hastings Sheltered Workshop

Hastings Sheltered Workshop. Located at the Brittania Enterprise Centre, the Hastings Sheltered Workshop provides work activities and training in a supportive environment. It can be used by any person who has, or is currently suffering from, mental health or stress related problems. It helps to develop skills and to regain lost confidence.

The types of activities available are varied and include woodwork, horticulture, upholstery and light craft work. Enquiries can be made by any professional involved in the person's care: e.g. GP, Social Worker, Occupational Therapist, or Community Mental Health Nurse. *Hours*: Mondays to Fridays 9.00am to 12.30pm and 2.00pm to 4.30pm. Fares for getting to the centre can be reimbursed. *Contact:* Peter Howard, project manager.

Address: Hastings Sheltered Work-shop, Britannia Enterprise Centre, Waterworks Road, Hastings, Sussex, TN34 1R. May 2000

National Organisations

Guideposts Trust

The GT develops Day Care Services Centres for people who have returned to the community after many years in an institution, and for people who have not been institutionalised, but need support. Contact: Clifford Upex, Director.

Address: Guideposts Trust, Two Rivers, Station Lane, Witney, Oxfordshire, OX8 6BH. *Tel*: 01993 772886. *Fax*: 01993 778160. Jul 2000

See also these chapters ...

Employment & Training, page 212.
Voluntary Work, page 266.

Rural Rother

People with mental health problems who happen to live in the country face problems of isolation far worse than those of their town cousins. For many, the 'Rural Rother Creative Care Network' has become a very welcome friend...

Local Organisations

Creative Care Network

The Rural Rother Creative Care Network has been set up to provide a support system for people who are recovering from, or are currently experiencing mental health distress. It is also open for carers. The Network aims to improve the mental health of members by encouraging socialisation and activity within a supportive environment.

What happens?

The Network consists of small groups of people that meet regularly in different villages, usually in community halls and pubs. Here people participate in activities such as art/crafts, photography, aromatherapy, trips out and guest speakers, or people just chat over coffee. People are encouraged to visit other villages and groups to 'network' and meet new people.

Newsletter

There is a newsletter produced which is contributed to by Network members and distributed throughout rural Rother. The newsletter is aimed to reach those people who don't feel able to come to a group but would like to feel part of a supportive network of people.

Who can join?

The Rural Rother Creative Care Network aims to be fully accessible to all people with mental health needs regardless of gender, ability, ethnic and religious background, sexuality, age, employment status or any other perceived difference. Anyone under 65 who is having/has had, experience of a mental health problem, or their carers.

How to join

Anyone may apply by simply telephoning Su Barnicoat during normal office hours, Monday to Friday. Unfortunately, the office is not open to the public. Messages will be taken if Su isn't there.

How much does it cost?

Group meetings are free, but pub and other outings need to be paid for by members.

Who pays for the service?

The important work of the Creative Care Network is financed jointly between the East Sussex Alliance of Mind Associations, SEEDA, Hastings and Rother NHS Trust and East Sussex Social Services.

Address: Rural Rother Creative Care Network, Admin Unit, Eversfield Hospital, West Hill Road, St Leonards, Sussex, TN38 0NG. *Tel:* 01424 710111. *Fax:*

01424 426858. May 2000

National Organisations

Rural Minds

The aims of this organisation are *to* promote better mental health for country people, developing innovative support and care networks.To provide information and training for volunteers and professionals, working in rural communities. To influence purchasing decisions to provide accessible rural mental health services. Publishes *Rural Minds Digest,* a monthly newsletter.

Address: Rural Minds, The Arthur Rank Centre, National Agricultural Centre, Stoneleigh Park, Warwickshire, CV8 2LZ. *Tel:* 01203 414366. *Fax:* 01203 414369. *E-mail:* ruralminds@ruralnet.org.uk 5271

See also ...

'Community Mental Health Teams' chapter for details of the Rural Rother Community Mental Health Team.

Acknowledgements
Our grateful thanks to Su Barnicoat of the Rural Rother Creative Care Network for editorial assistance with this chapter.

Social Services

Mental Health Services in Hastings and Rother are integrating with the Health Trust in 2000. Four multi-disciplinary teams are to be set up during the year 2000. May 2000

Social Workers
Social workers assess people's needs and provide counselling, advice, support, care planning and management. They can also help with benefit problems and arrange day care, breaks for carers, supported housing or residential care. They work closely with service users, carers and families.

Aprroved social workers
Mental Health social workers are usually 'approved social workers' (ASWs) who are qualified to assess whether or not someone needs to be admitted to hospital under the Mental Health Act. They work alongside other professionals in the community mental health teams. 5224

Day Centres
Social Services is responsible for two day centres: the 73a Centre in Bexhill and the Hastings Day Centre. Please see 'Day Centres' chapter, page 209, for more information.

Learning Disabilities
Social Services provides services for people with learning disabilities. For details, please see 'Learning disabilities' chapter, page 77.

Local Services

East Sussex Social Services
Director of Social Services: David Archibald; Assist. Director (adults): Heather Hill; Assistant Director (children & families): Mark Wheeler.

Address: East Sussex Social Services, County Hall, PO Box 5, St Anne's Crescent, Lewes, Sussex, BN7 1SW. *Tel:* 01273 481000. 5081 Jul 2000

Emergency Duty Service
Social Services Emergency Duty Service, for out of hours emergency cover (evenings, weekends and bank holidays). *Tel:* 01273 320202. *Fax:* 01273 814699. 5248, 5953

Healthcall
Provides an emergency service outside of normal office hours, including statutory mental health emergencies. Anyone can contact the Emergency Duty Team via Healthcall. *Hours:* Mondays to Fridays: 4.30 to 8.30pm; Weekends: 9.00am to 9.00pm. *Tel:* 01273 320202.

Information Line
A countywide information service about services to children and families, older people, people with disabilities and much more. *Information officers:* Nora Maunsell, Claudia Still, Liz Hutcheson.

Address: Information Line, Pinehill, 185, The Ridge, Hastings, TN34 2AE. *Tel:* 0845 601 0664. *Fax:* 01424 201946. *E-mail:* information.line@eastsussexcc.gov.uk 5953 Jul 2000

Social Services Assessment
Address: Social Services Contact Team for Adult Assessment, 11th Floor, Ocean House, 87-89, London Road, St Leonards-on-Sea, East Sussex, TN37 6DH. *Tel:* 01424 448555. [Jul 2000]

Rural Rother
Covering Battle, Rye and surrounding districts. *Address:* Saxonwood, Market Square, Battle, East Sussex, TN33 0XB. *Tel:* 01424 774355. *Fax:* 01424 775083. [Jul 2000]

St. Leonards
Address: Ocean House, 87-89, London Road, St Leonards-on-Sea, East Sussex, TN37 6DH. *Tel:* 01424 439714. [Jul 2000]

Contacts
Social Services divides its services for people with a mental health problem into two: one for those under 65 years of age and one for those over 65. The details given here are for those *under* 65. For information about Social Services for people *over* 65, please see the 'Elderly Mental Health' chapter, page 56. There are four areas covered for people under 65: Eastbourne & Seaford, Hastings & Rother, Lewes and Wealden. [5953]

Eastbourne & Seaford
Address: Eastbourne & Seaford Mental Health Team, 2-4, Birling Street, Eastbourne, East Sussex, BN21 1RL. *Tel:* 01323 532110. *Fax:* 01323 532118. [5953]

Hastings & Rother
Address: Hastings & Rother Mental Health Team, 8, London Road, Bexhill, East Sussex, TN39 3JU. *Tel:* 01424 730512. *Fax:* 01424 732249. [5953]

Lewes
Address: Lewes Mental Health Team, Newhaven Polyclinic, Church Hill, Newhaven, BN9 9HH. *Tel:* 01273 611838. *Fax:* 01273 512531. [5953]

Wealden
This area is served by two offices, one in Seaford and the other in Uckfield.

Address: Amberstone Hospital, Carters Corner, Hailsham, East Sussex, BN27 4HU. *Tel:* 01323 444101. *Fax:* 01323 844767.

Address: Millwood Unit, Uckfield Hospital, Uckfield, East Sussex, TN22 5AW. *Tel:* 01825 761177. *Fax:* 01825 766233. [5953]

Managers
The following people are all managers of the various departments within the Mental Health Section of Social Services.

Philip Gander
Group Manager. *Address*: Social Services Dept - Mental Health Section, County Hall, St Annes Crescent, Lewes, East Sussex, BN7 1SW. *Tel*: 01273 482195. *Fax*: 01273 481205. [5248]

James Johnson
Service Manager responsible for Countywide Substance Misuse and HIV/AIDS Services. *Address:* Social Services Dept - Mental Health Section, Ridgeway, 125, St Helens Down, Hastings, TN34 2AR. *Tel:* 01424 443893. [5993]

Christine Thomas
Service Manager responsible for Older People's Mental Health Services, Countywide. *Address:* Social Services Department, Mental Health Section, Social Services Dept - Mental Health Section, Ridgeway, 125, St Helens Down, Hastings, TN34 2AR. *Tel:* 01424 443893. [5993]

Kate Dawson
Operational Support Manager, CMHTs, day services, and community placement scheme. *Address:* Social Services Department, County Hall, St Anne's Crescent, Lewes, Sussex, BN7 1SW. *Tel:* 01273 482195. [5993]

Steve Metcalf
Development Manager responsible for Strategic Developments, Mental Health Services. *Address:* Social Services Department, Mental Health Section, County Hall, St Annes Crescent, Lewes, Sussex, BN7 1SW. *Tel:* 01273 481478. *Fax:* 01273 481205. [5248]

Further Information

The following publications are available free of charge from Social Services, Communications Unit, County Hall, Lewes, East Sussex. *Tel:* 0845 601 0664 (Information Line). Calls charged at local rate.

Charges for Miscellaneous Services.
April 1999. [5973]

Day Care & Home Care Services.
April 1999. [5978]

Confidentiality.
April 1999. [5972]

Direct Payments.
April 1999. [5983]

Gaining Access to Your Records.
April 1999. [5970]

How to make a Complaint.
April 1999. [5971]

Learning Disability Register.
April 1999. [5982]

Mental Illness

'Mental Illness - The Care Programme Approach'. April 1999. [5981]

Occupational Therapy Services.
April 1999. [5979]

Residential Care Services.
April 1999. [5977]

Sensory Impairment Services.
April 1999. [5980]

Services for Children & Families.
April 1999. [5975]

Social Services Department
General Information about Social Services. April 1999. [5969]

Voluntary Organisations in East Sussex.
April 1999. [5974]

Your Local Community Care Charter.
April 1999. [5976]

Health Information Service
The HIS is a free and confidential 24-hour service. You can speak to staff during office hours, and you can listen to any of hundreds of tapes at any time, e.g: *Social Work Services* (Tape 213).

Address: The College of Health, St Margaret's House, 21, Old Ford Road, London, E2 9PL. *Freephone:* 0800 66 55 44. [5367]

NOTES

References

Details of the numbered references in the text are given below. In each case the information is separated into eight fields divided by the 'slash' (/) symbol:

Number. Reference number used in the text.
Publisher. Publisher, organistion or individual producing the document.
Title. Title, if any, or description of reference.
Author. Author's, editor's or correspondent's name.
Chapter. The name of the chapter of the *Good Health Guide* in which the reference is used.
Pages. Number of pages, size, price, and other details, ('pp' means 'pages')
Publication. Date of publication or creation.
Receipt. Date of receipt of reference by editorial department at Hastings Mind .

142 / Mind Support Centre. / Hastings Mind Support Centre Leaflet / Unknown / Day Centres / 2 pp / ? / 17-Jun-99

143 / Eli Lilly & Company Limited. / Bereavement. Booklet. / Unknown / Bereavement / 2 pp / Jun-97 / 8-Jun-99

144 / Royal College of Psychiatrists / Schizophrenia. Booklet. / Unknown / Schizophrenia / 16 pp / Feb. 97 / 8-Jun-99

145 / Sleep Council / Sleeping Well. Booklet. / Unknown / Sleep / 16 pp / Mar. 98 / 8-Jun-99

146 / Eli Lilly & Company Limited. / Depression in the Elderly. Booklet. / Unknown / Elderly Mental Health / 16 pp / Jun. 97 / 8-Jun-99

147 / Royal College of Psychiatrists. / Manic Depressive Illness. Booklet. / Unknown / Manic Depression / 20 pp / Pub. 1997 / 8-Jun-99

148 / Eli Lilly & Company Limited. / Depression. Booklet. / Unknown / Depression / 20 pp / Jun. 1997 / 8-Jun-99

528 / NHS Hastings & Rother / Mental Health Services Directory 1998. / Anna Barnes / General / 96 pp / Jun-98 / May, 1999

530 / Mind. / Publications from Mind - Spring to Summer 1999. / Unknown / General / 4 pp / Spring/Summer 1999 / Oct. 1999

532 / Roebuck Medical Centre. / Surgery Information / Unknown / Docgors / 16 pp / ? / 1-Jun-99

533 / Carisbrooke House Surgery. / Surgery Information / Unknown / Doctors / 8 pp / ? / 11-Oct-99

534 / Mind in Barnet. / The Mental Health Guide for the London Borough of Barnet / Geraldine Cooney / General / 92 pp / Summer 1999. / 20-Oct-99

535 / Vermillion (Ebury Press) / The complete guide to psychiatric drugs - a layman's guide to anti-depressants, tranquillisers and other prescription drugs. / Ron Lacey / Medication / 172 pp / Pub. 1996 / 21-Dec-99

1566 / Mental Health Foundation / Fundamental Focus, Issue 13. / Rachel Clinton / General / 8 pp / Apr. 1999 / 4-Jun-99

1567 / Mental Health Foundation / Mental Health Foundation Annual Report 1997/98. / Mike Wilson / General / 24 pp / Apr. 1999 / 4-06-

1568 / Meridian Broadcasting / Talking about it. A booklet about your mental health. / Unknown / General / 40 pp / Oct. 1999 / 8-Jun-99

1569 / Meridian Broadcasting / Directory of Organisations. / Unknown / General / 16 pp / Oct. 1999 / 8-Jun-99

1570 / E. Sussex Social Services & ESBHHA. / East Sussex Community Care Plan, 1999-2002. / Anon. / Community Care Plan / 120 pp / Pub. 1999 / 7-Jun-99

1571 / Mental Health Foundation / The Fundamental Facts. ISBN 0-901-944-637 / Lisa Bird, researcher, Mental Health Foundation / General / 40 pp. £15.00 / Pub. 1999 / 19-Jun-99

5000 / Al-Anon / A merry-go-round named denial / Anon / Alcohol / 16 pp / ? / 26-Apr-00

5001 / Al-Anon / Freedom from despair / Anon / Alcohol / 4 pp / ? / 26-Apr-00

5002 / Al-Anon / Welcome / Anon / Alcohol / 6 pp / ? / 26-Apr-00

5003 / PSP Europe / Advocacy & Support leaflet and letter / Michael R. Koe / PSP / 7 pp / 17.01.00 / 18-Jan-00

5004 / Mental Health Foundation / All about bulimia nervosa / Charlotte Stark / Eating Disorders / 18 pp / . 1997 / 21-Oct-99

5005 / Mental Health Foundation / All about dementia / Dr. Sophie Zeman / Elderly Mental Health / 24 pp / . 1998 / 21-Oct-99

5006 / Mental Health Foundation / Because You Care / Dr. Katy Hinchliffe / Elderly Mental Health / 24 pp / . 1998 / 21-Oct-99

5007 / Mental Health Foundation / Understanding Schizophrenia / Dr. Sophie Zeman / Schizophrenia / 20 pp / . 1997 / 21-Oct-99

5008 / Mental Health Foundation / The Milk's in the Oven / Lizi Hann / Elderly Mental Health / 36 pp / . 1998 / 21-Oct-99

5009 / Migraine Trust / Taking Control of Your Migraine / Unknown / Migraine / 16 pp / . 1997 / 3-Jun-99

5010 / No Panic / Information sheets / Sian / Panic; Phobias; Obsessions; Compulsions / 7 pp / Oct. 1999 / 20-Oct-99

5011 / Trauma Aftercare Trust / Post Traumatic Stress - The Basics / Unknown / Trauma / 20 pp / ? / 26-Oct-99

5012 / Trauma Aftercare Trust / Information leaflet / Unknown / Trauma / 6 pp / ? / 26-Oct-99

5013 / No Panic / The Facts / Unknown / Obsessions; Compulsions / 8 pp / ? / 20-Oct-99

5014 / Down's Syndrome Association / Membership leaflet / Unknown / Learning Disabilities / 6 pp / ? / 3-Jun-99

5015 / First Steps to Freedom / Information pack / Sheila Harris / Phobias; Obsessions; Anxiety; Panic; Eating Disorders; Substance Misuse / 15 pp / ? / 20-Oct-99

5016 / Mind / Psychosis Factsheet / Kaaren Cruse / Paranoia /

11 pp / . 1998 / 22-Oct-99

5017 / NSPCC / Protecting Children Together - Annual Report / John Norton / Children & Young People / 24 pp / . 1998 / 5-Nov-98

5018 / SANE / About Sane / Unknown / Schizophrenia / 1 pp / . 1997 / 1-Jul-99

5019 / ADCESBH / Alcohol & Drugs Training Courses 2000-2001' / Unknown / Alcohol; Substance Misuse / 8 pp / ? / 10-Mar-00

5020 / Department of Health / The Children Act 1989 - An Introductory Guide for the NHS / June Thompson / Children & Young People / 58 pp / July, 99 / 22-Jan-00

5021 / Mind / Understanding the Psychological Effects of Street Drugs / Written by Terry Brown & edited by Sara Dunn / Substance Misuse / 12 pp / . 1998 / 21-Oct-99

5022 / Hastings & Rother Health Promotion Unit and Trinity Project, Hastings / XTC / Sam Allis, Catherine Pepper, Mark Reeves, Kyle James / Substance Misuse (Ecstasy) / 4 pp / ? / 3-Jun-99

5023 / Department of Health / Solvents - A Parent's Guide / Richard Ives / Substance Misuse (Solvents) / 16 pp / Mar-94 / 2-Feb-00

5024 / Mind / New Titles & Best Sellers from Mind / Unknown / Various / 4 pp / ? / 1-Jul-00

5025 / Huntington's Disease Association / All About the Huntington's Disease Association (Fact Sheet 1) / Unknown / Huntington's Disease / 4 pp / ? / 21-Oct-99

5026 / Huntington's Disease Association / General Information about Huntington's Disease (Fact Sheet 2) / Unknown / Huntington's Disease / 4 pp / ? / 21-Oct-99

5027 / Huntington's Disease Association / Predictive Testing for Huntington's Disease (Fact Sheet 3) / Unknown / Huntington's Disease / 12 pp / ? / 21-Oct-99

5028 / Huntington's Disease Association / Newsletter, Issue 55, Summer 1999. / Unknown / Huntington's Disease / 40 pp / Summer 99 / 21-Oct-99

5029 / Parentline Plus / Letter - corrections to entry / Esther Freeman / Family Problems / 1 pp / 30.06.00 / 3-Jul-00

5030 / PAX / Proof corrections / Alice Neville / Phobias; Obsessions; Anxiety; Panic; Eating Disorders; Substance Misuse / 2 pp / 8.05.00 / 3-Jul-00

5031 / HARC / Letter re: proof corrections / Sandra Lewis / Advice / 2 pp / 30.06.00 / 3-Jul-00

5032 / Mind / Openmind No. 104. July/August 2000. Article: Machismo & Misery / George Stewart / Men / 32 pp / July, 2000 / 1-Jul-00

5033 / South East Advocacy Projects / Proof corrections / Trudy Allen / Advocacy / 5 pp / 30.06.00 / 5-Jul-00

5034 / Roebuck House Surgery / Summer 2000 Newsletter / Unknown / Doctors / 2 pp / ? / 5-Jul-00

5035 / Samaritans Hastings / Letter / Harry 184 (volunteer) / Crises / 1 pp / 4.07.00 / 5-Jul-00

5036 / Agape Trust / Letter / Rev'd Kenn Baird / Family Problems / 1 pp / 3.07.00 / 5-Jul-00

5037 / Parenting Education & Support Forum / Information leaflet / Unknown / 1. Children 2. Family / 4 pp / ? / 5-Jul-00

5038 / Parenting Education & Support Forum / Supporting Parents & Children / ? / 1. Children 2. Family / 4 pp / Dec. 1996 / 5-Jul-00

5039 / Parenting Education & Support Forum / Newsletter number 6. / Hetty Einzig, editor / 1. Children 2. Family / 16 pp / Spring 1997 / 5-Jul-00

5040 / Boots Company plc / Prescription Collection Service / Unknown / Chemists / 4 pp / June, 2000 / 5-Jul-00

5041 / Boots Company plc / NHS Prescription Charges / Unknown / Chemists / 1 pp / March, 2000 / 5-Jul-00

5042 / Boots the Chemists, Priory Meadow / At Your Service / Unknown / Chemists / 4 pp / ? / 5-Jul-00

5043 / Al-Anon Family Groups / Letter / Sheila Ayriss / Alcohol / 1 pp / 4.07.00 / 7-Jul-00

5044 / Multiple Sclerosis society. / Leaflet. / Unknown / Multiple Sclerosis / 2 pp / ? / 5-Jun-99

5045 / Hastings & St Leonards Observer. / Article: Good News for Pregnant Women / Unknown / Women / 1 pp / Jun-99 / 11-Jun-99

5046 / Hastings & Rother Counselling Service. / Leaflet. / Unknown / Counselling / 6 pp / ? / 14-Jun-00

5047 / ESBHH. / You and your pharmacist. Leaflet. / Unknown / Chemists / 2 pp / ? / 23-Oct-99

5048 / NHS Hastings & Rother / Health News in Hastings & Rother NHS, Autumn 1999. / Unknown / NHS / 4 pp / ? / 3-Nov-99

5049 / BUPA. / Leaflet. / Unknown / Private Health Care / 6 pp / ? / 9-Nov-99

5050 / BUPA. / Letter. / Stephen Flanagan / Private Health Care / 1 pp / Oct-99 / 6-Nov-99

5051 / British Association for Counselling. / Information Office Fact Sheet C2. / Unknown / Counselling / 2 pp / ? / 11-Nov-99

5052 / Hastings & Rother Community Alcohol Team. / Counselling Services. / Unknown / Alcohol / 4 pp / ? / 12-Nov-99

5053 / British Association for Counselling. / Counselling & Psychotherapy Resource Directory. / Unknown / Counselling / 8 pp / ? / 11-Nov-99

5054 / British Association for Counselling. / Counselling & Psychotherapy Resources Directory, update sheet. / Unknown / Counselling / 3 pp / ? / 11-Nov-99

5055 / Hastings Voluntary Action. / Hastings Volunteer Bureau. Pamphlet. / Unknown / Voluntary Work / 2 pp / ? / 29.11.99

5056 / Daily Telegraph. / Making light work of illness. / Jane Alexander / Alternative Therapy. Colourpuncture / 1 pp / Dec-99 / 10-Dec-99

5057 / Daily Telegraph. / Homoeopathy. Article. / Nigel Summerley / Alternative Therapy. Homoeopathy / 1 pp / Nov-99 / 12-Nov-99

5058 / Focus on Mental Health. / Newsletter. / Unknown / Mental Health / 2 pp / ? / 12-Dec-99

5059 / National Institute of Medical Herbalists. / Register of Qualified Members, 1999/2000 with supplements. / Unknown / Alternative Therapy. Herbalism / 56 pp / ? / 15-Dec-99

5060 / Society of Homoeopaths. / Homeopathy simply explained. Leaflet. / Unknown / Alternative Therapy. Homoeopathy / 6 pp / ? / Dec. 1999

5061 / Society of Homoeopaths. / Register of Homeopaths. / Unknown / Alternative Therapy. Homoeopathy / 32 pp / Aug. 1999 / Dec. 1999

5062 / Friends of Homoeopathy. / Homeopathy for everyone. Leaflet. / Unknown / Alternative Therapy. Homoeopathy / 6 pp / ? / Dec. 1999

5063 / Friends of Homoeopathy. / Picture of Health, issue 11.

Newsletter. / Unknown / Alternative Therapy. Homoeopathy / 4 pp / ? / 17.12.99

5064 / Care for the Carers. / Who we are, what we do. Leaflet. / Unknown / Carers / 4 pp / ? / 13.12.99

5065 / Society of Teachers of the Alexander Technique. 1993. / An introduction to the Alexander Technique. Leaflet. / Unknown / Alternative Therapy. Alexander Technique / 6 pp / ? / 18-Dec-99

5066 / Society of Teachers of the Alexander Technique. / United Kingdom List of Teachers. / Unknown / Alternative Therapy. Alexander Technique / 60 pp / ? / 13-Dec-99

5067 / Manic Depression Fellowship / Working Matters, Edition 14. Leaflet. / Unknown / Manic Depression / 4 pp / ? / 18-Dec-99

5068 / Manic Depression Fellowship / Travel Insurance. Leaflet. / Unknown / Manic Depression / 2 pp / ? / 18-Dec-99

5069 / Manic Depression Fellowship / Pendulum, volume 15, number 4. / Unknown / Manic Depression / 16 pp / ? / 18-Dec-99

5070 / Mind. / Ten questions about compulsory treatment in the community. Leaflet. / Unknown / Mind Organisation / 4 pp / Dec-99 / 18-Dec-99

5071 / Hastings & St Leonards Observer. / Article: New Mental Health Unit Opens at the Conquest / Lanie Whiting / Hospitals / 1 pp / Dec-99 / 17-Dec-99

5072 / Clouds. / Collection of information leaflets. / Susanna Smith / Alcohol / 71 pp / June, 1999 / 18-Dec-99

5073 / London School of Classical Homoeopathy. / Prospectus. Booklet. / Unknown / Alternative Therapy. Homoeopathy / 46 pp / Autumn 1999 / 16-Dec-99

5074 / Focus on Mental Health. / Minutes of Meetings 30th November 1999. / Unknown / Mental Health / 2 pp / Dec. 1999 / 15-Dec-99

5075 / Hastings Borough Council Marketing Department 1999. / About, issue 6. Magazine. / HBC Marketing Dept. / Media / 16 pp / ? / 14-Dec-99

5076 / British Association for Counselling. / Invitation to membership. Booklet. / Unknown / Counselling / 45 pp / Apr-98 / 14-Dec-99

5077 / Hastings Voluntary Action. / Hastings Community News, issue 98. / Unknoqn / Voluntary Work / 4 pp / Nov. 1999 / 22-Nov-99

5078 / Multiple Sclerosis Society / MS on your mind - mental and emotional aspects of MS. Booklet. / Drs. Carolyn Young, Kieran O'Driscoll, Everard Thornton with Cynthia Benz. / Multiple Sclerosis / 12 pp / Summer 1999. / 18-Nov-99

5079 / Multiple Sclerosis Society / Publications Resume. Information sheet. / Unknown / Multiple Sclerosis / 9 pp / Autumn 1999 / Nov. 1999

5080 / Institute of Psychiatry. / Research Update, Maudsley Family Psychosis Study. Leaflet. / Unknown / Psychiatry / 4 pp / Autumn 1999 / 18-Nov-99

5081 / ESBHH. / Public Telephone Directory. / Unknown / Social Services / 11 pp / Nov-99 / 12-Nov-99

5082 / Multiple Sclerosis Society / What is MS? - what does it mean to be diagnosed with multiple sclerosis? Booklet. / Judy Graham / Multiple Sclerosis / 12 pp / Summer 1999. / 8-Nov-99

5083 / Multiple Sclerosis Society / Sources of Support - a signpost to specialised information and practical support. Booklet. / Judy Graham / Multiple Sclerosis / 12 pp / Spring 1999. / 8-Nov-99

5084 / Multiple Sclerosis Society / Making the most of life with MS - a new beginning. Booklet. / Rosalind Bayley / Multiple Sclerosis / 12 pp / Spring 1999. / 8-Nov-99

5085 / Multiple Sclerosis Society / Membership - acting together to make things better for people with MS and their families. Membership form leaflet. / Unknown / Multiple Sclerosis / 6 pp / Spring 1999. / 8-Nov-99

5086 / British Acupuncture Council. / Letter, including list of practitioners. / Enquiries Officer / Alternative Therapy. Acupuncture / 1 pp / Dec-99 / 23-Dec-99

5087 / British Acupuncture Council. / How can acupuncture help you? Leaflet. / Unknown / Alternative Therapy. Acupuncture / 6 pp / May, 1999 / 23-Dec-99

5088 / Mind. / New titles and best sellers from Mind. / Unknown / Mind Organisation / 4 pp / ? / Jan. 00

5089 / Hastings & Rother NHS Trust. / Eversfield Hospital - Queen Charlottes. Leaflet. / Unknown / Hospitals / 4 pp / ? / 3-Dec-99

5090 / ESBHHA / Working draft Health Improvement Programme. / Unknown / Community Health Councils / 72 pp / Oct-99 / 23-Dec-00

5091 / Mind. / Open Mind. Issue 101. / Unknown / Mind Organisation / 33 pp / Jan/Feb 2000 / 24-Dec-99

5092 / Manic Depression Fellowship / What next? Information leaflet. / MDF / Manic Depression / 6 pp / ? / 15-Nov-99

5093 / Penguin. / Dictionary of Psychology, 2nd edition. / Unknown / Psychology / 2 pp / 1985 & 1995 / 22-Dec-99

5094 / Focus on Mental health / Minutes of meeting / Unknown / Mental Health / 3 pp / ? / 13-Nov-99

5095 / NHS Hastings & Rother / Health in Hastings & Rother NHS. Leaflet. / Unknown / Health Authorities / 6 pp / Dec. 1999 / 4-Jan-00

5096 / APCMI / Befriending Scheme, Hastings. Leaflet. / Unknown / Befriending / 1 pp / ? / 4-Jan-00

5097 / Mental Health Media. / Shape the news about mental health. Advertising leaflet. / Unknown / Mental Health / 2 pp / ? / 24-Dec-99

5098 / Hastings Voluntary Action / Hastings Community News, No. 99. / Unknown / Voluntary Work / 4 pp / Dec. 1999 / 4-Jan-00

5099 / Mind in Barnet. / First National Standards for Mental Health. Press release. / Unknown / Mind Organisation / 6 pp / Oct-99 / 25-Oct-99

5100 / Hastings Voluntary Action. / Advocacy Services in East Sussex, Annual Report 1998-99. / Unknown / Voluntary Work / 25 pp / ? / 29-Nov-99

5101 / Department of Health. / Catalogue of free publications and information. / Communications Directorate Dept. of Health / Health Authorities / 33 pp / Jan. 1999 / 4-Nov-99

5102 / BUPA. / Your introduction to BUPA. / Unknown / Private Health Care / 6 pp / ? / 5-Nov-99

5103 / BUPA. / BUPA Information Brochure. / Unknown / Private Health Care / 19 pp / ? / 5-Nov-99

5104 / Association of British Insurers. / Are you buying private medical insurance? / Unknown / Private Health Care / 8 pp / ? / 3-Nov-99

5105 / BUPA. / Specially selected for you. List of BUPA hospitals. / Unknown / Private Health Care / 4 pp / ? / Nov. 1999

5106 / Mind. / Mind Publications Mail Order 1999. /

Unknown / Mind Organisation / 4 pp / ? / 5-Nov-99

5107 / Free Association Books. / New Books from FAB. Book list. / Unknown / Various / 6 pp / ? / Nov. 1999

5108 / Carfax Publishing. / Mental Health Religion & Culture. Leaflet. / Unknown / Various / 6 pp / ? / Nov. 1999

5109 / Mind / Creating accepting communities. Leaflet. / Unknown / Mental Health / 2 pp / ? / 5-Nov-99

5110 / Mind. / Open Mind, issue 100. / Carrie Viccars / Mental Health / 32 pp / Dec. 1999 / Nov. 1999

5111 / Times. / One cigarette shortens life by 11 minutes. Article. / Helen Rumbelow / Smoking / 1 pp / Dec-99 / 31-Dec-99

5112 / XS Health. / Stop-Loss, Private Medical Insurance - the Guide. Booklet. / Unknown / Insurance / 18 pp / ? / Oct. 1999

5113 / XS Health. / Warning - private medical insurance can seriously damage your wealth. Booklet. / Unknown / Insurance / 8 pp / ? / Oct. 1999

5114 / XS Health. / How little does XS Health cost? Leaflet. / Unknown / Insurance / 8 pp / ? / Oct. 1999

5115 / XS Health. / Application form. Leaflet. / Unknown / Insurance / 8 pp / ? / Oct. 1999

5116 / XS Health. / Letter. / Matthew Mills / Insurance / 1 pp / Jan-00 / Oct. 1999

5117 / Daily Telegraph. / Article: John McEnroe talks about his failed marriage / Jan Moir / Family Problems / 1 pp / Nov-99 / 30-Nov-99

5118 / Dr Michael Bott. / Letter. / Dr Michael Bott / Counselling / 3 pp / Nov-99 / 22-Nov-99

5119 / National Schizophrenia Fellowship / Leaflet. / Lynne / Schizophrenia / 1 pp / Jan. 2000 / 13-Jan-00

5120 / Hastings & Rother NSF. / Minutes of Meeting 15th September 1999. / Unknown / Schizophrenia / 1 pp / Sept. 1999 / 13-Jan-00

5121 / NARMI / Letter re residential care. / Pearl Baker / Residential Care / 1 pp / Dec-99 / 13-Jan-00

5122 / Hastings & Rother Manic Depression Fellowship. / Group meeting. Schedule. / Unknown / Manic Depression / 2 pp / ? / 13-Jan-00

5123 / Moat Care & Repair. / Advice & support for older and disabled people. / Unknown / Housing / 4 pp / ? / 13-Jan-00

5124 / Dr Bennett. / Letter. / Miss J J Lacey / Doctors / 1 pp / Oct-99 / 3-Nov-99

5125 / Cinque Ports House Surgery. / Correspondence / Karen Osborne / Doctors / 2 pp / Oct. 1999 / 15-Oct-99

5126 / Essenden Road Surgery. / Correspondence / Annette Taylor / Doctors / 2 pp / Oct. 1999 / 15-Oct-99

5127 / Little Common Surgery. / Correspondence / Judy Coates / Doctors / 2 pp / Oct. 1999 / 15-Oct-99

5128 / Stone Street Surgery. / Correspondence / Marion Nicholson / Doctors / 1 pp / Oct. 1999 / 19-Oct-99

5129 / Warrior Square Surgery. / Correspondence / Mrs Best / Doctors / 2 pp / Oct. 1999 / 14-Oct-99

5130 / Martins Oak surgery. / Correspondence / Anne Edmead / Doctors / 1 pp / Oct. 1999 / 14-Oct-99

5131 / Silver Spring surgery. / Correspondence / Malcolm Wright / Doctors / 2 pp / Oct. 1999 / 15-Oct-99

5132 / Fairfield Surgery. / Correspondence / Stephen Fowler / Doctors / 1 pp / Oct. 1999 / 15-Oct-99

5133 / Reedswood Road Surgery. / Correspondence / Linda Cox / Doctors / 3 pp / Oct. 1999 / 20-Oct-99

5134 / Main Street Surgery, Northiam. / Correspondence / Linda Cox / Doctors / 2 pp / Oct. 1999 / 13-Oct-99

5135 / Old Town Surgery. / Correspondence / Tricia Busbridge / Doctors / 1 pp / Oct. 1999 / 14-Oct-99

5136 / Lower Glen Surgery. / Correspondence / Mrs C Smith / Doctors / 1 pp / Oct. 1999 / 14-Oct-99

5137 / Churchwood Surgery. / Correspondence / Sharon Hitchman / Doctors / 1 pp / Oct. 1999 / 14-Oct-99

5138 / Beaconsfield Road Surgery. / Correspondence / Mrs Bowditch / Doctors / 2 pp / Oct. 1999 / 16-Oct-99

5139 / Fernhill Centre. / Correspondence / Monica Jephcott / Counselling / 2 pp / Oct. 1999 / 8-Nov-99

5140 / Mel Stockdale. / Correspondence / Mel Stockdale / Counselling / 2 pp / Oct. 1999 / 4-Nov-99

5141 / Clare Crellin. / Correspondence / Clare Crellin / Counselling / 2 pp / Oct. 1999 / 29-Oct-99

5142 / Dr M Botha. / Correspondence / Dr M E Botha / Counselling / 2 pp / Oct. 1999 / 29-Oct-99

5143 / Boots the Chemists, Bexhill. / Correspondence / Janet Crawford, consultant pharmacist / Chemists / 3 pp / Oct. 1999 / 15-Dec-99

5144 / Hastings Befrienders. / Correspondence / Lewis / Befriending / 1 pp / ? / 15-Dec-99

5145 / Brighton & Hove Mind. / Correspondence / Andy Porter / Mind Organisation / 2 pp / Oct. 1999 / 29-Nov-99

5146 / Mind Shop, Bexhill. / Correspondence / Lynne Collins / Mind Organisation / 2 pp / Oct. 1999 / 23-Nov-99

5147 / Get It While You Can. / Correspondence / Robyn Rimmell / Legal Matters / 1 pp / Oct. 1999 / 27-Oct-99

5148 / Get It While You Can Project. / Arrest referral and support for substance misuers. Leaflet. / Unknown / Legal Matters / 5 pp / Oct. 1999 / 27-Oct-99

5149 / Bensons Chemists. / Correspondence / Unknown / Chemists / 2 pp / Oct. 1999 / 9-Nov-99

5150 / Andersens Pharmacy / Correspondence / Unknown / Chemists / 2 pp / Oct. 1999 / 27-Oct-99

5151 / Boots the Chemists, Battle. / Correspondence / Unknown / Chemists / 2 pp / Oct. 1999 / 16-Oct-99

5152 / Marsh Chemists. / Correspondence / Unknown / Chemists / 2 pp / Oct. 1999 / 15-Oct-99

5153 / Collis Chemists. / Correspondence / Unknown / Chemists / 2 pp / Oct. 1999 / 15-Oct-99

5154 / Martel Ltd. / Correspondence / Unknown / Chemists / 1 pp / Oct. 1999 / 23-Oct-99

5155 / Safeways Pharmacy / Correspondence / Unknown / Chemists / 2 pp / Oct. 1999 / 23-Oct-99

5156 / MDFF. / Correspondence / Mrs Maureen Baines / Manic Depression / 2 pp / Oct. 1999 / 20-Oct-99

5157 / Steve Clifford / Correspondence / Steve Clifford / Counselling / 3 pp / Nov. 1999 / 23-Nov-99

5158 / Joanna Beazley Richards. / Correspondence / Joanna Beazley Richards / Counselling / 2 pp / Oct. 1999 / 20-Oct-99

5159 / John Roylance. / Correspondence / John Roylance / Counselling / 1 pp / Oct. 1999 / 27-Oct-99

5160 / Leslie Ironside. / Correspondence / Leslie Ironside / Counselling / 3 pp / Oct. 1999 / 22-Oct-99

5161 / Hazel Redsull / Correspondence / Hazel Redsull /

Counselling / 2 pp / Oct. 1999 / 22-Oct-99

5162 / Sandy Adey. / Correspondence / Sandy Adey / Counselling / 1 pp / Oct. 1999 / 22-Oct-99

5163 / Counselling Centre / Correspondence / Ron Fellows / Counselling / 2 pp / Oct. 1999 / 19-Oct-99

5164 / A J Anderson. / Correspondence / A J Anderson / Counselling / 2 pp / Oct. 1999 / 18-Oct-99

5165 / Kay Thomson. / Correspondence / Kay Thomson / Counselling / 2 pp / Oct. 1999 / 19-Oct-99

5166 / Peter Sanders. / Correspondence / Peter Sanders / Counselling / 3 pp / Oct. 1999 / 19-Oct-99

5167 / Peter Sanders. / Correspondence / Peter Sanders / Counselling / 1 pp / Oct. 1999 / 19-Oct-99

5168 / Janet McDonald / Correspondence / Janet McDonald / Counselling / 2 pp / Oct. 1999 / 19-Oct-99

5169 / Christine Cox. / Correspondence / Christine Cox / Counselling / 2 pp / Oct. 1999 / 18-Oct-99

5170 / Jen Popkin. / Correspondence / Jen Popkin / Counselling / 2 pp / Oct. 1999 / 20-Oct-99

5171 / KCPU. / Correspondence / Val / Counselling / 2 pp / Oct. 1999 / 18-Oct-99

5172 / Hastings & Rother NHS Trust. / Use of illicit drugs and alcohol. Leaflet. / Unknown / Substance Misuse / 4 pp / ? / 14-Jan-00

5173 / Joy Oakley. / Letter. / Joy Oakley / Counselling / 1 pp / ? / 14-Jan-00

5174 / PPP Healthcare. / Your membership agreement. Booklet / Unknown / Private Healthcare / 15 pp / ? / 14-Jan-00

5175 / PPP Healthcare. / Letter. / John DuBois / Private Healthcare / 1 pp / Jan-00 / 14-Jan-00

5176 / Obsessive Action. / Letter. / Andrew Ravensdale / Obsessions / 1 pp / Jan-00 / 14-Jan-00

5177 / Obsessive Action. / Obsessions or Compulsions. Leaflet. / Unknown / Obsessions / 6 pp / ? / 14-Jan-00

5178 / Obsessive Action. / Challenging OCD. Leaflet. / Unknown / Obsessions / 6 pp / Autumn, 1999 / 14-Jan-00

5179 / Mental Health Foundation / Understanding Depression. Booklet. / Unknown / Manic Depression / 23 pp / ? / 21-Oct-99

5180 / Mental Health Foundation / All about anorexia nervosa. Booklet. / Unknown / Eating Disorders / 18 pp / ? / 21-Oct-99

5181 / Mental Health Foundation / All about anxiety. Booklet. / Unknown / Anxiety / 27 pp / ? / 21-Oct-99

5182 / Sussex Autistic Society. / What is autism? Leaflet. / Unknown / Autism / 7 pp / ? / 30-Oct-99

5183 / Sussex Autistic Society. / Practical workshops for teachers of children with autism. Leaflet. / Unknown / Autism / 12 pp / ? / 30-Oct-99

5184 / Sussex Autistic Community Trust Ltd. / Asperger Support Groups. Leaflet. / Unknown / Autism / 6 pp / ? / 30-Oct-99

5185 / Daily Telegraph. / Answers to anxiety. Article. / Unknown / Anxiety / 1 pp / Dec-99 / 22-Dec-99

5186 / Shiatsu Society. / Practitioners' Register. List. / Unknown / Alternative Therapy. Shiatsu / 2 pp / ? / 20-Jan-00

5187 / Cruse Bereavement Care. / Letter / John Dilley / Bereavement / 2 pp / Jan-00 / 20-Jan-00

5188 / Blue Cross Pet Bereavement Support Service. / After The Death of someone Very Close / Unknown / Bereavement / 14 pp / ? / 20-Jan-00

5189 / APCMI. / Correspondence / Lynn / Befriending / 3 pp / Jan-00 / 20-Jan-00

5190 / National Association of Bereavement Services. / Correspondence / Carole Lambert / Bereavement / 2 pp / ? / 21-Jan-00

5191 / Outside in, Cambridge. / Letter, catalogue and brochure. / Letter: Steve Hayes / Seasonal Affective Disorder / 34 pp / ? / 21-Jan-00

5192 / Daily Telegraph. / Article: Osteopathy, the way the Japanese do it / Rosalyn Lewis / Alt. Therapy. / 1 pp / Jan-00 / 21-Jan-00

5193 / Counselling Partnership. / Correspondence / Frances Rae / Counselling / 2 pp / Oct. 1999 / 22-Nov-99

5194 / Daily Telegraph. / Article: Putting It Out Without Putting It On / Amanda Ursell / Smoking / 1 pp / Jan-00 / 24-Jan-00

5195 / Daily Telegraph. / Article: Bulletin / Celia Hall / Alternative Therapy / 1 pp / Jan-00 / 3-Jan-00

5196 / Hastings & St Leonards Observer. / Article: Hospitals stub out smoking / Unknown / Smoking / 1 pp / Jan-00 / 4-Jan-00

5197 / Daily Telegraph. / Connected. / Unknown / General / 1 pp / Jan-00 / 13-Jan-00

5198 / Godden Green Clinic / Letter. / Penny Barr / Hospitals & Clinics / 2 pp / Oct-99 / 15-Oct-99

5199 / Ore Clinic. / Correspondence / Trevor Cossen / Hospitals & Clinics / 1 pp / Oct. 1999 / 14-Oct-99

5200 / BUPA Hospital, Hastings. / Correspondence / Judith Bonner / Private Healthcare / 2 pp / Oct. 1999 / 14-Oct-99

5201 / Social Misfit Society. / Leaflets. / Unknown / Social Exclusion / 9 pp / ? / 19-Jan-00

5202 / Priory Healthcare. / Alcohol, social use? Mild abuse? Totally hooked? Brochure. / Unknown / Alcohol / 14 pp / ? / 19-Jan-00

5203 / Hastings Borough Council. / List of Councillors. / Unknown / Complaining / 4 pp / ? / 10-Feb-00

5204 / Daily Telegraph. / Article: Medicine by mouse / Christine Doyle / Medication / 1 pp / Feb-00 / 9-Feb-00

5205 / Daily Telegraph. / Article: Cigarettes are as addictive as hard drugs / Robert Ward / Smoking / 1 pp / Feb-00 / 9-Feb-00

5206 / Hastings & Rother NHS Trust. / Woodlands. Leaflet. / Unknown / Hospitals / 4 pp / ? / 19-Jan-00

5207 / Cruse Bereavement Care. / Letter & data entry form / Charles Croft / Bereavement / 2 pp / Feb-00 / 16-Feb-00

5208 / Daily Telegraph. / Article: Love conquered my food phobia / Antony King-Deacon / Eating Disorders / 1 pp / Feb-00 / 18-Feb-00

5209 / Hastings Voluntary Action / Hastings Community News Issue 100 / Unknown / Voluntary Work / 4 pp / Jan/Feb 2000 / 11-Feb-00

5210 / Daily Telegraph. / Article: A place for families to share eating disorders / Unknown / Eating Disorders / 1 pp / Jan-00 / 19-Feb-00

5211 / NHS Hastings & Rother / Letter / Lynne Bingham / Schizophrenia / 1 pp / ? / 10-Feb-00

5212 / Hastings & St Leonards Observer. / Article: Patricia takes the high road in Peru / Unknown / Cerebral Palsy / 1 pp / Feb-00 / 18-Feb-00

5213 / Daily Telegraph. / Article: Trust me, I'm a doctor / Unknown / General / 1 pp / Feb-00 / 17-Feb-00

5214 / Citizens Advice Bureau Hastings & Rother / Leaflet / Unknown / CABs / 6 pp / ? / 25-Feb-00

5215 / Focus on Mental Health / Focus on mental health / Unknown / Mental Health / 6 pp / ? / 25-Feb-00

5216 / Creativity & Mental Health / Information Sheet / Unknown / Mental Health / 1? / ? / ?

5217 / Margaret Taylor / Art therapy information sheet / Margaret Taylor / Alternative Therapy. Art / 2 pp / ? / 25-Feb-00

5218 / User Q Group / Quality monitoring of mental health services. / Unknown / Mental Health / 12 pp / ? / 25-Feb-00

5219 / MDFF. / Proposed dates for meetings / Unknown / Manic Depression / 1 pp / ? / 25-Feb-00

5220 / NHS Executive / The Care Programme Approach / Unknown / Carers / 6 pp / ? / 25-Feb-00

5221 / Focus on Mental Health / Meeting. Talk by Christine Lockwood / Unknown / Mental Health / 1 pp / ? / ?

5222 / MDF Hastings & Rother / Leaflet / Unknown / Manic Depression / 1 pp / June, 1999 / ?

5223 / Society for Manic Depression (USA) / Program for remission (web-site) / Unknown / Manic Depression / 1 pp / ? 1999 / ?

5224 / Mind in Barnet / Mental Health Guide / Unknown / Mental Health / 2 pp / ? 1999 / ?

5225 / Seitai Association UK / List of Registered Practitioners / Craig McConnell / Alternative Therapy. Seitai / 1 pp / ? / 2-Feb-00

5226 / Rural Rother Creative Care Network / Information Sheet / Unknown / Rural Rother / 1 pp / Jan-00 / 1-Feb-00

5227 / NHS Hastings & Rother / Patient Factsheet 6: Cognitive Therapy / Unknown / Counselling & Therapy / 3 pp / ? / 29-Feb-00

5228 / Hastings & Rother NHS Trust. / Patient Factsheet 1: Tranquilisers & Anti-Depressants / Unknown / Medication / 4 pp / ? / 29-Feb-00

5229 / Daily Telegraph. / Article: Safety alert over herbal remedy for depression / Sandra Laville & Tara Womersley / Alternative Therapy. Herbalism / 1 pp / Mar-00 / 2-Mar-00

5230 / National Institute of Medical Herbalists / Herbal Medicine - a caring profession / Unknown / Alternative Therapy. Herbalism / 4 pp / ? / 15-Dec-99

5231 / Mind in Barnet / First National Standards in Mental Health / Unknown / Mind Organisation / 1 pp / Sep. 1999 / Sep. 1999

5232 / NHS Hastings & Rother / Patient Factsheet 2. The Psychiatric Team / Unknown / Psychiatry / 3 pp / ? / 29-Feb-00

5233 / NHS Hastings & Rother / Patient Factsheet 5. Lithium Therapy / Unknown / Medication / 4 pp / ? / 29-Feb-00

5234 / NHS Hastings & Rother / Patient Factsheet 4. Depot Anti-psychotic medication / Unknown / Medication / 4 pp / ? / 29-Feb-00

5235 / NHS Hastings & Rother / Health News in Hastings & Rother / Unknown / General / 4 pp / Summer 99 / 29-Feb-00

5236 / Margaret Taylor / Correspondence / Margaret Taylor / Alt. Art therapy / 5 pp / Mar-00 / 2-Mar-00

5237 / National Society for Epilepsy / Explaining Epilepsy / Unknown / Epilepsy / 6 pp / Feb. 1997 / 2-Feb-00

5238 / National Society for Epilepsy / Epilepsy & Work / Unknown / Epilepsy / 6 pp / Nov-98 / 2-Feb-00

5239 / National Society for Epilepsy / We are all you need to know / Unknown / Epilepsy / 6 pp / Jul. 1997 / 2-Feb-00

5240 / RTFB Publishers / What should I do? / E van der Does / Doctors / 64 pp / Dec-97 / 3-Mar-00

5241 / Social Misfit Society. / Bulletin Issue No 2 / Claire / Social Exclusion / Letter & form & bulletin / Mar-00 / 2-Mar-00

5242 / Anti-Bullying Campaign / Website / Unknown / Bullying / Internet site / Mar-00 / 4-Mar-00

5243 / Pupiline / Website / Unknown / Bullying / Internet site / Mar-00 / 4-Mar-00

5244 / Kidscape / Website / Unknown / Bullying / Internet site / Mar-00 / 4-Mar-00

5245 / Department of Health NHS / Prescriptions - Claiming free prescriptions. Important news. / Unknown / Chemists / 6 pp / Mar-99 / 2-Mar-00

5246 / Hastings Voluntary Action / Hastings Community News - issue 101 / Unknown / Voluntary Work / 4 pp / Feb. 2000 / 1-Mar-00

5247 / Migraine Trust / Taking Control of Your Migraine / Unknown / Migraine / 16 pp / Jan. 1997 / 2-Feb-00

5248 / Social Services Mental Health / Correspondence / Philip Gander / Social Exclusion / 4 pp / Feb. 2000 / 6-Mar-00

5249 / Mind Fields Seminars / Understanding Anxiety / Joe Griffin / Anxiety / 4 pp / ? / 6-Mar-00

5250 / Mind / Seminars, training consultancy / Unknown / Mind Organisation / 16 pp / Feb.2000 / 6-Mar-00

5251 / Mind / New Titles & Best Sellers from Mind / Unknown / Mind Organisation / 4 pp / ? / 6-Mar-00

5252 / Athlone Press / Publications List / Unknown / Mind Organisation / 2 pp / ? / 6-Mar-00

5253 / ESBHHA / Drug Abuse chapter correspondence / Simon Scott / Substance Misuse / 4 pp / Feb. 2000 / 6-Mar-00

5254 / AD/HD Support Network / Attention Deficit / Judith Guest / Attention Deficit / 2 pp / Feb. 2000 / 2-Mar-00

5255 / Hastings & Rother Federation of Information Providers / Y2K Info. Day 12 April 2000 / Katy Burbridge / Information / 2 pp / ? / 4-Mar-00

5256 / Focus on Mental Health / Minutes of Meeting 11 Feb 2000 / Unknown / Mental Health / 2 pp / Feb-00 / 4-Mar-00

5257 / Mind / Open Mind 102 / Unknown / Mental Health / 32 pp / Mar-00 / 6-Mar-00

5258 / Henderson Hospital / Dialogue, issue 1 / Unknown / Personality Disorder / 6 pp / Summer 99 / 8-Mar-00

5259 / Henderson Hospital / Dialogue, issue 2 / Unknown / Personality Disorder / 6 pp / Autumn 99 / 8-Mar-00

5260 / Henderson Hospital / Dialogue, issue 3 / Unknown / Personality Disorder / 6 pp / Winter 99 / 8-Mar-00

5261 / T.R. Beckett Newspapers / Citizens' Guide 2000 / Unknown / General / 48 pp / Mar-00 / 10-Mar-00

5262 / Christine Lockwood / Correspondence / Christine Lockwood / Care Programme Approach / 3 pp / Mar. 2000 / 10-Mar-00

5263 / Henderson Hospital / Correspondence / Sue Ryan /

Personality Disorder / 2 pp / Mar. 2000 / 14-Mar-00

5264 / Cavendish Clinics / Information sheets & letter / Clive Looker / Smoking / 5 pp / ? / 14-Mar-00

5265 / Linda Mooncie / Bereavement. Chapter & Intro. / Linda Mooncie / Bereavement / E-mail / Mar-00 / 13-Mar-00

5266 / Daily Telegraph. / Alternative answers online / Jane Feinmann / Alternative Therapy / 1 pp / Mar-00 / 10-Mar-00

5267 / Hastings Voluntary Action / Voluntary Work / Rose Austen / Voluntary Work / Letter & form & bulletin / Mar-00 / 15-Mar-00

5268 / Mind / Publications from Mind. Autumn 99/Spring 2000 / Unknown / Mind Organisation / A5 booklet / Aut/Spr. 1999/2000 / 10-Mar-00

5269 / Mind / Mindlink Information Sheets / Unknown / Mind Organisation / 12 pp / ? / 10-Mar-00

5270 / Mind / Factsheets Order Form / Unknown / Mind Organisation / 12 pp / Feb-00 / 10-Mar-00

5271 / Mind / Rural Minds Information Sheet / Unknown / Mind Organisation / A4 leaflet / ? / 10-Mar-00

5272 / APCMI / Befriending Chapter Corrections / Lynn Jenkins / Befriending / 5 pp / Mar-00 / 16-Mar-00

5273 / Oasis / Information Sheet / Unknown / Advice / 6 pp / ? / 16-Mar-00

5274 / BUPA / BUPA Care Membership guide / Unknown / Private Health Care / 50 pp / Jul-99 / 16-Mar-00

5275 / BUPA / Letter / Linda Theobald / Private Health Care / Letter & form & bulletin / Mar-00 / 16-Mar-00

5276 / Daily Telegraph. / Article: Meditation / Sarah Brewer / Alternative Therapy. Mediation / Article / Nov-99 / Nov. 1999

5277 / Mind / Diverse Minds / Unknown / Mind Organisation / Leaflet A4 / ? / 10-Mar-00

5278 / Mind / Open Mind - the mental health magazine / Unknown / Mind Organisation / Leaflet A4 / ? / 10-Mar-00

5279 / Mind / Mind InfoLine / Unknown / Mind Organisation / Leaflets A4 / ? / 10-Mar-00

5280 / Ash / Factsheet 1. Smoking Statistics / Unknown / Smoking / 4 pp / ? / 16-Mar-00

5281 / Ash / Factsheet 3. Young people & smoking / Unknown / Smoking / 3 pp / ? / 16-Mar-00

5282 / Daily Telegraph. / Cerebral Palsy / Barbara Lantin / Cerebral Palsy / 1 pp / Mar-00 / 9-Mar-00

5283 / ME Association / Chronic Fatigue Syndrome - A Doctor's Guide / Charles Shepherd / Chronic Fatigue / 16 pp / ? / 18-Mar-00

5284 / ME Association / Chronic Fatigue Syndrome - Information sheet. / Colin Barton / Chronic Fatigue / 1 pp / Mar-00 / 18-Mar-00

5285 / Scope / What is cerebral palsy? / Unknown / Cerebral Palsy / 2 pp / ? / 20-Mar-00

5286 / ABC ESBH / Alcohol & Drugs Training Courses / Unknown / Alcohol / 2 pp / ? / 10-Mar-00

5287 / CHC / Election of Voluntary Sector Members 2000 / Carmen Winch / Community Health Councils / 13 pp / Mar-00 / 23-Mar-00

5288 / Hastings Voluntary Action / Voluntary Work chapter & letter / Rose Austen / Voluntary Work / A4 letter / Mar-00 / 23-Mar-00

5289 / Ben Edwards / Herbalism chapter corrections / Ben Edwards / Alternative Therapy. Herbalism / 6 pp / Mar. 2000 / 24-Mar-00

5290 / British Autogenic Society / Life Force Management for the rest of your life / Unknown / Alternative Therapy. Autogenic / 6 pp / ? / 24-Mar-00

5291 / Basingstome & Alton Mental Health Carers Empowerment Forum / Information for carers of people with mental health problems / Unknown / Carers / 1 pp / May, 2000 / 7-May-00

5292 / Priory Road Surgery / Correspondence / Mrs Godden / GPs' Surgeries / 7 pp / Mar. 2000 / 28-Mar-00

5293 / Buckhurst Road Surgery / Correspondence / Unknown / GPs' Surgeries / 7 pp / Mar. 2000 / 28-Mar-00

5294 / Essenden Road Surgery / Correspondence / Annette Tayan / GPs' Surgeries / 7 pp / Mar. 2000 / 28-Mar-00

5295 / Wellington Square Medical Centre / Correspondence / C. Proudlock / GPs' Surgeries / 7 pp / Mar. 2000 / 28-Mar-00

5296 / Belmont Surgery / Correspondence / Mrs Pilbeam / GPs' Surgeries / 7 pp / Mar. 2000 / 28-Mar-00

5297 / Collington Surgery / Correspondence / Mrs Jill Jarrett / GPs' Surgeries / 7 pp / Mar. 2000 / 28-Mar-00

5298 / MDF / Pendulum. Vol. 16; No. 1 / Unknown / Manic Depression / 22 pp / Spring 2000 / 27-Mar-00

5299 / Trudy Allen / Learning Difficulties chapter. Letter / Trudy Allen / Learning Disabilities / 2 pp / Mar-00 / 28-Mar-00

5300 / Hastings & St Leonards Observer / Job vacancies / Hastings & St Leonards Observer / Media Issues / 2 pp / Mar-00 / 17-Mar-00

5301 / Beaconsfield Road Surgery / Correspondencecc / Mrs C Bowditch / GPs' Surgeries / 7 pp / Mar. 2000 / 29-Mar-00

5302 / Martins Oak Surgery / Correspondencecc / Anne Edmead / GPs' Surgeries / 7 pp / Mar. 2000 / 29-Mar-00

5303 / High Street Ninfield Surgery / Correspondencecc / Unknown / GPs' Surgeries / 7 pp / Mar. 2000 / 29-Mar-00

5304 / Old Town Surgery Bexhill / Correspondencecc / Tricia Busbridge / GPs' Surgeries / 7 pp / Mar. 2000 / 29-Mar-00

5305 / Roebuck Surgery / Correspondencecc / Mrs G Brooks / GPs' Surgeries / 7 pp / Mar. 2000 / 30-Mar-00

5306 / Albert Road Surgery Bexhill / Correspondencecc / Mrs Haslett / GPs' Surgeries / 7 pp / Mar. 2000 / 30-Mar-00

5307 / Sea Road Surgery Bexhill / Correspondencecc / Kay Davey / GPs' Surgeries / 7 pp / Mar. 2000 / 30-Mar-00

5308 / Main Street Surgery Northiam / Correspondencecc / Linda Cox / GPs' Surgeries / 7 pp / Mar. 2000 / 30-Mar-00

5309 / Carisbrooke House Surgery / Correspondencecc / Mrs D Reddie / GPs' Surgeries / 7 pp / Mar. 2000 / 30-Mar-00

5310 / North Ridge Surgery / Correspondencecc / Miss L Adamson / GPs' Surgeries / 7 pp / Mar. 2000 / 30-Mar-00

5311 / Carisbrooke House Surgery / Correspondencecc / Mrs D Reddie / GPs' Surgeries / 7 pp / Mar. 2000 / 30-Mar-00

5312 / Fairfield surgery / Correspondencecc / Stephen Fowler / GPs' Surgeries / 1 pp / Mar. 2000 / 30-Mar-00

5313 / Wish Valley Surgery / Correspondencecc / Christine Paddock / GPs' Surgeries / 7 pp / Mar. 2000 / 30-Mar-00

5314 / Cinque Ports House Surgery / Correspondencecc / Karen Osborne / GPs' Surgeries / 7 pp / Mar. 2000 / 30-Mar-00

5315 / Harold Road Surgery / Correspondencecc / Mrs G Williams / GPs' Surgeries / 7 pp / Mar. 2000 / 31-Mar-00

5316 / Little Common Surgery / Correspondencecc / Judy Coates / GPs' Surgeries / 7 pp / Mar. 2000 / 2-Apl-00

5317 / National Society for Epilepsy / Correspondence / Anna Parikh / Epilepsy / 4 pp / Mar. 2000 / 31-Mar-00

5318 / Mary Cairns / Correspondence / Mary Cairns / Counselling & Therapy / 2 pp / Mar-00 / 31-Mar-00

5319 / Ben Edwards / Correspondence / Ben Edwards / Alternative Therapy. Autogenic / 4 pp / Mar-00 / 30-Mar-00

5320 / Jenny Hart / Correspondence / Jenny Hart / Alternative Therapy / 50 pp / Mar. 2000 / 27-Mar-00

5321 / NHS in Hastings & Rother / Health News in Hastings & Rother NHS / Unknown / Health Authorities / 4 pp / Mar-00 / 4-Apl-00

5322 / Trefoil Guild / Letter / Eileen Bolster / Learning Disabilities / 1 pp / Apr. 2000 / 2-Apl-00

5323 / Survivors' Poetry / Promoting Poetry by survivors of mental distress / Unknown / Poetry & Writing / 10 pp / ? / 30-Mar-00

5324 / Focus on Mental Health / Minutes of Meeting 10 Mar. 2000 / Unknown / Mental Health / 2 pp / Mar-00 / 3-Apr-00

5325 / Hastings Voluntary Action / Hastings Community News / Unknown / Voluntary Work / 4 pp / Mar./Apr. 2000 / 2-Apr-00

5326 / Partners in Advocacy / Correspondence / Trudy Allen / Advocacy / 5 pp / Apr. 2000 / 5-Apr-00

5327 / Barbara Hardcastle / Correspondence / Barbara Hardcastle / Information / 2 pp / Mar. 2000 / 5-Apr-00

5328 / Anna Barnes / Correspondence / Anna Barnes / Mental Health / 300 pp / Mar. 2000 / 5-Apr-00

5329 / Jenny Hart / Correspondence / Jenny Hart / Various / 20 pp / Mar. 2000 / 6-Apr-00

5330 / Hastings Lifeline / Correspondence / Michael Daly / Mental Health / 4 pp / 29 Jun. 1998 / 5-Apr-00

5331 / Hastings & Rother NHS Trust / Core Brief / Simon Purkiss / Smoking / 3 pp / 20 Mar. 2000 / 5-Apr-00

5332 / Sarah Holmes-Smith / Correspondence / Sarah Homes-Smith / Community Mental Health Teams / 1 pp / 4 Apr. 2000 / 5-Apr-00

5333 / Ann Cox / Correspondence / Ann Cox / Eating Disorders / A4 8pp + photo / Mar. 2000 / 8-Apr-00

5334 / Barbara Hardcastle / Correspondence / Barbara Hardcastle / Various / e-mail 1p / 7 Apr. 2000 / 7-Apr-00

5335 / NSF Hastings & Rother / AGM notice 20-Apr-00 / Lynne Bingham / Schizophrenia / 4 pp / Apr. 2000 / 11-Apr-00

5336 / ESBHHA etc / Community Mental Health Teams - draft / Unknown / Community Mental Health Teams / 14 pp / Sep.99 / 11-Apr-00

5337 / ESBHHA etc / CMHT News / Unknown / Community Mental Health Teams / 2 pp / Jun.99 / 11-Apr-00

5338 / Higher Nature / A4 magazine & leaflets / Unknown / Alternative Therapy / 76 pp / Autumn/Winter 1999 / 12-Apr-00

5339 / Mary Cairns / Correspondence / Mary Cairns / Counselling / 40 pp / Mar. 2000 / 31-Mar-00

5340 / International Network of Esoteric Healing / Information brochure / Unknown / Alternative Therapy / 4 pp / ? / 12-Apr-00

5341 / South Saxons House Surgery / Correspondence / Mrs Avril Chambers / GPs' Surgeries / 8 pp / Mar. 2000 / 13-Apr-00

5342 / Lower Glen Surgery / Doctors chapter corrections / Mrs S Hitchman / GPs' Surgeries / 8 pp / Mar. 2000 / 13-Apr-00

5343 / Anna Barnes / Community Mental Health Teams - draft / Anna Barnes / Community Mental Health Teams / 1 pp / ? / 12-Apr-00

5344 / Anna Barnes / Substance Abuse / Anna Barnes / Alcohol / 1 pp / ? / 12-Apr-00

5345 / Young Minds / Correspondence & Information Sheets / Unknown / Children & Young People / 19 pp / ? / 14-Apr-00

5346 / Health Promotion / Mental Health Media Resources Pack / Barbara Hardcastle / Media Issues / 28 pp / ? / 15-Apr-00

5347 / Samaritans / Media Guidelines on the Portrayal of Suicide / Unknown / Media Issues / 20 pp / Oct. 97 / 15-Apr-00

5348 / NUJ / Mental Health in the Media / Unknown / Media Issues / 12 pp / ? / 15-Apr-00

5349 / Press Standards Board of Finance / Code of Practice / Unknown / Media Issues / 1 pp / Nov-97 / 15-Apr-00

5350 / Depression Alliance / Young Person's Guide to Stress / Unknown / Children & Young People / 24 pp / ? / 17-Apr-00

5351 / Depression Alliance / About Depression Alliance / Unknown / Depression / 24 pp / ? / 17-Apr-00

5352 / Hastings & Rother NHS Trust / Mental Health Liaison Operation Policy & Background / Sarah Tindall / Health Authorities / 11 pp / ? / 17-Apr-00

5353 / Anna Barnes / Mental Health Guide April 2000 / Anna Barnes / General / 300pp / Apr-00 / 17-Apr-00

5354 / ESBHHA / GPs. Bexhill & Rother PCG / ESBHHA / Doctors / 5 pp / Apr-00 / 15-Apr-00

5355 / ESBHHA / GPs Hastings & Rother PCG / ESBHHA / Doctors / 5 pp / Apr-00 / 15-Apr-00

5356 / Dept. of Clinical Psychology / Eating Disorders Service / Unknown / Eating Disorders / 4 pp / ? / 18-Apr-00

5357 / Margaret Moss / User Groups chapter corrections / Margaret Moss / User Groups / 3 pp / Apr-00 / 18-Apr-00

5358 / MDF / Pendulum. Spring 97 / Unknown / Mood Diaries / A4 / Spring 1997 / ?

5359 / Hambleden Herbs / Organic Herb Catalogue 2000 / Unknown / Alternative Therapy. Herbalism / 12 pp / Spring 2000 / 19-Apr-00

5360 / Ellen Harley / Racial Issues chapter corrections / Ellen Harley / Racial Issues / 6 pp / Apr-00 / 19-Apr-00

5361 / Turkey Road Surgery / Doctors chapter corrections / Mrs Haslett / Doctors / 7 pp / Apr-00 / 11-Apr-00

5362 / Anna Barnes / Mental Health Guide / Anna Barnes / General / E-Mail 2pp / Apr-00 / 18-Apr-00

5363 / Barbara Hardcastle / Liaison Nurse Service / Barbara Hardcastle / Suicide / 1 pp / Apr-00 / 18-Apr-00

5364 / Ben Edwards / Autogenic Therapy corrections / Ben Edwards / Alternative Therapy. Autogenic / 2 pp / April / 25-Apr-00

5365 / Jenny Hart / Proofreading Chemists to Counselling (part) / Jenny Hart / Chemists to Counselling / 36 pp / April / 25-Apr-00

5366 / Ann Cox / Eating Disorders corrections / Ann Cox / Eating Disorders / 6 pp / April / 26-Apr-00

5367 / College of Health / Health Information Service / Unknown / General / 24 pp / ? / 26-Apr-00

5368 / Woodlands / Woodlands corrections / Jacqui Wilson / Woodlands / 6 pp / April / 27-Apr-00

5369 / Hastings Mind / Mind Organisation chapter / Franco Di Francesco / Mind Organisations / 2 pp / April / 28-Apr-00

5370 / ESBHHA / Health Promotion / Unknown / Health Authorities / 24 pp A4 / Jan. 99 / 13-Apr-00

5371 / Mary Dawson / Correspondence / Mary Dawson / Alternative Therapies / 9 pp / Apr-00 / 20-Apr-00

5372 / Mary Dawson / Correspondence / Mary Dawson / Children & Young People / 5 pp / Apr-00 / 20-Apr-00

5373 / Mary Dawson / Correspondence / Mary Dawson / Family Problems / 8 pp / Apr-00 / 20-Apr-00

5374 / Family Support Practitioners / Information sheet / Unknown / Family Problems / 1 pp / ? / 20-Apr-00

5375 / ESCC / A-Z ofProviders. All large homes / Unknown / Residential Care / 5 pp / Apr-00 / 21-Apr-00

5400 / Community Alcohol Team / Client Information / Andrea Crawford / Alcohol / 2 pp / Apr-00 / 29-Apr-00

5401 / Community Alcohol Team / Counselling Services / Unknown / Alcohol / 4 pp / ? / 29-Apr-00

5402 / Focus on Mental Health / Minutes of meeting. 7 April 2000 / Unknown / User Groups / 2 pp / Apr-00 / 29-Apr-00

5403 / Wallace. Alternative / Wallace Alternative Medical Practice / Unknown / Alternative Therapy. Clinics / 2 pp / ? / 25-Apr-00

5404 / ESBHHA / Joint Investment Plan & Community Care Plan. Progress Statement 2000-2001 / Unknown / Health Authorities / 20 pp / 13 Dec. 99 / 25-Apr-00

5405 / NHS Confederation / Who we are / Unknown / Health Authorities / 4 pp / Apr-00 / 30-Apr-00

5406 / Westfield Surgery / Correspondence / Mrs J Collins / GPs' Surgeries / 8 pp / April / 28-Apr-00

5407 / Mind / Peace of Mind / Unknown / Legal Matters / 1 pp / ? / 2-May-00

5408 / Madeleine Iddison / Community Mental Health Teams / Madeleine Iddison / Community Mental Health Teams / 1 pp / April / 28-Apr-00

5409 / UKCP / Register / Unknown / Counselling & Therapy / 12 pp / Apr-00 / 28-Apr-00

5410 / Madeleine Mayhew / Media Issues correspondence / Madeleine Mayhew / Media Issues / 7 pp / Apr-00 / 29-Apr-00

5411 / Press Complaints Commission / Code of Practice / Unknown / Media Issues / 3 pp / Dec-99 / 29-Apr-00

5412 / Elizabeth Downs / Correspondence / Elizabeth Downs / Alternative Therapy. Aromatherapy / 1 pp / Mar. 2000 / 3-May-00

5413 / Karen Sedgewick / Correspondence / Karen Sedgewick / Housing / 2 pp / May-00 / 3-May-00

5414 / MS Society / Corresponence / Gladys Stewart / Multiple Sclerosis / 1 pp / May-00 / 3-May-00

5415 / Al-Anon / News & Views, March 2000 / Unknown / Alcohol / 18 pp / Mar-00 / 3-May-00

5416 / Al-Anon / Poster. Alcoholism Can Tear a Family Apart / Unknown / Alcohol / 1 pp / ? / 3-May-00

5417 / Association of Carers / Information sheet / Unknown / Carers / 2 p A4 / ? / 3-May-00

5418 / Chemical Dependency Centre / Sharp programme / Unknown / Alcohol / 4 pp A4 / ? / 29-Apr-00

5419 / Anna Barnes / Health Improvement Programmes / Unknown / Health Authority / 2 pp / ? / 25-Apr-00

5420 / Anna Barnes / Joint Planning Discussion Paper / Unknown / Health Authority / 8 pp / August 1999 / 25-Apr-00

5421 / Anna Barnes / Bexhill & Rother PC Group Newsletter / Unknown / Health Authority / 2 pp / Sep-98 / 25-Apr-00

5422 / Anna Barnes / Primary Care Groups / Unknown / Health Authority / 4 pp / ? / 25-Apr-00

5423 / Madeleine Iddison / Social Services corrections / Madeleine Iddison / Social Services / 4 pp / Mar-00 / 20-Apr-00

5424 / Talking Life / Catalogue / Unknown / Various / 12 pp / ? / 2-May-00

5425 / Mind / Open Mind, 103. May 2000 / Various / Various / 32 pp / May-00 / 2-May-00

5426 / Press Complaints Commission / Correspondence / Laura Perito / Media Issues / 2 pp / May-00 / 4-May-00

5427 / Hastings & Rother NHS Trust / Child & Adolescent Mental Health Service / Unknown / Children & Young People / 6 pp / ? / 4-May-00

5428 / St Michael's Hospice / Correspondence / Unknown / Hospitals / 2 pp / May, 2000 / 5-May-00

5429 / Gingerbread, London / Correspondence / Tim Holt / Family / 1 pp / May, 2000 / 5-May-00

5430 / CHC, Eastbourne / Correspondence / Unknown / Community Health Councils / 1 pp / May, 2000 / 5-May-00

5431 / Barchester Towers / Correspondence / Unknown / Elderly Mental Health / 1 pp / May, 2000 / 5-May-00

5432 / Assoc. of Carers / Correspondence / Yvonne Hartnoll / Carers / 2 pp / May, 2000 / 5-May-00

5433 / Anna Barnes / Community Mental Health Teams / Anna Barnes / Community Mental Health Teams / 1 pp / May, 2000 / 5-May-00

5434 / Springfield Centre / Correspondence / Jen Popkin / Alternative Therapy. Clinics / 3 pp / May, 2000 / 5-May-00

5435 / H & Rother NHS Consumer Relations / Correspondence / Frances Bates / Complaining / 2 pp / May, 2000 / 5-May-00

5436 / NARMI / Correspondence / Pearl Baker / Carers / 2 pp / May, 2000 / 5-May-00

5437 / Learning Disability Forum / Correspondence / John McManus / Learning Disabilities / 2 pp / May, 2000 / 5-May-00

5438 / Council & Care / Correspondence / Unknown / Counselling / 2 pp / May, 2000 / 5-May-00

5439 / Crossroads / Correspondence / Jan Cackett / Carers / 3 pp / May, 2000 / 5-May-00

5440 / Relate / Correspondence / Anne Deas / Family Problems / 2 pp / May, 2000 / 5-May-00

5441 / Sleep Disorder Clinic / An end to problem snoring / S. Byrne / Miscellaneous. Sleeping / 7 pp / May, 2000 / 5-May-00

5442 / Hastings & Rother Counselling Service / Correspondence / Rose Webster / Counselling & Therapy

/ 1 pp / May, 2000 / 6-May-00

5443 / No Panic / Correspondence / Colin M Elles / Panic / 1 pp / May, 2000 / 6-May-00

5444 / Moat Care & Repair / Correspondence / Ann Smith / Housing; Elderly Mental Health / 3 pp / May, 2000 / 6-May-00

5445 / AD/HD Adult Support Network / Correspondence / Judith Guest / Attention Deficit / 4 pp / May, 2000 / 6-May-00

5446 / Nat. Phobics Society / Correspondence / N. Lidbetter / Phobias / 5 pp / May, 2000 / 6-May-00

5447 / Assoc. of Brit. Insurers / Correspondence / Mary Wooden / Private Health Care / 5 pp / May, 2000 / 6-May-00

5448 / Brit. Acupuncture Council / Correspondence / Jocelyn Gray / Alternative Therapy. Acupuncture / 6 pp / May, 2000 / 6-May-00

5449 / UKCP / Correspondence / Unknown / Counselling & Therapy / 2 pp / May 200 / 2-May-00

5450 / Mencap / Correspondence / Pauline Fletcher / Learning Disabilities / 1 pp / May, 2000 / 6-May-00

5451 / Backcare / Correspondence / Emma Tait / Miscellaneous / 1 pp / May, 2000 / 6-May-00

5452 / Henderson Hospital / Correspondence / Sue Ryan / Personality Disorder / 1 pp / May, 2000 / 6-May-00

5453 / Families Need Fathers / Correspondence / T. Rait / Family Problems / 1 pp / May, 2000 / 6-May-00

5454 / Cruse Bereavement Care / Correspondence / kKristy Craig / Bereavement / 2 pp / May, 2000 / 6-May-00

5455 / Mount Denys / Correspondence / L. Lambert / Elderly / 2 pp / May, 2000 / 6-May-00

5456 / East. & Wealden Social Services / Correspondence / Unknown / Learning Disabilities / 1 pp / May, 2000 / 6-May-00

5457 / PPP Healthcare / Correspondence / Peter Roach / Private Health Care / 2 pp / May, 2000 / 6-May-00

5458 / Social Services. Eastbourne / Correspondence / Unknown / Learning Disabilities / 1 pp / May, 2000 / 6-May-00

5459 / Mental Health Review Trib. / Correspondence / A. Archard / Mental Health Act / 1 pp / May, 2000 / 6-May-00

5460 / Alzheimer's Society / Correspondence / Unknown / Elderly Mental Health / 1 pp / May, 2000 / 6-May-00

5461 / Psychiatry Research Trust / Correspondence / Unknown / Psychiatry / 2 pp / May, 2000 / 6-May-00

5462 / Matthew Trust / Correspondence / Jean Bailie / Legal Matters / 2 pp / May, 2000 / 6-May-00

5463 / Memorial Care Centre / Correspondence / Unknown / Hospitals / 1 pp / May, 2000 / 6-May-00

5464 / St Michael's Bereavement Service / Correspondence / Veronica Bishop / Bereavement / 3 pp / May, 2000 / 6-May-00

5465 / Mental Health Act Commission / Correspondence / Mat Kinto / Mental Health Act / 2 pp / May, 2000 / 6-May-00

5466 / Fernside Family Centre / Correspondence / E. Cowper / Family Problems / 3 pp / May, 2000 / 6-May-00

5467 / Crossroads / Correspondence / Jan Cackett / Residential & Respite / 2 pp / May, 2000 / 6-May-00

5468 / My Choice / Correspondence / Trudy Allen / Learning Disabilities / 3 pp / May, 2000 / 6-May-00

5469 / Alan Mooncie / Manic Depression chapter / Alan Mooncie / Manic Depression / 6 pp / May, 2000 / 6-May-00

5470 / Mind / Find Peace of Mind / Unknown / Legal Matters / 16 pp / May, 1998 / 6-May-00

5471 / Mind / Making Provision / Unknown / Legal Matters / 16 pp / ? / 6-May-00

5472 / Battle Against Tranquilisers / Correspondence / Una Corbett / Substance Misuse / 3 pp / May, 2000 / 6-May-00

5473 / Aromatherapy Organisations Council / Correspondence / Sylvia Baker / Alternative Therapy. Aromatherapy / 8 pp / May, 2000 / 6-May-00

5474 / HCHA / Correspondence / Unknown / Housing / 2 pp / May, 2000 / 6-May-00

5475 / Parentline Plus / Correspondence / E. Freeman / Family / 1 pp / May, 2000 / 8-May-00

5476 / International Eating Disorder Centre / Correspondence / Beryl Foy / Eating Disorders / 3 pp / May, 2000 / 8-May-00

5477 / Priory Ticehurst House / Correspondence / Amy Hanham / Hospitals / 2 pp / May, 2000 / 8-May-00

5478 / Shiatsu Society / Correspondence / Ian Macwhinnie / Alternative Therapy. Shiatsu / 4 pp / May, 2000 / 8-May-00

5479 / St Michael's Bereavement Service / Correspondence / K.J. Brunger / Bereavement / 1 pp / May, 2000 / 8-May-00

5480 / Alzheimer's Society / Correspondence / Unknown / Elderly Mental Health / 1 pp / May, 2000 / 8-May-00

5481 / Manic Depression Fellowship / Correspondence / Ben Wit / Manic Depression / 1 pp / May, 2000 / 8-May-00

5482 / Eastbourne & County Healthcare / Correspondence / Duncan Barton / Legal Matters / 1 pp / May, 2000 / 8-May-00

5483 / Counselling & Involuntary Tranquiliser Addiction / Correspondence / Paul Entwistle / Substance Misuse / 3 pp / May, 2000 / 8-May-00

5484 / Independent Television Commission / Correspondence / Unknown / Media Issues / 5 pp / May, 2000 / 8-May-00

5485 / Suzie Sanderson / Correspondence / Suzie Sanderson / Alternative Therapy. Alexander Technique / 2 pp / May, 2000 / 8-May-00

5486 / Children's Legal Centre / Correspondence / Unknown / Children / 1 pp / May, 2000 / 8-May-00

5487 / Mental Health Directorate / Correspondence / Sarah Holmes Smith / Health Authorities / 2 pp / May, 2000 / 8-May-00

5488 / Relate / Correspondence / Maureen Anstey / Family Problems / 2 pp / May, 2000 / 8-May-00

5489 / Robert Parry / Correspondence / Robert Parry / Alternative Therapy. Acupuncture / 1 pp / May, 2000 / 8-May-00

5490 / Clare Hughes / Correspondence / Clare Hughes / Alternative Therapy. Alexander Technique / 1 pp / May, 2000 / 8-May-00

5491 / Manic Depression Fellowship / Information sheets / Unknown / Manic Depression / 18 pp / Feb. 2000 / 8-May-00

5492 / NHS Confederation / Understanding the NHS Confederation / Unknown / Health Authorities / 8 pp / Jan. 2000 / 4-May-00

5493 / Peter Howard / Correspondence / Peter Howard / Employment / 1 pp / Apr-00 / 5-May-00

5494 / Firstbridge / Information sheet / Unknown / Employment / 1 pp / ? / 5-May-00

5495 / Anna Taylor / Correspondence / Anna Taylor / Alternative Therapy. Homoeopathy / 1 pp / May, 2000 / 9-May-00

5496 / Broadcasting Standards Commission / Correspondence / Lorraine Miller / Media Issues / 2 pp / May, 2000 / 9-May-00

5497 / Sussex Private Clinic / Correspondence / Nichola Cox / Private Health / 4 pp / May, 2000 / 9-May-00

5498 / Sedlescombe Surgery / Correspondence / Judy Collins / Doctors / 3 pp / May, 2000 / 9-May-00

5499 / Brit. Psychological Society / Correspondence / S. White / Counselling / 3 pp / May, 2000 / 9-May-00

5500 / Gillian Smith / Correspondence / G. Smith / Psychiatry / 1 pp / May, 2000 / 9-May-00

5501 / Psychiatry Research Trust / Correspondence / Unknown / Counselling / 1 pp / May, 2000 / 9-May-00

5502 / Jane Sloan / Correspondence / Jane Sloan / Alternative Therapy. Homoeopathy / 2 pp / May, 2000 / 9-May-00

5503 / Arc Healthcare / Correspondence / Jon elster / Residential Care / 1 pp / May, 2000 / 9-May-00

5504 / Bohemia Trust / Correspondence / C. Beaumont / Money Matters / 2 pp / May, 2000 / 9-May-00

5505 / Ouse Valley PCG / Correspondence / Denise Rendell / Primary Care Group / 2 pp / May, 20 / 9-May-00

5506 / Bexhill CaringCommunity / Correspondence / J. Halsall / Carers / 3 pp / May, 2000 / 9-May-00

5507 / Ore Clinic / Correspondence / Babs Martin / Hospitals & Clinics / 3 pp / May, 2000 / 9-May-00

5508 / Both Parents Forever / Correspondence / John Bell / Families / 1 pp / May, 2000 / 9-May-00

5509 / Colin Griffith / Correspondence / Colin Griffith / Alternative Therapy. Homoeopathy / 3 pp / May, 2000 / 9-May-00

5510 / Godden Green Clinic / Correspondence / Abi Munnery / Private Health / 2 pp / May, 2000 / 9-May-00

5511 / Trinity Project / Correspondence / Unknown / Advice / 1 pp / May, 2000 / 9-May-00

5512 / Eastbourne Clinic of Natural Medicine / Correspondence / Harry Boys / Alternative Therapy / 4 pp / May, 2000 / 9-May-00

5513 / Employment Medical Advisory Service / Correspondence / Unknown / Employment / 1 pp / May, 2000 / 9-May-00

5514 / HARC / Correspondence / Unknown / Residential / 1 pp / May, 2000 / 9-May-00

5515 / Holiday Care / Correspondence / D. Moore / Residential / 1 pp / May, 2000 / 9-May-00

5516 / Sohami Gonzalez / Correspondence / S. Gonzalez / Alternative Therapy / 2 pp / May, 2000 / 9-May-00

5517 / Get it While You Can / Correspondence / Unknown / Substance Misuse / 2 pp / May, 2000 / 9-May-00

5518 / ME Association / Correspondence / Colin Barton / Chronic Fatigue / 3 pp / May, 2000 / 9-May-00

5519 / Brit. Brain & Spine Foundation / Correspondence / Victoria Murray / Brain Injury / 3 pp / May, 2000 / 9-May-00

5520 / Job Centre. Bexhill / Correspondence / N. Baker / Employment / 1 pp / May, 2000 / 10-May-00

5521 / Job Centre. Hastings Castle / Correspondence / N. Baker / Employment / 1 pp / May, 2000 / 10-May-00

5522 / Job Centre. Hastings Ashdown / Correspondence / N. Baker / Employment / 1pp / May, 2000 / 10-May-00

5523 / Stone Street Surgery / Correspondence / Unknown / Doctors / 1 pp / May, 2000 / 10-May-00

5524 / Sea Road Surgery / Correspondence / Kay Davey / Doctors / 10 pp / May, 2000 / 10-May-00

5525 / Vietnamese Mental Health / Correspondence / Nx Cam / Racial / 1 pp / May, 2000 / 10-May-00

5526 / London School of Classical Homoeopathy / Correspondence / Unknown / Alternative Therapy. Homoeopathy / 1 pp / May, 2000 / 10-May-00

5527 / Bexhill & Rother PCG / Correspondence / Unknown / Primary Care / 1 pp / May, 2000 / 10-May-00

5528 / Bexhill & Rother CAB / Correspondence / Unknown / Citizens Advice Bureaux / 3 pp / May , 2000 / 10-May-00

5529 / National Association of CABs / Correspondence / Unknown / Citizens Advice Bureaux / 2 pp / May, 2000 / 10-May-00

5530 / Bexhill Old Town Surgery / Correspondence / Unknown / Doctors / 3 pp / May, 2000 / 10-May-00

5531 / Sussex Police / Correspondence / C.S. Wratten / Miscellaneous / 2 pp / May, 2000 / 10-May-00

5532 / Fellowship of Depressives Anonymous / Correspondence / Pat Freya / Depression / 1 pp / May, 2000 / 10-May-00

5533 / ESCC Hailsham / Correspondence / Jackie Bennett / Learning Disabilities / 2 pp / May, 2000 / 10-May-00

5534 / Karen Sedgewick / Correspondence / Karen Sedgewick / Housing / 3 pp / May, 2000 / 10-May-00

5535 / Albert Road Surgery, Bexhill / Correspondence / Mrs Haslett / Doctors / 2 pp / May, 2000 / 10-May-00

5536 / Sea Road Surgery, Bexhill / Correspondence / Unknown / Doctors / 2 pp / May, 2000 / 10-May-00

5537 / Ninfield surgery / Correspondence / Unknown / Doctors / 1 pp / May, 2000 / 10-May-00

5538 / Bexhill Hospital / Correspondence / Jane Tolofson / Hospitals / 2 pp / May, 2000 / 10-May-00

5539 / High Weald PCG / Correspondence / Unknown / Primary Care Groups / 2 pp / May, 2000 / 10-May-00

5540 / Eastbourne District Hospital / Correspondence / Julie Perrin / Hospitals / 5 pp / May, 2000 / 10-May-00

5541 / Traumatic Stress Clinic / Correspondence / Unknown / Trauma / 1 pp / May, 2000 / 10-May-00

5542 / ACHCEW / Correspondence / Unknown / Community Health Councils / 2 pp / May, 2000 / 10-May-00

5543 / Audrey Wright / Correspondence / Audrey Wright / Alternative Therapy. Herbalism / 2 pp / May, 2000 / 10-May-00

5544 / Cornwallis Garden Surgery / Correspondence / Dr G.G. Bennett / Doctors / 1 pp / May, 2000 / 10-May-00

5545 / Fellowship of St Nicholas / Correspondence / Stephanie Edmonds / Children / 2 pp / May, 2000 / 10-May-00

5546 / Lynn Jackson / Telephone call / Lynn Jackson / Counselling / 1 pp / May-00 / 10-May-00

5547 / Sussex Police / Correspondence / Judy Fougere / Miscellaneous / 2 pp / May, 2000 / 11-May-00

5548 / Volunteer Bureau / Correspondence / Rose Austen /

Voluntary Work / 1 pp / May, 2000 / 11-May-00

5549 / Brit. Assoc. for Counselling / Correspondence / Denise Cherylin / Counselling Organisations / 1 pp / May, 2000 / 11-May-00

5550 / UK Register of Counsellors / Correspondence / Helen C. Wales / Counselling Organisations / 1 pp / May, 2000 / 11-May-00

5551 / Crossroads Association / Correspondence / Unknown / Carers / 1 pp / May, 2000 / 11-May-00

5552 / Kym Murden / Correspondence / Kym Murden / Alternative Therapy. Herbalism / 1 pp / May, 2000 / 11-May-00

5553 / Amberstone / Correspondence / Gareth Miller / Hospitals / 2 pp / May, 2000 / 11-May-00

5554 / St Anne's Centre / Correspondence / Martin Faulkner / Elderly Mental Health / 2 pp / May, 2000 / 11-May-00

5555 / Times / Correspondence / Roger Wood / Media Issues / 3 pp / May-00 / 11-May-00

5556 / Dr Sally Paget / Correspondence / Dr Sally Paget / Doctors / 2 pp / May, 2000 / 11-May-00

5557 / NCH Action for Children / Correspondence / Unknown / Children / 2 pp / May, 2000 / 11-May-00

5558 / Battle Road Surgery / Correspondence / Unknown / Doctors / 1 pp / May, 2000 / 11-May-00

5559 / Trauma Help Line / Correspondence / Unknown / Trauma / 1 pp / May, 2000 / 11-May-00

5560 / Mel Stockdale / Correspondence / Mel Stockdale / Counselling / 1 pp / May, 2000 / 11-May-00

5561 / Hazelbrae / Correspondence / Diana Fowler / Residential / 2 pp / May, 2000 / 11-May-00

5562 / Louis Appleby / Correspondence / Louis Appleby / Mental Health / 1 pp / May, 2000 / 11-May-00

5563 / Radio Authority / Correspondence / J. McCatty / Media Issues / 2 pp / May, 2000 / 11-May-00

5564 / SHARP / Correspondence / Sue Mercer / Substance Misuse / 2 pp / May, 2000 / 11-May-00

5565 / Eastbourne Downs PCG / Correspondence / Unknown / PC Groups / 1 pp / May, 2000 / 11-May-00

5566 / Compassionate Friends / Correspondence / P.J. Hunt / Bereavement / 2 pp / May, 2000 / 11-May-00

5567 / Warden Housing Assoc. / Correspondence / Glynis Gatenby / Housing / 2 pp / May, 2000 / 11-May-00

5568 / Buckhurst Road Surgery / Correspondence / Unknown / Doctors / 1 pp / May, 2000 / 11-May-00

5569 / Royal College of Psychiatrists / Correspondence / Unknown / Counselling / 2 pp / May, 2000 / 11-May-00

5570 / Bexhill Health Clinic / Correspondence / Hazel Brooks / Hospitals & Clinics / 1 pp / May, 2000 / 11-May-00

5571 / NSPCC / Correspondence / Unknown / Children / 6 pp / May, 2000 / 11-May-00

5572 / Eating Disorders Service / Correspondence / Dr Busattil / Eating Disorders / 2 pp / May, 2000 / 11-May-00

5573 / WPF Counselling & Therapy / Correspondence / Simon Pike / Counselling / 1 pp / May, 2000 / 11-May-00

5574 / Newmarket House Clinic / Correspondence / Unknown / Eating Disorders / 2 pp / May, 2000 / 11-May-00

5575 / Postern Gate, Rye / Correspondence / Mrs S.J. Harris / Doctors / 2 pp / May, 2000 / 11-May-00

5576 / Braeburn House / Correspondence / Unknown / Residential / 1 pp / May, 2000 / 11-May-00

5577 / National Viewers' & Listeners' Association / Correspondence / John Beyer / Media Issues / 1 pp / May, 2000 / 11-May-00

5578 / Mr Noakes / Correspondence / S. Noakes / Alternative Therapy. Herbalism / 1 pp / May, 2000 / 11-May-00

5579 / Nat. Assoc. Premenstrual Syndrome / Correspondence / C.G. Baker / Women's Issues / 2 pp / May, 2000 / 11-May-00

5580 / Care for the Carers / Correspondence / Unknown / Carers / 4 pp / May, 2000 / 11-May-00

5581 / National Viewers' & Listeners' Association / Directory 2000 / Unknown / Media Issues / 1 pp / May, 2000 / 11-May-00

5582 / Gudi Schipokat / Correspondence / Gudi Schipokat / Alternative Therapy. Alexander Technique / 1 pp / May, 2000 / 11-May-00

5583 / Eating Disorders Recovery via Self Help / Correspondence / Ann Cox / Eating Disorders / 2 pp / May, 2000 / 11-May-00

5584 / Jen Popkin / Correspondence / Jen Popkin / Counselling / 1 pp / May, 2000 / 12-May-00

5585 / ISMA (UK) / Information Sheet / Unknown / Stress / 1 pp / May, 2000 / 11-May-00

5586 / ISMA (UK) / Correspondence / David Moore / Stress / 2 pp / May, 2000 / 11-May-00

5587 / Mind in Barnet / E-Mail / Mike O'Sullivan / Good Health Guide / 1 pp / May-00 / 10-May-00

5588 / Obsessive Action / Correspondence / Mrs Mirna Honeyman / Obsession / 6 pp / May, 2000 / 10-May-00

5589 / XS Health / E-Mail / Tony Hayman / Private Health / 1 pp / May-00 / 8-May-00

5590 / Al-Anon / Literature Order Form / Unknown / Alcohol / 2 pp / Jan. 2000 / 10-May-00

5591 / ECT Anonymous / E-Mail / Pat / ECT / 20 pp / May-00 / 8-May-00

5592 / Today Programme / E-Mail / John Humphries / General / 1 pp / May-00 / 9-May-00

5593 / ECT Anonymous / E-Mail / Pat Butterfield / ECT / 1 pp / May-00 / 4-May-00

5594 / MS Society / Correspondence / Unknown / Multiple Sclerosis / 1 pp / May, 2000 / 12-May-00

5595 / North Ridge Surgery / Correspondence / Unknown / Doctors / 1 pp / May, 2000 / 12-May-00

5596 / Hastings Drug Dependency Unit / Correspondence / Kate Barry / Substance Misuse / 1 pp / May, 2000 / 12-May-00

5597 / Simon Howell / Correspondence / Simon Howell / Counsellors & Therapists / 1 pp / May, 2000 / 12-May-00

5598 / Families Anonymous / Correspondence / Unknown / Family Problems / 1 pp / May, 2000 / 12-May-00

5599 / Wellington Square Surgery / Correspondence / Malcolm Wright / Doctors / 1 pp / May, 2000 / 12-May-00

5600 / Tusker House / Correspondence / Unknown / Residential & Respite Care / 1 pp / May, 2000 / 12-May-00

5601 / Christine Cox / Correspondence / Christine Cox / Counsellors & Therapists / 1 pp / May, 2000 / 12-May-00

5602 / Prue Doherty / Correspondence / Prue Doherty / Counsellors & Therapists / 1 pp / May, 2000 / 12-May-00

5603 / SHAH Housing Aid Centre / Correspondence /

Unknown / Housing / 1 pp / May, 2000 / 12-May-00

5604 / Deborah Birnie / Correspondence / Deborah Birnie / Alternative Therapy / 1 pp / May, 2000 / 12-May-00

5605 / London Road Residential Home / Correspondence / Mr & Mrs J Walton / Residential & Respite Care / 1 pp / May, 2000 / 12-May-00

5606 / Carisbrooke House / Correspondence / Mrs D Reddie / Doctors / 1 pp / May, 2000 / 12-May-00

5607 / Sue Cook / Correspondence / Sue Cook / Counsellors & Therapists / 1 pp / May, 2000 / 12-May-00

5608 / Dr Michael Bott / Correspondence / Dr Michael Bott / Psychiatry / 1 pp / May, 2000 / 12-May-00

5609 / Anti-Bullying Campaign / Correspondence / Pauline Hasler / Bullying / 1 pp / May, 2000 / 12-May-00

5610 / Genevieve Picquart / Correspondence / Genevieve Picquart / Counsellors & Therapists / 1 pp / May, 2000 / 12-May-00

5611 / Northiam Surgery / Correspondence / Linda Cox / Doctors / 1 pp / May, 2000 / 12-May-00

5612 / Kenilworth Surgery / Correspondence / Dr & Mrs Das / Doctors / 1 pp / May, 2000 / 12-May-00

5613 / Hastings Age Concern / Correspondence / Angela Colburn / Elderly Mental Health / 1 pp / May, 2000 / 12-May-00

5614 / Institute of Psychiatry / Correspondence / Muriel Walshe / Schizophrenia / 2 pp / May-00 / 12-May-00

5615 / Parkinson's Disease Society / Information Sheet / Unknown / Elderly Mental Health / 3 pp / Apl. 1999 / 12-May-00

5616 / Premenstrual Society / Correspondence / Dr Michael Brush / Women's Issues / 1 pp / May, 2000 / 13-May-00

5617 / HVA Volunteer Bureau / Correspondence / Katy Burbridge / Voluntary Work / 1 pp / May, 2000 / 13-May-00

5618 / Wendy Lidster / Correspondence / Wendy Lidster / Counsellors & Therapists / 1 pp / May, 2000 / 13-May-00

5619 / Warrior Square Surgery / Correspondence / Mrs Val Best / Doctors / 3 pp / May, 2000 / 13-May-00

5620 / Bexhill Community Mental Health Team / Correspondence / J.P. Parmainteny / Community Mental Health Teams / 1 pp / May, 2000 / 13-May-00

5621 / Re-Solv / Correspondence / Unknown / Substance Misuse / 1 pp / May, 2000 / 13-May-00

5622 / Social Services / Correspondence / Unknown / Learning Disabilities / 1 pp / May, 2000 / 13-May-00

5623 / Scope / Correspondence / Jaime Burbridge / Cerebral Palsy / 1 pp / May, 2000 / 13-May-00

5624 / Joy Cobban / Correspondence / Joy Cobban / Counsellors & Therapists / 1 pp / May, 2000 / 13-May-00

5625 / ESCC / Correspondence / Kate Dawson / Social Services / 1 pp / May, 2000 / 13-May-00

5626 / Collis Pharmacy / Correspondence / Unknown / Chemists / 1 pp / May, 2000 / 13-May-00

5627 / Boots, Rye. / Correspondence / Unknown / Chemists / 1 pp / May, 2000 / 13-May-00

5628 / Gordon Barr Assoc. / Michael Bulman / Dee Barr / Counsellors & Therapists / 1 pp / May, 2000 / 13-May-00

5629 / Cruse Bereavement Bexhill / Correspondence / Charles Croft / Bereavement / 2 pp / May, 2000 / 13-May-00

5630 / Roger Powe / Correspondence / Roger Powe / Counsellors & Therapists / 1 pp / May, 2000 / 13-May-00

5631 / Cumberland Court / Correspondence / Unknown / Residential & Respite Care / 1 pp / May, 2000 / 13-May-00

5632 / Andersen's Pharmacy / Correspondence / Unknown / Chemists / 1 pp / May, 2000 / 13-May-00

5633 / Youth Access / Correspondence / Amber Collingwood / Children & Young People / 1 pp / May, 2000 / 13-May-00

5634 / Debbie Rimmer / Correspondence / Debbie Rimmer / Occupational Therapy / 2 pp / May, 2000 / 13-May-00

5635 / Home Truths (Radio 4) / Stammering / Unknown / Stammering / 1 pp / ? / 14-May-00

5636 / Chateau Fleur de Lys / Correspondence / Mrs B Dendy / Residential & Respite Care / 3 pp / May, 2000 / May, 2000

5637 / Bupa Hospital, Hastings / Correspondence / J. Bonner / Hospitals & Clinics / 1 pp / May, 2000 / 13-May-00

5638 / Jenny Hart / Proofreading / Jenny Hart / Alternative Therapy; Depression / 22 pp / May, 2000 / 15-May-00

5639 / Jenny Hart / Proofreading corrections / Jenny Hart / Counselling & Therapy / 29 pp / May, 2000 / 15-May-00

5640 / Black & Ethnic / Correspondence / Nadimeh Zeytoun / Race / 1 pp / May, 2000 / May, 2000

5641 / Pinehill / Corespondence / Pinehill Day Centre / Elderly Mental Health / 1 pp / May, 200 / 12-May-00

5642 / Beryl Hope / Correspondence / Beryl Hope / Counsellors & Therapists / 1 pp / May, 2000 / 15-May-00

5643 / Ombudsman / Correspondence / Hilary Pook / Complaining / 1 pp / May, 200 / 15-May-00

5644 / Assoc. for Post Natal Illness / Correspondence / J Cummins / Women's Issues / 1 pp / May-00 / 15-May-00

5655 / ESBHHA / Correspondence / Sally Allen / Health Authorities / 2 pp / May, 2000 / 15-May-00

5656 / Juliet Cox / Correspondence / Juliet Cox / Alternative Therapy / 1 pp / May, 200 / 15-May-00

5657 / Arrow FM / Correspondence / M. Buxton / Media / 2 pp / May-00 / 15-May-00

5658 / Wendy Clyde Elliott / Correspondence / Wendy Clyde Elliott / Counsellors & Therapists / 1 pp / May, 200 / 15-May-00

5659 / Brook / Correspondence / Paula Currie / Sex / 1 pp / May-00 / 15-May-00

5660 / Profession Centre / Correspondence / Richard Eaton / Alternative Therapy / 1 pp / May, 2000 / 15-May-00

5661 / Greensleeves / Correspondence / Unknown / Residential & Respite Care / 1 pp / May, 2000 / 15-May-00

5662 / Jill Halpin / Correspondence / Jill Halpin / Alternative Therapy / 1 pp / May, 2000 / 15-May-00

5663 / Ore Village Pharmacy / Correspondence / Unknown / Chemists / 1 pp / May, 2000 / 15-May-00

5664 / Peter Saunders / Correspondence / Peter Saunders / Counselling & Therapy / 1 pp / May, 2000 / 15-May-00

5665 / Sanctuary / Correspondence / Mr G. Body / Crises / 1 pp / May, 2000 / 15-May-00

5666 / Susan Chiswell Jones / Correspondence / Susan Chiswell Jones / Counselling & Therapy / 1 pp / May, 2000 / 15-May-00

5667 / Wish Valley, Hawkhurst / Correspondence / Christine Paddock / Doctors / 1 pp / May, 2000 / 15-May-00

5668 / Young Minds / Correspondence / Dr Mike Birkett /

Psychiatry / 2 pp / May, 2000 / 13-May-00

5669 / Bupa / Correspondence / Adam Lewis / Private Health Care / 1 pp / May, 2000 / 16-May-00

5670 / Trinity Project / Correspondence / Karen Brooker / Substance Misuse / 1 pp / May, 2000 / 16-May-00

5671 / Hastings Sheltered Workshop / Correspondence / Peter Howard / Rehabilitation / 1 pp / May, 2000 / 16-May-00

5672 / Social Services / Correspondence / Unknown / Social Services / 1 pp / May, 2000 / 16-May-00

5673 / Social Services / Correspondence / Unknown / Community Care / 1 pp / May, 2000 / 16-May-00

5674 / Pauline Mackay-Danton / Correspondence / Pauline Mackay-Danton / Counselling & Therapy / 1 pp / May, 2000 / 16-May-00

5675 / Pamela Embden / Correspondence / Pamela Embden / Alternative Therapy / 1 pp / May, 2000 / 16-May-00

5676 / Frances Rae / Correspondence / Frances Rae / Counselling & Therapy / 1 pp / May, 2000 / 16-May-00

5677 / All Wales User & Survivor Network / Correspondence / Steve Craine / Self-Harm / 1 pp / May, 2000 / 16-May-00

5678 / Elizabeth Hemmings / Correspondence / Elizabeth Hemmings / Alternative Therapy / 1 pp / May, 2000 / 16-May-00

5679 / Oaklands Residential Home / Correspondence / Mr Danny Rickaby / Learning Disabilities / 1 pp / May, 2000 / 16-May-00

5680 / Hastings Multiple Sclerosis Society / Correspondence / Mrs Beryl Carr / Multiple Sclerosis / 1 pp / May, 2000 / 16-May-00

5681 / Leslie Ironside / Correspondence / Leslie Ironside / Counsellors & Therapists / 1 pp / May, 2000 / 16-May-00

5682 / Hospital Radio, Hastings / Correspondence / Unknown / Media / 1 pp / May, 2000 / 16-May-00

5683 / Counselling Centre / Correspondence / Ron Fellows / Counselling & Therapy / 1 pp / May, 2000 / 16-May-00

5684 / Drug Dependency Unit / Correspondence / Unknown / Substance Misuse / 1 pp / May, 2000 / 16-May-00

5685 / Rural Rother Creative Care / Correspondence / Su Barnicoat / Rural Rother / 1 pp / May, 2000 / 16-May-00

5686 / BIBC / Correspondence / Unknown / Brain Injury / 4 pp / May, 2000 / 17-May-00

5687 / British Assoc. of Psychotherapists / Correspondence / G. Rusbridger / Counselling & Therapy / 3 pp / May, 2000 / 17-May-00

5688 / Hazel Redsull / Correspondence / Hazel Redsull / Counselling & Therapy / 1 pp / May, 2000 / 17-May-00

5689 / Jocelyn Jones / Correspondence / Jocelyn Jones / Counselling & Therapy / 1 pp / May, 2000 / 17-May-00

5690 / Philipa Cannan / Correspondence / Philipa Cannan / Counselling & Therapy / 1 pp / May, 2000 / 17-May-00

5691 / Frankie Sidhu / Correspondence / Frankie Sidhu / Counselling & Therapy / 4 pp / May, 2000 / 17-May-00

5692 / Edna Murdoch / Correspondence / Edna Murdoch / Counselling & Therapy / 1 pp / May, 2000 / 17-May-00

5693 / Health Promotion / Correspondence / Barbara Hardcastle / Health Authorities; Information / 2 pp / May, 2000 / 17-May-00

5694 / Graham Molyneux / Correspondence / Graham Molyneux / Counselling & Therapy / 1 pp / May, 2000 / 17-May-00

5695 / Peter Stehle / Correspondence / Peter Stehle / Counselling & Therapy / 1 pp / May, 2000 / 17-May-00

5696 / Dr Malik / Correspondence / Dr Malik / Psychiatry / 3 pp / May, 2000 / 17-May-00

5697 / Mental Health Act Commission / Correspondence / Unknown / Woodlands / 3 pp / May, 2000 / 17-May-00

5698 / Hastings Furniture Service / Correspondence / Nick Bellis / Housing / 2 pp / May, 2000 / 17-May-00

5699 / Migraine Support Group / Correspondence / June Gavin / Migraine / 2 pp / May, 200- / 17-May-00

5700 / Mary Wagner / Correspondence / Mary Wagner / Alternative Therapy. Herbalism / 2 pp / May, 200 / 17-May-00

5701 / Lorna Couldrick / Correspondence / Lorna Couldrick / Counselling & Therapy / 3 pp / May, 2000 / 17-May-00

5702 / ESBHHA / Correspondence / Madeleine Mayhew / Health Authorities / 3 pp / May 15, 2000 / 17-May-00

5703 / Paul Hambly / Correspondence / Paul Hambley / Alternative Therapy. Herbalism / 3 pp / May, 2000 / 17-May-00

5704 / Mental Health Advocacy / Correspondence / Allison Peterson / Advocacy / 2 pp / May, 2000 / 17-May-00

5705 / John Rignall / Correspondence / John Rignall / Counselling & Therapy / 1 pp / May, 2000 / 17-May-00

5706 / Care for the Carers / Correspondence / Jeanette Howlett / Carers / 1 pp / May, 2000 / 17-May-00

5707 / Tesco / Correspondence / Unknown / Chemists / 1 pp / May, 2000 / 17-May-00

5708 / Anthony Anderson / Correspondence / Anthony Anderson / Counselling & Therapy / 1 pp / May, 2000 / 17-May-00

5709 / Sussex Autistic Society / Correspondence / Philippa Erasmus / Autism / 6 pp / May, 2000 / 17-May-00

5710 / Nigel Short / Correspondence / Nigel Short / Counselling & Therapy / 1 pp / May, 2000 / 17-May-00

5711 / Hastings & Bexhill Youth Service / Correspondence / Kerry Smith / Children & Young People / 4 pp / May, 2000 / 17-May-00

5712 / Esperance Hospital / Correspondence / Frances Melville-Brown / Hospitals / 1 pp / May, 2000 / 17-May-00

5713 / Arthur Blackman Clinic / Correspondence / Unknown / Miscellaneous / 2 pp / May, 2000 / 18-May-00

5714 / Stephen Clifford / Correspondence / Stephen Clifford / Counselling; Depression / 3 pp / May, 2000 / 18-May-00

5715 / Mountside / Correspondence / Unknown / Residential Care / 3 pp / May, 2000 / 18-May-00

5716 / Direct Debt Line / Correspondence / Maggie Kirkpatrick / Money / 1 pp / May, 2000 / 18-May-00

5717 / ESCC- Learning Disability / Correspondence / Unknown / Learning Disabilities / 2 pp / May, 2000 / 18-May-00

5718 / Little Common Surgery / Correspondence / Judy Coates / Doctors / 4 pp / May, 2000 / 18-May-00

5719 / Voice UK / Correspondence / Jane Mather / Learning Disabilities / 2 pp / May, 200 / 18-May-00

5720 / Philip Holmes / Correspondence / Philip Holmes / Alternative Therapy. Acupuncture / 1 pp / May, 2000 / 18-May-00

5721 / Triumph over Phobia / Triumph Over Phobia Can Help / Unknown / Phobias / 2 pp / ? / 18-May-00

5722 / Careline / Correspondence / Angela Sharp / Carers / 1 pp / May, 2000 / 18-May-00

5723 / Clare Crellin / Correspondence / Clare Crellin / Counselling & Therapy / 2 pp / May, 2000 / 18-May-00

5724 / Women's Therapy Centre / Correspondence / Amber Djemal / Women's Issues / 1 pp / May, 2000 / 18-May-00

5725 / Priory Ticehurst House / Correspondence / Amy Hanham / Hospitals / 2 pp / May, 2000 / 18-May-00

5726 / Lesley King / Correspondence / Lesley King / Alternative Therapy. Homoeopathy / 2 pp / May, 2000 / 18-May-00

5727 / Boots the Chemists / Correspondence / Ann Cherry / Chemists / 2 pp / May, 2000 / 18-May-00

5728 / Francesca Inskipp / Correspondence / Francesca Inskipp / Counselling & Therapy / 1 pp / May, 2000 / 18-May-00

5729 / John Reading / Correspondence / John Reading / Alcohol / 8 pp / May, 2000 / 18-May-00

5730 / Age Concern / Correspondence / Unknown / Elderly / 2 pp / May, 2000 / 19-May-00

5731 / Dave Flewett / Correspondence / Dave Flewett / Counselling & Therapy / 2 pp / May, 2000 / 19-May-00

5732 / Swiss Life / Correspondence / Srosalind Pearson / Private Health Care / 5 pp / May, 2000 / 19-May-00

5733 / Seaview Projects / Creative Thinking For The New Millennium' / John Evans / Day Centres / 4 pp / May, 2000 / 19-May-00

5734 / Joanna Beazley Richards / Correspondence / Joanna Beazley Richards / Counselling & Therapy / 4 pp / May, 2000 / 19-May-00

5735 / APCMI / Correspondence / Claire Jowett / Befriending / 3 pp / May, 2000 / 19-May-00

5736 / Lawrence Suss / Correspondence / Lawrence Suss / Counselling & Therapy / 1 pp / May, 2000 / 19-May-00

5737 / Churchwood Medical Practice / Correspondence / Unknown / Doctors / 2 pp / May, 2000 / 19-May-00

5738 / Community Link Nurses / Correspondence / Unknown / Rehabilitation / 1 pp / May, 2000 / 19-May-00

5739 / Rock Clinic Assoc. / Correspondence / Melanie Withers / Counselling & Therapy / 1 pp / May, 2000 / 19-May-00

5740 / Melanie Withers / Correspondence / Melanie Withers / Counselling & Therapy / 1 pp / May, 2000 / 19-May-00

5741 / La Chenerie / Correspondence / Unknown / Residential Care / 1 pp / May, 2000 / 19-May-00

5742 / Michael Bulman / Correspondence / Michael Bulman / Counselling & Therapy / 3 pp / May, 2000 / 19-May-00

5743 / Christine Coxhead / Correspondence / Christine Coxhead / Counselling & Therapy / 2 pp / May, 2000 / 19-May-00

5744 / HACT / Correspondence / Jean Fletcher / Miscellaneous / 1 pp / May-00 / 19-May-00

5745 / Essenden Road Surgery / Correspondence / Annette Tayan / Doctors / 2 pp / May, 2000 / 19-May-00

5746 / British Complementary Medicine Association / Correspondence / Unknown / Alternative Therapy / 1 pp / May, 2000 / 19-May-00

5747 / Safeways Supermarket / Correspondence / Unknown / Chemists / 1 pp / May, 2000 / 19-May-00

5748 / Alan Crook / Correspondence / Alan Crook / Alternative Therapy. Homoeopathy / 2 pp / May, 2000 / 19-May-00

5749 / Bradley Carr-Hopkins / Correspondence / Bradley Carr-Hopkins / Alternative Therapy. Acupuncture / 1 pp / May, 2000 / 19-May-00

5750 / Social Services / Correspondence / M. Iddison / Social Services / 3 pp / May, 2000 / 19-May-00

5751 / British Autogenic Society / Correspondence / Elizabeth Ogilvie Davies / Alternative Therapy. Autogenic / 3 pp / May, 2000 / 19-May-00

5752 / Prof. Graham Thornicroft / E-Mail / Prof. Graham Thornicroft / National Service Framework / 1 pp / May, 2000 / 19-May-00

5753 / Family Service Units / Correspondence / H. Evans / Family / 1 pp / May-00 / 19-May-00

5754 / Department of Health / National Service Framework for Mental Health' / Unknown / National Service Framework / 6 pp / Sep-99 / 8-May-00

5755 / Al-Anon / News & Views / Anon / Alcohol / 20 pp / May, 2000 / 3-May-00

5756 / Department of Health / National Service Framework for Mental Health' / Unknown / National Service Framework / 150 pp / Sept. 1999 / 8-May-00

5757 / Department of Health / National Service Framework. Exec. Summary / Unknown / National Service Framework / 32 pp / Sept. 1999 / 8-May-00

5758 / Trefoil Guild / Correspondence / Eileen Bolster / Learning Disabilities / 2 pp / May, 2000 / 20-May-00

5759 / MACA / Correspondence / John McElvie / Day Centres / 1 pp / May, 2000 / 20-May-00

5760 / ESCC- Learning Disability / East Sussex Libraries Hastings & Rother / Unknown / General / 2 pp / May, 2000 / 20-May-00

5761 / Care for the Carers / Correspondence / Anna Geall / Carers / 2 pp / May, 2000 / 20-May-00

5762 / St Dominics Resid. Home / Correspondence / M. Dempsey / Residential Care / 1 pp / May, 2000 / 20-May-00

5763 / Beech Group / Correspondence / M.J. Richardson / Counselling & Therapy / 4 pp / May, 2000 / 20-May-00

5764 / Pema Sanders / Correspondence / Pema Sanders / Counselling & Therapy / 1 pp / May, 2000 / 23-May-00

5765 / Margaret Taylor / Correspondence / Margaret Taylor / Art Therapy / 3 pp / May, 2000 / 23-May-00

5766 / Val Simanowitz / Correspondence / Val Simanowitz / Counselling & Therapy / 2 pp / May, 2000 / 23-May-00

5767 / Anna Barnes / Correspondence / Anna Barnes / Woodland. Hospitals / 3 pp / May, 2000 / 20-May-00

5768 / ESCC Libraries / Correspondence / Unknown / Mailing Lists / 10 pp / May, 2000 / 22-May-00

5769 / Oasis / Telephone call / Clare Croft / Advice / 1 call / May-00 / 22-May-00

5770 / Peter Dale / E-Mail / Peter Dale / Counselling & Therapy / 1 pp / May-00 / 21-May-00

5771 / Turning Point / Correspondence / Benedict Knox / Substance Misuse / 2 pp / May, 2000 / 22-May-00

5772 / KCPU / Correspondence / Valerie Cunningham / Counselling & Therapy / 2 pp / May, 2000 / 22-May-00

5773 / National Autistic Society / Correspondence / Denis Cunningham / Autism / 4 pp / May, 2000 / 22-May-00

5774 / Ruth Venner / Correspondence / Ruth Venner / Counselling & Therapy / 2 pp / May, 2000 / 22-May-00

5775 / Debbie Rimmer / Correspondence / Debbie Rimmer /

Occupational Therapy / 1 pp / May, 2000 / 22-May-00

5776 / Christine Terris / Correspondence / Christine Terris / Counselling & Therapy / 1 pp / May, 2000 / 22-May-00

5777 / Hugh Maxwell / Correspondence / Hugh Maxwell / Counselling & Therapy / 1 pp / May, 2000 / 24-May-00

5778 / Streatfield House / Correspondence / Unknown / Residential Care / 2 pp / May, 2000 / 24-May-00

5779 / Toria Horner / Correspondence / Toria Horner / Alternative Therapies / 2 pp / May, 2000 / 24-May-00

5780 / Nicola Rejbakoz / Correspondence / Nicola Rejbakoz / Children & Young People / 1 pp / May, 2000 / 24-May-00

5781 / Leah Landau / Correspondence / Leah Landau / Alternative Therapy. Alexander Technique / 1 pp / May-00 / 24-May-00

5782 / Marta Vazquez Rio / Correspondence / Marta Vazquez Rio / Alternative Therapy. Alexander Technique / 1 pp / May-00 / 24-May-00

5783 / Dr Raj / E-Mail / Dr Raj / Psychiatrists / 1 pp / May-00 / 24-May-00

5784 / Sally McLaughlin / Correspondence / Sally McLaughlin / Counselling & Therapy / 1 pp / May-00 / 25-May-00

5785 / Lower Glen Family Practice / Correspondence / Unknown / Doctors / 3 pp / May-00 / 25-May-00

5786 / Bill O'Meara / Correspondence / Bill O'Meara / Alt. Homoeopathy / 1-Jan-00 / May-00 / 25-May-00

5787 / Sarah Child / Correspondence / Sarah Child / Alt. Alexander / 2 pp / May-00 / 25-May-00

5788 / McGuire Programme / Correspondence / Unknown / Stuttering / 10 pp / May-00 / 24-May-00

5789 / Celia O'Brien / Correspondence / Celia O'Brien / Counselling & Therapy / 1 pp / May, 2000 / 26-May-00

5790 / Women's Therapy Centre / Correspondence / Amber Djemal / Counselling & Therapy / 1 pp / May, 2000 / 26-May-00

5791 / Jenny Deadman / Correspondence / Jenny Deadman / Counselling & Therapy / 2 pp / May, 2000 / 26-May-00

5792 / Oldwood Surgery / Correspondence / Unknown / Doctors / 1 pp / May, 2000 / 26-May-00

5793 / Gillian Rock / Correspondence / Gillian Rock / Counselling & Therapy / 3 pp / May, 2000 / 26-May-00

5794 / Focus on Mental Health / Newsletter 2 / Unknown / General / 2 pp / May, 2000 / 26-May-00

5795 / Focus on Mental Health / Minutes 5-05-00 / Unknown / General / 2 pp / May, 2000 / 26-May-00

5796 / ASH / E-Mail / Karl Brookes / Smoking / 1 pp / May-00 / 26-May-00

5797 / Ashesonthesea / Internet Site / Unknown / Substance Misuse / 6 pp / May-00 / 26-May-00

5798 / Brit. Confed. Of Psychotherapists / Alphabetical list of practitioners / Unknown / Counselling & Therapy / 13 pp / May-00 / 25-May-00

5799 / Brit. Confed. Of Psychotherapists / Correspondence / Susan Lucks / Counselling & Therapy / 1 pp / May-00 / 25-May-00

5800 / Brit. Assoc. Psychotherapists / Clinical Service, etc. / ? / Counselling & Therapy / 14 p / ? / 25-May-00

5801 / Hastings College / Correspondence / Unknown / Employment / 4 pp / May-00 / 27-May-00

5802 / Threshold / Correspondence / Anne Guildford / Women's Issues / 6 pp / ? / 27-May-00

5803 / Henderson Hospital / Correspondence / Unknown / Personality Disorder / 2 pp / May-00 / 27-May-00

5804 / Jilly Hall / Correspondence / Jilly Hall / Counselling & Therapy / 1 pp / May, 2000 / 27-May-00

5805 / Kilncroft Residential Home / Correspondence / V. Riedel / Residential Care / 3 pp / May-00 / 27-May-00

5806 / Norton Lodge Residential Home / Correspondence / Unknown / Residential Care / 1 pp / ? / 27-May-00

5807 / Little Ridge / Correspondence / Unknown / Doctors / 1 pp / ? / 27-May-00

5808 / Seitai Assoc. / Correspondence / J. Kuszmar / Alt. Seitai / 1 pp / May-00 / 27-May-00

5809 / National Soc. Epilepsy / Correspondence / Unknown / Epilepsy / 1 pp / May, 2000 / 27-May-00

5810 / Carla Sher / Correspondence / Unknown / Alternative Therapy. Energy Field / 2 pp / May, 2000 / 18-May-00

5811 / Mind / Surviving Working Life / Unknown / Employment / 20 p / May, 2000 / 18-May-00

5812 / Tamarisk / Correspondence / Unknown / Residential Care / 1 pp / May, 2000 / 30-May-00

5813 / Marie Botha / Correspondence / Marie Botha / Counselling & Therapy / 1 pp / May, 2000 / 30-May-00

5814 / Lloyds Pharmacy / Correspondence / Margaret Geering / Chemists / 1 pp / May-00 / 30-May-00

5815 / Tunbridge Wells Counselling Centre / Correspondence / Marilyn Foster / Counselling & Therapy / 1 pp / May-00 / 30-May-00

5816 / Guestling Surgery / Correspondence / Unknown / Doctors / 8 pp / ? / 31-May-00

5817 / Roebuck Surgery / Correspondence / Unknown / Doctors / 1 pp / ? / 31-May-00

5818 / Roebuck Surgery / Correspondence / Unknown / Doctors / 13 p / ? / 31-May-00

5819 / Parents' Helpline / Correspondence / Sheila C. Summerton / Family / 3 pp / May-00 / 31-May-00

5820 / Hastings College of Arts & Technology / Correspondence / A. C. Russell / Education / 2 pp / May-00 / 31-May-00

5821 / Carol Geer / Correspondence / Carol Geer / Counselling & Therapy / 1 pp / May-00 / 31-May-00

5822 / Katheryne Kavanagh / Correspondence / Katheryne Kavanagh / Counselling & Therapy / 2 pp / May-00 / 31-May-00

5823 / Clouds / Correspondence / Heather Whitmore / Alcohol / 6 pp / May-00 / 30-May-00

5824 / Exeter Healthcare / Letter & Brochure / Jane Darke / Private Health / 36 pp / May-00 / 31-May-00

5825 / Leage of Friends of Eversfield Hospital / Correspondence / Mrs S Holt / Hospitals / 2 pp / May-00 / 1-Jun-00

5826 / Sandy Adey / Correspondence / Sandy Adey / Counselling & Therapy / 1 pp / May, 2000 / 1-Jun-00

5827 / Jen Bridges / Correspondence / Jen Bridges / Alternative Therapy. Alexander Technique / 1 pp / May-00 / 1-Jun-00

5828 / Phoenix House / Correspondence / C. Reddington / Substance Misuse / 4 pp / May, 2000 / 1-Jun-00

5829 / Standard Life / Correspondence / Debbie Chapman / Private Health / 2 pp / May-00 / 1-Jun-00

5830 / Eastbourne & County Health Care / Correspondence / Martin Corfe / Legal / 1 pp / May-00 / 1-Jun-00

5831 / Westwood Centre Dept. of Psychology / Correspondence / Mary Locke / Counselling & Therapy /

1 pp / May-00 / 17-May-00

5832 / Anna Barnes / Correspondence / Anna Barnes / Introduction / 1 pp / Mar-00 / 30-May-00

5833 / Hastings Vol. Act. News / Hastings Community News, 103. / Unknown / Various / 4 pp / May, 2000 / 26-May-00

5834 / British Stammer Assoc. / A World that Understands Stammering' / ?/ Stammering / 2 pp / ? / 18-May-00

5835 / Jenny Hart / Doctors, etc. corrections. / Jenny Hart / Various / 45 pp / May, 2000 / 2-Jun-00

5836 / H & RCS / Correspondence / Rose Webster / Counselling / 1 pp / ? / 2-Jun-00

5837 / Draper House / Correspondence / Unknown / Residential Care / 1 pp / ? / 2-Jun-00

5838 / Brit. Autogenic Soc. / Correspondence / Janet Marshall / Alternative Therapy. Autogenic / 2 pp / ? / 2-Jun-00

5839 / Sue Cottrell / Correspondence / Sue Cottrell / Counselling / 3 PP / May-00 / 2-Jun-00

5840 / The Children's Society / Correspondence / Unknown / Children & Young People / 2 pp / ? / 3-Jun-00

5841 / Hastings College of Arts & Technology / Part-time courses starting September 20000 / Unknown / Alternative Therapy / 52 pp / ? / 3-Jun-00

5842 / Rock Clinic / Correspondence / Robert Withers / Counselling / 2 pp / Jun-00 / 5-Jun-00

5843 / Local Government Ombudsman / Complaint about the Council / Unknown / Complaining / 8 pp / March, 2000 / 15-Jun-00

5844 / Mary Jenkins / Correspondence / Mary Jenkins / Counselling / 1 pp / May-00 / 6-Jun-00

5845 / Francoise Hutton / Correspondence / Francoise Hutton / Counselling / 3 pp / ? / 6-Jun-00

5846 / Sussex Carers Service / "Hastings Careers Centre" / Unknown / Employment / 2 pp / ? / 6-Jun-00

5847 / John Stedman / Correspondence / John Stedman / Counselling / 2 pp / Jun-00 / 6-Jun-00

5848 / Crisis Response Service / Correspondence / Matt Fribbens / Crises / 2 pp / May-00 / 6-Jun-00

5849 / Francesca Inskipp / Correspondence / Francesca Inskipp / Counselling / 30 pp / / 6-Jun-00

5850 / National Asthma Campaign / Information Sheets / KJ / Asthma / 6 pp / July, 1999 / 7-Jun-00

5851 / Mind Alliance / E-Mail / Sue Brown / Mental Health / 1 PP / May-00 / 31-May-00

5852 / Anna Barnes / Meeting at St Anne's / Anna Barnes / NHS & Social Services / 2 pp / May, 2000 / 7-Jun-00

5853 / Peter Nolan Lawrence / Impressive Depressives / Peter Nolan Lawrence / Miscellaneous / 96 pp / ? / 19-May-00

5854 / Lindsay Miller / Correspondence / Lindsay Miller / Counselling / 2 pp / Jun-00 / 8-Jun-00

5855 / Eastbourne & County Health Care / Correspondence / G.J. Weppner / Legal Matters / 2 pp / Jun-00 / 8-Jun-00

5856 / June Broadhurst / Correspondence / June Broadhurst / Counselling / 2 pp / Jun-00 / 8-Jun-00

5857 / Clare Tredgold / Correspondence / Clare Tredgold / Counselling / 1 pp / ? / 8-Jun-00

5858 / Sleep Apnoea Trust Assoc. / Information sheets / Mrs Wilma Govan / Sleep / 4 pp / Jun-00 / 8-Jun-00

5859 / Nina Russell / Correspondence / Nina Russell / Counselling / 3-Jun-00 / June, 2000 / 9-Jun-00

5860 / John Lofts / Correspondence / John Lofts / Alternative Therapy. Alexander Technique / 1 pp / Jun-00 / 9-Jun-00

5861 / Hastings Sheltered Workshop / Correspondence / Peter Howard / Employment / 2 pp / Jun-00 / 9-Jun-00

5862 / P. Chedgey / Correspondence / P. Chedgey / Alternative Therapy. Herbalism / 1 pp / ? / 9-Jun-00

5863 / Ron Fellows / Correspondence / Ron Fellows / Counselling / 5 pp / ? / 9-Jun-00

5864 / Narcotics Anonymous / "Global Society of Recovering Addicts" / Unknown / Substance Misuse / 2 pp / ? / 9-Jun-00

5865 / Narcotics Anonymous / Where to find NA meetings / Unknown / Substance Misuse / 32 pp / ? / 9-Jun-00

5866 / Cedar Health / Healthcare Naturally / Unknown / Alternative Therapy. Herbalism / 6 pp / ? / 9-Jun-00

5867 / HVA / Directory of Local Voluntary & Community Resources / Unknown / Voluntary Work / 40 pp / May, 2000 / 9-Jun-00

5868 / Geoffrey Ward / Correspondence / Geoffrey Ward / Counselling / 2 pp / June, 2000 / 10-Jun-00

5869 / Age Concern East Sussex / Correspondence / Dorothy Smith / Elderly / 1 pp / May-00 / 10-Jun-00

5870 / Lewes District & Wealden Mind / User Q Project / Peter Nicholls / User Groups / 3 pp / Jun-00 / 10-Jun-00

5871 / HARC / Correspondence / Sandra Lewis / Advice / 1 pp / Jun-00 / 10-Jun-00

5872 / Beaconsfield Surgery / Correspondence / Unknown / Doctors / 1 pp / ? / 12-Jun-00

5873 / Boots the Chemists / Correspondence / J.M. Crawford / Chemists / 1 pp / ? / 12-Jun-00

5874 / Impact Income Maximisation / Correspondence / Julie O'Brien / Not in Guide / 4 pp / Jun-00 / 9-Jun-00

5875 / CAIT / Correspondence / Sally Carr / Advocacy / 4 pp / Jun-00 / 12-Jun-00

5876 / Daily Telegraph / "Stop Smoking Drug" / Tara Womersley / Smoking / 1 pp / Jun-00 / 12-Jun-00

5877 / Francesca Inskipp / Chapter corrections / Francesca Inskipp / Counselling / 34 pp / June, 2000 / 10-Jun-00

5878 / Information Centre / Correspondence / Marilyn Wrench / Information / 1p / June, 2000 / 13-Jun-00

5879 / Well Man Clinic / Male Impotence & its Treatment / Unknown / Sex / 8 pp / ? / 13-Jun-00

5880 / Hastings Lifeline / Correspondence / D. Nugent / Housing / 1 pp / May-00 / 13-Jun-00

5881 / Anne Simpson / Correspondence / Anne Simpson / Counselling / 1 pp / Jun-00 / 14-Jun-00

5882 / Jessica Fox / Correspondence / Jessica Fox / Counselling / 2 pp / Jun-00 / 14-Jun-00

5883 / UKCC / Correspondence / Richard Bradshaw / Not known / 1 pp / Jun-00 / 14-Jun-00

5884 / Ayurvedic Company / Ayurveda' / Unknown / Alternative Therapies / 13 p / June, 2000 / 14-Jun-00

5885 / Daily Mail / Top Ten Retreats' / Unknown / Alternative Therapies / 1 pp / Jun-00 / 14-Jun-00

5886 / Families Anonymous / Information literature / Jean Howe / Substance Misuse / 12 pp / June, 2000 / 15-Jun-00

5887 / Frances Neilson / Correspondence / Frances Neilson / Counselling / 1 pp / June, 2000 / 15-Jun-00

5888 / Peach / Information pack / Carrie Haslett / Autism / 44 pp / June, 2000 / 16-Jun-00

5889 / Peter Baker / E-mail / Peter Baker / Learning Disability / 2 pp / Jun-00 / 12-Jun-00

5890 / BLAGH / Corrections / Steve Noakes / Sex / 1 pp / ? / 17-Jun-00

5891 / 73a Centre / Corrections / Dave Harris / Day Centres / 2 pp / ? / 16-Jun-00

5892 / Silverhill Natural Health Centre / Correspondence / Unknown / Alternative Therapies / 1 pp / ? / 16-Jun-00

5893 / Daily Telegraph / Committed Quitters Programme / David Derbyshire / Smoking / 1 pp / Jun-00 / 15-Jun-00

5894 / Hastings Befrienders / Correspondence / Lewis Nicholls / Sex / 1 pp / ? / 19-Jun-00

5895 / British Snoring & Sleep Apnoea Association / Catalogue / Marianne Davey / Sleep / 21 pp / Jun-00 / 19-Jun-00

5896 / 73a Centre / Corrections / Andrew Joyce / Day Centres / 2 pp / Jun-00 / 19-Jun-00

5897 / Hastings CHC / Correspondence / Patricia Marston / CHCs / 3 pp / Jun-00 / 20-Jun-00

5898 / Eastbourne CHC / Correspondence / Unknown / CHCs / 1 pp / ? / 20-Jun-00

5899 / Conquest Hospital League of Friends / Correspondence / K. Clarke / Hospitals / 3 pp / Jun-00 / 21-Jun-00

5900 / Community Learning Disability Service / Correspondence / Peter Baker / Learning Disability / 2 pp / Jun-00 / 21-Jun-00

5901 / Anne Tyndale / Correspondence / Anne Tyndale / Counselling / 2 pp / Jun-00 / 21-Jun-00

5902 / Rosemary Dixon-Nuttall / Correspondence / Rosemary Dixon-Nutall / Counselling / 2 pp / Jun-00 / 21-Jun-00

5903 / Shorelink Comm. Writers / Correspondence / Unknown / Poetry & Writing / 2 pp / Jun-00 / 21-Jun-00

5904 / Sussex Tinnitus Association / Correspondence / Mavis A. Constable / Tinnitus / 1 pp / Jun-00 / 21-Jun-00

5905 / Xpress Advocacy / Correspondence / Unknown / Children / 4 pp / Jun-00 / 22-Jun-00

5906 / Jenny Hart / Proof corrections / Jenny Hart / Health to Manic Depression / 36 pp / Jun-00 / 22-Jun-00

5907 / H&RCS / Proof corrections / Rose Webster / Counselling / 3 pp / Jun-00 / 22-Jun-00

5908 / Scope East Sussex / Proof corrections / Mrs Brazier / Cerebral Palsy / 2 pp / June, 2000 / 22-Jun-00

5909 / Hazel Redsull / Proof corrections / Hazel Redsull / Counselling / 1 pp / Jun-00 / 22-Jun-00

5910 / Havacare / Proof corrections / Helen Mitchell / Health Authorities / 2 pp / June, 2000 / 22-Jun-00

5911 / Parent Link / Proof corrections / Unknown / Children / 3 pp / Jun-00 / 22-Jun-00

5912 / Scope / Proof corrections / Beryl Cross / Cerebral Palsy / 2 pp / Jun-00 / 22-Jun-00

5913 / Focus on Mental Health / Minutes 2/6/00 / Unknown / User Groups / 2 pp / June, 2000 / 22-Jun-00

5914 / Children's Society / Proof corrections / Unknown / Children / 1 pp / June, 2000 / 22-Jun-00

5915 / Frances Neilson / Proof corrections / Frances Neilson / Counselling / 1 pp / Jun-00 / 23-Jun-00

5916 / Family Matters / Proof corrections / Revd. K. Baird / Family Problems / 6 pp / Jun-00 / 23-Jun-00

5917 / Al-Anon / Understanding Ourselves & Alcoholism / Anon / Alcohol / 10 pp / Jun-00 / 23-Jun-00

5918 / Richard Morgan-Jones / Proof corrections / Richard Morgan-Jones / Counsellors & Therapists / 1 pp / June, 2000 / 23-Jun-00

5919 / Hastings College of Art & Technology - Students Union / Proof corrections / Anon / Employment / 2 pp / Jun-00 / 23-Jun-00

5920 / Young Carers Project / Proof corrections / C. Stevenson / Carers / 3 pp / Jun-00 / 24-Jun-00

5921 / Hastings CHC / Proof corrections / Patricia Marston / CHCs / 3 pp / Jun-00 / 24-Jun-00

5922 / Centre for Stress Management / Proof corrections / Peter Ruddell / Stress / 1 pp / Jun-00 / 24-Jun-00

5923 / My Choice / Proof corrections / Trudy Allen / Advocacy / 3 pp / Jun-00 / 27-Jun-00

5924 / Lloyds Pharmacy / Proof corrections / B.C. Hunt / Chemists / 2 pp / Jun-00 / 27-Jun-00

5925 / Manic Depression Fellowship / Corrections / Alan Mooncie / Manic Depression / 6 pp / Jun-00 / 27-Jun-00

5926 / Madeleine Iddison / Chapter corrections / Madeleine Iddison / Community Mental Health Teams; NHS & Social Services Section / 39 pp / Jun-00 / 28-Jun-00

5927 / Christine Lockwood / Chapter corrections / Christine Lockwood / Care Programme Approach / 3 pp / Jun-00 / 28-Jun-00

5928 / Madeleine Mayhew / Chapter corrections / Madeleine Mayhew / NHS & Social Services Section / 39 pp / Jun-00 / 28-Jun-00

5929 / Su Barnicoat / Section corrections / Su Barnicoat / Rural Rother / 2 pp / Jun-00 / 29-Jun-00

5930 / Barbara Hardcastle / Section corrections / Barbara Hardcastle / NHS & Social Services / 39 pp / Jun-00 / 29-Jun-00

5931 / Eating Disorders Association / Directory information / Steve Bloomfield / Eating Disorders / 3 pp / Jun-00 / 29-Jun-00

5932 / Westwood Centre. Dept. of Clinical Psychology / Chapter corrections / Mary Locke / Psychology / 1 pp / Jun-00 / 29-Jun-00

5933 / McGuire Programme / Chapter corrections / Bernadette Bailey / Stammering / 3 pp / Jun-00 / 29-Jun-00

5934 / Manic Depression Fellowship / Aims & Values / Marcia Brown / Manic Depression / 3 pp / Jun-00 / 29-Jun-00

5935 / South East Advocacy Service / Proof corrections / Alison Peterson / Advocacy / 3 pp / Jun-00 / 29-Jun-00

5936 / Focus on Mental Health / Minutes of Meeting, 14 January 2000 / Margaret Moss / User Groups / 2 pp / Jan-00 / 5-Feb-00

5937 / Harcourt Brace & Co / Medical Hypotheses. Schizophrenia: the illness that made us human / D.F. Horrobin / Schizophrenia / 20 pp / Pub. 1998 / Oct. 1999

5938 / Sane / Sanetalk / Unknown / Schizophrenia / 16 PP / Spring 1999 / 22-Mar-99

5939 / Hastings Voluntary Action / Hastings Community News, No. 80 / Katy Burbridge / General / 4 pp / Dec. 1997 / Jan. 1998

5940 / Hastings Voluntary Action / Hastings Community News, No. 88 / Katy Burbridge / General / 4 pp / Oct. 1998 / Nov. 1999

5941 / Hastings Voluntary Action / Hastings Community News No. 92 / Katy Burbridge / General / 4 pp / Mar/Apr 1999 / 28-Aug-99

5942 / Hastings Voluntary Action / Hastings Community News No. 94 / Katy Burbridge / General / 4 pp / June/July 1999 / 8-Sep-99

5943 / Hastings Voluntary Action / Hastings Community News No. 95 / Katy Burbridge / General / 4 pp / July/Aug 1999 / 20-Aug-99

5944 / Hastings Voluntary Action / Hastings Community News No. 96 / Katy Burbridge / General / 4 pp / Aug/Sep 1999 / 8-Sep-99

5945 / Hastings Voluntary Action / Hastings Community News No. 97 / Katy Burbridge / General / 4 pp / Oct. 1999 / 11-Oct-99

5946 / Mind / Open Mind No. 92 / Sara Dunn / General / 28 pp / July/Aug 1998 / 3-Jul-98

5947 / Mind / Open Mind No. 93 / Sara Dunn / General / 28 pp / Sep/Oct 1998 / 4-Sep-98

5948 / Mind / Open Mind No. 94 / Sara Dunn / General / 28 pp / Nov/Dec 1998 / 5-Nov-98

5949 / Mind / Open Mind No. 96 / Sara Dunn / General / 28 pp / Mar/Apr 1999 / 6-Mar-99

5950 / Mind / Open Mind No. 97 / Sara Dunn / General / 28 pp / May/Jun 1999 / 7-May-99

5951 / Mind / Open Mind No. 98 / Sara Dunn / General / 28 pp / Jul/Aug 1999 / 9-Jul-99

5952 / Mind / Open Mind No. 99 / Sara Dunn / General / 28 pp / Sep/Oct 1999 / 8-Sep-99

5953 / East Sussex County Council / Proof corrections (e-mail) / Kate Griffiths / Social Services; Learning Disabilities; Learning Difficulties / 3 pp / Jun-00 / 29-Jun-00

5954 / Manic Depression Fellowship / Parenthood & Manic Depressive Illness / Alison Clements & Dr R Kumar / Manic Depression / 4 pp / Apr-92 / 8-Jun-99

5955 / Manic Depression Fellowship / Comfort for Carers / Unknown / Manic Depression / 4 pp / ? / 8-Jun-99

5956 / Manic Depression Fellowship / Why Did My World Have to Change? / Unknown / Manic Depression / 4 pp / ? / 8-Jun-99

5957 / Manic Depression Fellowship / Drug Treatment of Manic Depression / Anne Cole / Manic Depression / 4 pp / Feb-94 / 8-Jun-99

5958 / East Sussex County Library / Help in Hand / Unknown / General / 296 pp / Jul-97 / 14-Jan-00

5959 / Manic Depression Fellowship / Pendulum, vol. 14, No. 1 / Polly Mortimer / Manic Depression / 16 pp / Spring 1998 / 14-Apr-98

5960 / Manic Depression Fellowship / Pendulum, Vvol. 14, No. 2 / Kirsty White / Manic Depression / 16 pp / Summer 1998 / 27-Jun-98

5961 / Manic Depression Fellowship / Pendulum, Vol. 14, No. 3 / Poly Mortimer / Manic Depression / 16 pp / Autumn 1998 / 19-Oct-98

5962 / Manic Depression Fellowship / Pendulum, Vol. 15, No. 1 / Polly Mortimer / Manic Depression / 16 pp / Spring 1999 / 1-Apr-99

5963 / Manic Depression Fellowship / Pendulum, Vol. 15, No. 2 / Poly Mortimer / Manic Depression / 16 pp / Summer 1999 / 2-Jul-99

5964 / Manic Depression Fellowship / Pendulum, Vol. 15, No. 3 / Poly Mortimer / Manic Depression / 16 pp / Autumn 1999 / 27-Sep-99

5965 / Department of Health / Contact - Update / Unknown / General / 54 pp / Apr-97 / 21-Oct-98

5966 / Mind / Publications from Mind Spring/Summer 2000 / Ann McCarthy / General / 40 pp / Pub. 2000 / 30-Mar-00

5967 / Manic Depression Fellowship / Annual Report 1998 / Jacki Reason / Manic Depression / 12 pp / Pub. 1999 / 19-Aug-99

5968 / Hearing Voices Network / Information Sheets / Michael de Valda / Hearing Voices / 10 pp / Pub. 1999 / 19-Oct-99

5969 / Social Services / Information leaflet/Social Services; 1. General information / Unknown / Social Services / 12 pp / Apr-99 / 13-Apr-00

5970 / Social Services / 2. Gaining Access to Your Records / Unknown / Social Services / 6 pp / Apr-99 / 13-Apr-00

5971 / Social Services / 3. How to Make a Complaint / Unknown / Social Services / 6 pp / Apr-99 / 13-Apr-00

5972 / Social Services / 4. Confidentiality / Unknown / Social Services / 6 pp / Apr-99 / 13-Apr-00

5973 / Social Services / Information leaflet. 5. Charges for Miscellaneous Services / Unknown / Social Services / 8 pp / Apr-99 / 13-Apr-00

5974 / Social Services / 6. Voluntary Organisations in East Sussex / Unknown / Social Services / 8 pp / Apr-99 / 13-Apr-00

5975 / Social Services / 7. Services for Families & Children / Unknown / Social Services / 12 pp / Apr-99 / 13-Apr-00

5976 / Social Services / 9. Your Local Community Care Charter / Unknown / Social Services / 16 pp / Apr-99 / 19-Jan-00

5977 / Social Services / 10. Residential Care Services / Unknown / Social Services / 16 pp / Apr-99 / 13-Apr-00

5978 / Social Services / 11. Day Care & Home Services / Unknown / Social Services / 12 pp / Apr-99 / 13-Apr-00

5979 / Social Services / 12. Occupational Therapy Services / Unknown / Social Services / 6 pp / Apr-99 / 13-Apr-00

5980 / Social Services / 13. Sensory Impairment Services / Unknown / Social Services / 16 pp / Apr-99 / 13-Apr-00

5981 / Social Services / 14. Mental Illness - The Care Approach Programme / Unknown / Social Services / 6 pp / Apr-99 / 13-Apr-00

5982 / Social Services / 15. Learning Disability Register / Unknown / Social Services / 8 pp / Apr-99 / 13-Apr-00

5983 / Social Services / 16. Direct Payments / Unknown / Social Services / 6 pp / Apr-99 / 13-Apr-00

5984 / Manic Depression Fellowship / Manic Depressive Disorder / Unknown / Manic Depression / 4 pp / Dec. 1994 / 8-Jun-99

5985 / MACA / About MACA / Unknown / Day Centres / 6 pp / ? / 25-Feb-00

5986 / Westminster Pastoral Foundation / Counselling Services / Unknown / Counselling & Therapy / 20 pp / ? / 12-May-00

5987 / Gay Helpline in Hastings / Proof corrections / Lewis Nicholls / 1. Sex 2. Befriending / 3 pp / 25.06.00 / 25-Jun-00

5988 / Frances Neilson / Proof corrections / Frances Neilson / Counselling & Therapy / 2 pp / 25.06.00 / 26-Jun-00

5989 / Salvation Army Day Centre / Proof corrections / Unknown / Day Centres / 1 pp / 17.06.00 / 30-Jun-00

5990 / Family Matters / Proof corrections / Kenn Baird / Family Problems / 3 pp / 29.06.00 / 30-Jun-00

5991 / Hastings Voluntary Action / Hastings Community News 104 / ?/ General / 4 pp / June/July 2000 / 1-Jul-00

5992 / Debbie Rimmer / Section corrections / Debbie Rimmer / NHS & Social Services / 4 pp / 23.06.00 / 1-Jul-00

5993 / Phil Gander & Steve Metcalf / Section corrections / Phil Gander / NHS & Social Services / 9 pp / 23.06.00 / 30-Jun-00

5994 / Candice Miller / Section corrections / Candice Miller / NHS & Social Services / E-mail 1 page / 29.06.00 / 29-Jun-00

5995 / PSP Association / Unite to Fight / Unknown / PSP / 6 pp / ? / 13-Apr-00

5996 / Alzheimer's Disease Society / Information leaflet / ?/ Elderly Mental Health / 6 pp / Apr-92 / 13-Apr-00

5997 / DAIS / Information leaflet / Unknown / Substance Misuse / 1 pp / ? / 19-Oct-99

5998 / Re-Solv / Stop Solvent Abuse Problems / Unknown / Substance Misuse / 6 pp / ? / 25-Oct-99

5999 / Fellowship of Depressives Anonymous / Newsletter 102 / ? / Depression / 30 pp / May/June 1999 / 27-Oct-99

6000 / Jenny Hart / Proof reading. Manic Depression to Your Rights / Jenny Hart / Various / 167 pp / Jun-00 / 10-Jul-00

6001 / Brit. Confederation of Psychotherapists / Corrections to proof entry / Susan Lucks / Counselling & Therapy / 3 pp / 14.06.00 / 17-Jul-00

6002 / College of Health / Healthline Service / Marianne Rigg / Information / 3 pp / ? / 20-Jul-00

6003 / Headway Hurstwood Park / Proof corrections / E.J. Squires / Brain Injury / 3 pp / 19.06.00 / 21-Jul-00

6004 / Jean Mulvey / Proof corrections / Jean Mulvey / Counselling & Therapy / 1 pp / 13.07.00 / 14-Jul-00

6005 / General Medical Council /Corrections / Katherine Vale / Complaining / 3 pp / 19.07.00 / 21-Jul-00

6006 / Langford Clinic / Proof corrections / Unknown / Hospitals & Clinics / 2 pp / 27.06.00 / 10.07.00

6007 / Margaret Taraz / Proof corrections / Margaret Taraz / Alexander Tech. / 1 pp / 5.07.00 / 10-Jul-00

6008 / Nick Muriel / Proof corrections / Nick Muriel / Counselling & Therapy / 2 pp / 27.06.00 / 10-Jul-00

6009 / McGuire Programme / Proof corrections / Heidi Bristow / Stammering / 3 pp / Jun-00 / 12-Jul-00

6010 / Alegra Garner / Proof corrections / Alegra Garner / Counselling & Therapy / 2 pp / 6.07.00 / 12-Jul-00

6011 / MACA / Tenby House corrections / Judy Hobbs / Residential & Respite Care / 1 pp / 11.07.00 / 13-Jul-00

6012 / Dept. of Health & BBC / Contact - a directory for mental health / Unknown / General / 106 pp / Apl 95 / 25-Jul-98

6013 / Focus on Mental Health / Minutes 7 Jul 2000 / Margaret Moss / Various / 2 pp / 7.07.00 / 25-Jul-00

6014 / Focus on Mental Health / Newsletter Autumn 99 / Unknown / Various / 4 pp / Autumn 99 / 28-Aug-99

6015 / Community Service Volunteers / Proof corrections / Jules Payne / Voluntary Work / 2 pp / 20.07.00 / 27-Jul-00

6016 / NHS / A Primary Care Trust in Hastings & St Leonards / Dr Greg Wilcox / Primary Care Groups / ? / Jul-00 / 27-Jul-00

6017 / Herringtons Solicitors / Letter / David Harding / Legal Matters / 2 pp / 26.07.00 / 27-Jul-00

6018 / Hastings & Rother NHS Trust / Letter / Sarah Holmes-Smith / Health Authorities / 1 pp / 30.06.00 / 5-Jul-00

6019 / Hastings & Rother NHS Trust / Proof corrections. NHS & Social Service section / Anna Barnes / Various / 39 pp / 4.07.00 / 13-Jul-00

6020 / Hastings Voluntary Action / Hastings Community News Issue No. 105 / Unknown / Various / 2 pp / Jul-00 / 28-Jul-00

6021 / Assn of CHCs for England & Wales / Patients' Rights / Anon / Your Rights / 16 pp / Apr-99 / 13-Apr-00

6022 / Assn of CHCs for England & Wales / CHCs / Anon / Community Health Councils / 6 pp / ? / 13-Apr-00

6023 / Assn of CHCs for England & Wales / Your Rights - Making Choices / Anon / Your Rights / 6 pp / Dec-98 / 13-Apr-00

6024 / Assn of CHCs for England & Wales / Your Rights - On the Record / Anon / Your Rights / 6 pp / Jun-98 / 13-Apr-00

6025 / Assn of CHCs for England & Wales / Your Rights - Going into Hospital / Anon / Your Rights / 6 pp / Jun-96 / 13-Apr-00

6026 / Assn of CHCs for England & Wales / Your Rights - Care in the Community / Anon / Your Rights / 6 pp / Aug-98 / 13-Apr-00

6027 / Assn of CHCs for England & Wales / Your Rights - Family Doctors / Anon / Your Rights / 6 pp / Apr-98 / 13-Apr-00

6028 / Mental Health Foundation / Publications Catalogue / Unknown / Various / 28 pp / ? / 21-Oct-99

6029 / East Sussex County Council Social Services / Learning Disability Services Structure Chart / Keith Hinkley / Learning Disabilities / 2 pp / 28.02.00 / 4-Mar-00

6030 / Department of Health / The Patients' Charter & You / Unknown / Patients' Charter / 32 pp / Jun-99 / 22-Jan-00

6031 / Hastings & Rother NHS Trust / Annual Report 1997-1998 / ?/ Health Authorities / 16 pp / ? / 11-Oct-99

6032 / NHS in Hastings & Rother / Health News in Hastings & Rother NHS / Unknown / Hospitals / 4 pp / Mar-00 / 2-Apr-00

6033 / ECT Anonymous / Information Sheets EA8, EA9, EA10, EA11, EA12 / Unknown / ECT / 16 pp / Jan-97 / 15-Jan-00

6034 / ECT Anonymous / Reprints & correspondence / Unknown / ECT / 11 pp / various / 15-Jan-00

6035 / Hastings & Rother NHS Trust / A Volunteers' Guide / Unknown / Hospitals / 54 pp / ? / 22-Oct-99

6036 / Blue Cross / Pet Bereavement Service / Jo-Ann Dono / Bereavement / 1 pp / 30.07.00 / 1-Aug-00

6037 / Al Anon / Understanding Ourselves & Alcoholism (E-mail) (permission) / Caryn Johnson / Alcohol / 2 pp / 7.07.00 / 7-Jul-00

6038 / Society of Homeopaths / Proof corrections / Unknown / Homoeopathy / 1 pp / Jul-00 / 2-Aug-00

6039 / Eastbourne & County Healthcare / Eastbourne Patients' Council / Ian Watling / User Groups / 3 pp / 1.08.00 / 2-Aug-00

6040 / Brenda Riley / Corrections to proof entry / Brenda Riley / Counselling & Therapy / 2 pp / 2.08.00 / 2-Aug-00

6041 / Angelgate Foundation / Treatments & Training Courses / Gill Ayres / Alternative Therapy / 5 pp / 2.08.00 / 3-Aug-00

6042 / Daily Telegraph / Future of the NHS' / Celia Hall / Patients' Charter / 92 pp / 28.07.00 / 28-Jul-00

6043 / Hastings & Rother Inter Agency Mental Health Action Group / Action Plan 1999 - 2000 / Unknown / NHS & Social Services / 9 pp / ? / 22-Nov-99

6044 / Carers National Assn. / Benefits: What's available & how to get them / ?/ Carers / 16 pp / . 1997 / 12-May-99

6045 / Carers National Assn. / How do I get help? / Camilla Parker / Carers / 24 pp / Mar-99 / 12-May-99

6046 / Carers National Assn. / Taking a break / Sheila White / Carers / 20 pp / . 1997 / 12-May-99

6047 / Carers National Assn. / Correspondence / Max Beckerman / Carers / 6 pp / 10.05.99 / 12-May-99

6048 / Samaritans / Time to talk / ?/ Crises / 4 pp / ? / 13-Apr-00

6049 / NHS Executive / Advocacy - a code of practice / Edna Conlan & others / Advocacy / 36 pp / Feb-00 / 7-Feb-00

6050 / Kings College London / National Practice Development Network / ?/ Hospitals / 2 pp / ? / 18-Jan-00

6051 / MACA / Living at Tenby House / Unknown / Residential & Respite Care / 20 pp / ? / 25-Feb-00

6052 / Hastings & Rother NHS Trust / Crisis Card / Unknown / Crises / 2 pp / ? / 19-Oct-99

6053 / Samaritans / 1999 Review / Unknown / Crises / 6 pp / ? / 13-Apr-00

6054 / Age Concern / Advocacy Service / Unknown / Elderly People / 2 pp / ? / 13-Apr-00

6055 / APCMI / Befriending Scheme / Unknown / Befriending / 2 pp / ? / 13-Apr-00

6056 / Hastings & Rother NHS Trust / Mental Health Weekend Crisis Line / ?/ Crises / 4 pp / ? / 8-Jun-99

6057 / Albany Trust / Counselling, Psychotherapy Consultancy / Carol Zimmerman / Counselling & Therapy / 5 pp / 19.10.99 / 22-Oct-99

6058 / Befrienders International / Face to Face Annual Report 97-98 / Unknown / Befriending / 20 pp / . 1998 / 2-Nov-98

6059 / Befrienders International / Website pages / Unknown / Befriending / 4 pp / 4.08.00 / 4-Aug-00

6060 / Mind in Barnet / Your local mental health charity / Unknown / Mind Organisations / 2 pp / Aug-00 / 2-Aug-00

6061 / NSF / Carers' Support / Suzy Levy / Schizophrenia / 2 pp / Aug-00 / 2-Aug-00

6062 / Department of Health / Drug & Solvent Misuse / Unknown / Substance Misuse / 32 pp / Oct-95 / 4-Aug-00

6063 / Hastings & Rother Health Promotion / LSD Trips / Ben Wileman / Substance Misuse / 2 pp / ? / 4-Aug-00

6064 / Social Services / Day Care Services / Unknown / Elderly Mental Health / 2 pp / Jun-98 / 13-Apr-00

6065 / Help the Aged / Managing your medicines / Dr Peter Rivers / Medication / 12 pp / Summer 99 / 2-Feb-00

6066 / Women's Aid / Women's Aid National Helpline / Maggie / Women / 1 pp / ? / 14-Jul-00

6067 / Shaw Trust / Releasing potential of disabled people / ? / Employment & Training / 12 pp / ? / 21-Oct-99

6068 / Shaw Trust / Opportunities for all - Annual Review 97/98 / Tim Pape / Employment & Training / 20 pp / ? / 21-Oct-99

6069 / Henderson Hospital / Dialogue No. 4 / Sue Ryan / Personality Disorder / 6 pp / Spring 2000 / 24-Jul-00

6070 / Outside In (Cambridge) / Letter & brochure SAD / Unknown / Seasonal Affective Disorder / 3 pp / Jul-00 / 17-Jul-00

6071 / Alzheimer's Society / A Rough Guide to the new NHS / Dr Shona Arora / Elderly Mental Health / 48 pp / Jan-00 / 13-Jul-00

6072 / Alzheimer's Society / Letter / Jenny Hogarth / Elderly Mental Health / 1 pp / 10.07.00 / 13-Jul-00

6073 / Alzheimer's Society / Newsletter, June 2000 / Janice Brown / Elderly Mental Health / 8 pp / Jun-00 / 13-Jul-00

6074 / DrugScope / Informing policy, reducing risk / Unknown / Substance Misuse / 8 pp / ? / 13-Jul-00

6075 / DrugScope / Combining ISDD, SCODA and You / Unknown / Substance Misuse / 6 pp / ? / 13-Jul-00

6076 / DrugScope / Publications & Services / Unknown / Substance Misuse / 28 pp / ? / 13-Jul-00

6077 / Mental Health Foundation / Brochure SAD / Lindsey Clarke / Mental Health / 1 pp / 19.10.99 / 21-Oct-99

6078 / British Confederation of Psychotherapists / Finding a therapist & other literature / Susan Lucks / Counselling & Therapy / 16 pp / Jul-00 / 17-Jul-00

6079 / Boots the Chemist / Give up Smoking / Unknown / Smoking / 12 pp / Dec-99 / 5-Jul-00

6080 / Mind / Understanding Personality Disorders / Janet Gorman / Personality Disorder / 12 pp / . 1997 / 9-Aug-00

6081 / Henderson Hospital / Main House and Webb House / Unknown / Personality Disorder / 12 pp / ? / 9-Aug-00

6082 / ESCC Social Services / Corrections to proof entry / Christine Thomas / Social Services / 4 pp / Aug-00 / 9-Aug-00

6083 / Department of Health / Antibiotics - don't wear me out / Unknown / Medication / 2 pp / Sep-99 / 8-Aug-00

6084 / ESBHHA / Prepayment Certificates / Tracy Mitchell / Chemists / 2 pp / ? / 8-Aug-00

6085 / MDF / Pendulum Vol 16 No. 2 / Polly Mortimer / Various / 20 pp / summer 00 / 23-Jun-00

6086 / ECT Anonymous / What is ECT / Pat Butterfield / ECT / 4 pp / Aug-00 / 10-Aug-00

6087 / Fiona Rankine / Movement & Arts Therapy / Fiona Rankine /Movement & Arts / 2 pp / ? / 13-Apr-00

6088 / Department of Health / Professor Louis Applyby / Manjeet Sidher / Mental Health / 1 p + photo / Aug-00 / 11-Aug-00

6089 / Agape Trust / Sharing the care of profoundly disabled people / Unknown / Learning Disabilities / 2 pp / Aug-00 / 11-Aug-00

6090 / Clouds / Mission Statement / Heather Whitmore / Alcohol / 3 pp / 26.07.00 / 11-Aug-00

6091 / Gillian Smith / An Invitation to Reiki Training / Gillian Smith / Reiki / 2 pp / ? / 13-Apr-00

6092 / Focus on Mental Health / Minutes of Meeting / Unknown / User Groups / 2 pp / 4.08.00 / 15-Aug-00

6093 / Daily Telegraph / Smokers swallow the pill / Dr Sarah Brewer / Smoking / 1 pp / 16.08.00 / 16-Aug-00

6094 / Ben Mooncie / Correspondence re entry / Ben Mooncie / Counsellors & Therapists / 1 pp / Aug-00 / 17-Aug-00

6095 / Ben Edwards / Correspondence re entry / Ben Edwards / Autogenic Therapy / 3 pp / Aug-00 / 17-Aug-00

6096 / Obsessive Action / Annual Conference 2000 / David Veale / Obsessions / 4 pp / Aug-00 / 17-Aug-00

6097 / British Hypnotherapy Association / Greenguide / ? / Hypnotherapy / 16 pp / Pub 1994 / 18-Aug-00

Index